Engaging
Bodies

Engaging Bodies

The Politics and Poetics of Corporeality

ANN COOPER ALBRIGHT

WESLEYAN UNIVERSITY PRESS

MIDDLETOWN, CONNECTICUT

Wesleyan University Press

Middletown CT 06459

www.wesleyan.edu/wespress

© 2013 Ann Cooper Albright

Manufactured in the United States of America

Designed by Katherine Kimball

Typeset in Sabon by Alice W. Bennett

Wesleyan University Press is a member of the Green
Press Initiative. The paper used in this book meets
their minimum requirement for recycled paper.

Hardcover ISBN: 978-0-8195-7410-7

Paperback ISBN: 978-0-8195-7411-4

Ebook ISBN: 978-0-8195-7412-1

Library of Congress Cataloging-in-Publication Data
available upon request

5 4 3 2 1

for my students

Contents

Preface

Although it represents a quarter-century of writing on dance, this collection evolved over a period of two years. It began during the time I was working on a contribution to a special issue of *Dance Research Journal* focused on critical reappraisals of dance and phenomenology. That piece, "Situated Dancing: Notes from Three Decades in Contact with Phenomenology," traces several intellectual shifts in dance studies over the past three decades, using my own educational trajectory (from a BA in philosophy to an MFA in choreography to a PhD in performance studies) as a point of departure. That retrospective essay, which serves as a conceptual introduction to this book, gave me the opportunity to articulate the connections between my own approach to writing about movement training and choreography and the critical influence of feminist theory and cultural studies on the development of dance scholarship in the late twentieth and early twenty-first centuries. The writings collected here also reflect that blend of personal experience, theoretical inquiry, and historical context.

Last year, as I was going through my mother's things in the process of moving her to an assisted-living situation, I came across a folder with some of my first published dance reviews and early performance criticism. Most of these articles were from a pre-digital era and I had long since thrown out the manuscripts and lost the tear sheets for these pieces. As I reread them, I began to realize how important these early forays into dance criticism were to my development both as a writer and a dancer. Even before I thought about the possibility of going to graduate school, I practiced honing my descriptive skills in order to try and capture the choreographic dynamism and new paradigms of virtuosity on display in much of the contemporary dancing I was surrounded by in Philadelphia, New York, and later in Cleveland. I see now that reviewing dance performances in my mid-twenties was a crucial first step in understanding my own perspective as a scholar. Writing about the dancing I was seeing in lofts and theaters was a way for me to connect the dual pleasures of thinking and moving, and I found the experience of transcribing movement into words extremely satisfying.

Like many of my generation, I was influenced by two different approaches to thinking about dance. The first was Laban Movement Analysis, particularly the descriptive language of effort/shape; the second was the plethora of scholarly discussions of the body throughout the late 1980s and 1990s. Although I first encountered Labanotation while studying one summer at the Laban Centre in England, I did not really explore the language of effort/

shape until several years later when I began to study dance composition and write about dance performances for a local paper. Those Laban-based categories of kinesthetic qualities, movement initiation, spatial directionality, force, and flow were helpful in parsing out the various dynamic elements within a dance. As my attention to motion became more intentional, I delighted in trying to translate my perceptions into language. I was fortunate at this point to be able to take short writing workshops from two renowned dance critics: Marcia Siegel and Deborah Jowitt.

Elaborate movement descriptions by themselves, however, do not articulate the layers of cultural meaning in a dance. One of the conundrums that I faced as I became more committed to a life in dance was the sad fact that most people (including my very own brother) did not understand how to look at most modern dance. The high-energy, full-body dancing that was a hallmark of contemporary choreography in the 1980s and 1990s wowed the public to be sure, but its particular blend of movement abstraction left little more than a vague impression of physical virtuosity on the audience. The meaning of the dancing was elusive to most people, and this situation contributed, I believed, to the cultural marginalization of dance. I wanted to think deeply about the dances I was seeing and articulate the importance of live, moving bodies. My sense of urgency grew as the AIDS crisis and the culture wars began to heat up in the early 1990s.

Inspired by many of the new ideas and critical methodologies concerning the study of the body from disciplines across the humanities, I decided to shift my energies from making dances to thinking and writing about dancing bodies. Yet my ongoing involvement with the act of dancing—training, teaching, performing—claimed its own allegiance as I tried to keep the material experience of dancing bodies at the core of my theoretical analyses. Because I have continued to dance throughout my academic career, I perceive dancing differently. This gut-reality was clear to me even before the latest neurological research in mirror neurons confirmed that fact. For me, dancing is a physical inquiry, a way of experiencing and participating in the world, and my writing reflects that conviction.

I have tried to write with an awareness of the person on the other end of the process—the one who picks up my article or book and begins to read my description and analysis of a dance. The materials collected in this book were originally written for a variety of audiences, including those who read local newspapers (*Dance Dialogue,* the *Cleveland Reader*) regional arts magazines (*Dialogue Magazine for the Arts*), artist-based publications (*Movement Research Journal, Contact Quarterly*), scholarly journals (*Dance Research Journal* and *Women and Performance,* among others), as well as fellow dancers and scholars at conference panels and keynote presentations. Despite the wildly different venues that sponsored the original circumstances of these writings, my hope is that *Engaging Bodies: The Politics and Poetics of Corporeality* creates a coherent, if multifaceted, vision of the cultural vitality of dancing bodies. I have always enjoyed reading smart academic books that also reveal the intriguing ways that ideas tend to emerge from the ground of someone's life passions and pursuits. The writing here charts an intertwined trajectory of moving and thinking, and I am particularly hopeful that this blend of cultural theory and personal circumstance will be useful and inspiring for emerging scholars and young dancers looking for a model of writing about dance that thrives on the interconnectedness of watching and doing, gesture and thought.

As I chose the individual pieces as well as the organizational categories for this collection of writings, I was interested in gathering together a selection of essays and reviews that was representative of the breadth of my interests as well as the evolution of those different perspectives over time. Thus, each section—Performance Writings, Feminist Theories, Dancing Histories, Contact Improvisation, Pedagogy, and Occasional Pieces—contains my work from the early 1990s, as well as something from the last few years, although this distribution is not necessarily evenly balanced. For instance, most of the writings on performance in Feminist Theories are from the 1990s, when I was most keen on using insights from feminist thought to draw out critical issues about physical bodies and cultural identities in contemporary dance. Nonetheless, some of my later work on Loïe Fuller's early twentieth-century spectacles directly incorporates feminist scholarship and perspectives, and therefore I have included a piece on Fuller's Salome performances in the Feminist Theories section, rather than in Dancing Histories.

Because I started my career reviewing and thinking about contemporary dance, historical research is a more recent adventure of mine. And yet, while looking through my writing over the past two decades, I found a talk on issues of audience reception and historical reconstruction from the beginning of my academic career that I have included in the history section. It was intriguing for me to see how an early foray into questions of historical reconstruction laid the foundation for a project focused on embodied research a decade later. Over the course of several months rereading, selecting, and organizing my earlier writings, it has been similarly interesting to recognize how the beginning threads of a theoretical argument can often be traced back to the first discussions of a particular performance in my early dance reviews. While I created the thematic sections in order to provide some coherence and easy reference, they are quite permeable. For instance, the first essay in the section on pedagogy centers on my teaching of contact improvisation, but because it was written specifically for a special issue of *Women and Performance* focused on that topic, I have included it in Pedagogy instead of Contact Improvisation. Although the section titles are mostly self-explanatory, I have written short introductions for each category, hoping to give the reader a sense of the original contexts for the various writings presented in that cluster.

It is an odd exercise in forced self-reflection to reread talks and essays that I wrote many, many years ago. And it is enlightening to have to confront the aspects of my intellectual history I may have overlooked. For instance, even though I wrote *Modern Gestures: Abraham Walkowitz Draws Isadora Duncan Dancing* in 2010, I realized that I was talking about Walkowitz's sketches and watercolors of Duncan all the way back in 1989 when I first began thinking deeply about the conjunction of movement, drawing, and text in an essay called "Writing the Moving Body." The autobiographical exchanges of Duncan's writing and dancing also created the frame for another early essay, "Auto-Body Stories," which looks at the intersection of dance and autobiography from late twentieth-century choreography, particularly in the work of African-American choreographer Blondell Cummings. And predictably, Duncan pops up again in some of my later work on Loïe Fuller. Nonetheless, if someone had asked me just last month if I thought of myself as a Duncan scholar, I would have said no. It is funny what we fail to recognize sometimes.

Another theme that runs throughout the individual sections in *Engaging Bodies* is my interest in bodies that cross over stylistic, geographic, and historical boundaries, complicating the cultural categories of health, ability, race, class, gender, and sexuality. In many of the writings included in this collection, I analyze the different ways that various performances call static definitions of identity into question while at the same time presenting a somatically cohesive body. I also draw from those theoretical inquiries to propose intentional and unconventional ways of crossing over these boundaries while teaching a variety of bodies. Recently, I have been teaching a series of workshops for VSA—a national organization focused on bringing the arts to disabled populations—and that work is part of a continuum of theory and practice across which I find myself moving daily.

The title of this collection, *Engaging Bodies,* reflects my commitment to thinking seriously about the meshing of cultural representation and material circumstance that constitutes our experience of embodiment. I use the term "engaging" as a conscious reference to the mid-twentieth-century French notion of politically engaged literature, as well as the sense of deeply connecting with another person in contact improvisation. For me, this kind of engaged seeing and thinking about dance is a form of witnessing. To witness something is to involve oneself energetically—to stake one's body as the place of that connection. It implies a responsiveness that I articulate as a kind of responsibility—literally an ability to respond to the experience at hand. The particular conjunction of politics and poetics in the subtitle attests to this double vision of mine. In my engagement as both a dancer and a scholar, I draw on my kinesthetic sensibilities and my intellectual knowledge as I strive to evoke the poetic immediacy of the dancing as well as the political implications of that embodied commotion.

Acknowledgments

Because this book is a collection of previously published or performed work and was not researched as a separate project, there are no usual lists of librarians and fellow researchers to thank. Those acknowledgments were given in the original source. I want to thank Suzanna Tamminen for her support of my work over the last two decades, and Nadine George-Graves for her invaluable comments on an earlier version of the manuscript. This project was brought to fruition with the aid of two remarkable young women. My student assistant, Alyssa Marcum, helped secure permissions and typed up early writings for which I had no digital copies. For her patience and her embracing of my scholarly projects (including the marvelous tattoo of Duncan on her back), I thank her profusely. Thanks also to Sabrina Paskewitz-Drew, who helped me ready the manuscript for publication.

My daughter, Isabel Albright Newlin, was indispensable in the preparation of this manuscript. Not only did she advise me on the selection of pieces, help copyedit, and type in the text and footnotes that got lost in software translations, but she graciously listened to the many stories of how my work and her life intersected—including the moment when, nine months pregnant, I finally sent off a manuscript and gave her permission to be born. (She came on her own good time, a week later.) Her presence in my life over the past twenty-one years is part of the ground of family and friends who have supported my full-time, full-bodied engagement with dance. Most of the writing contained in these pages happened while raising Isabel and her brother Cyrus, and even though I never found the perfect balance of academic career and parenting, they have survived my multitasking with a grace and resiliency that is truly inspiring. For Isabel's willingness to spend a month of her summer helping me to bring this project to fruition—all the while learning to tango with me—I am deeply grateful.

Engaging
Bodies

Introduction

Situated Dancing

Dance Research Journal 43, no. 2, Fall 2011.

Notes from Three Decades in Contact with Phenomenology

I began to study philosophy at the same time that I began to study dance, at college in the early 1980s. Both of these choices surprised me at first, as I had originally planned on studying politics and becoming a civil-rights lawyer after college. I see now that these two areas of inquiry were routes towards figuring out how to bridge the divides between my academic self and my increasingly explosive physicality. Divided into day and night, my academic experience and the club scene I thrived in were separated by geographic distance and differing class values—a study in the cultural bifurcation produced by the hierarchies of brain and brawn. But these body/mind boundaries were always porous for me, and they became increasingly so as I explored the epistemological origins of the Cartesian split in my survey of Western philosophy course while also taking my first modern-dance class. My desire was to become both verbally and physically articulate, and I savored those moments when vague impulses or ideas found the right expressive gesture or crucial wording. By the time I was a senior, I was choreographing a quartet and writing a thesis on Maurice Merleau-Ponty's *The Phenomenology of Perception* (1962). Somewhere along the way, philosophy and dance leaned into one another, beginning a duet that would lead to a life spent thinking and moving.

This essay is just that—an attempt to situate and reflect on the various intersections of phenomenology and dance that have captured my curiosity over the past three decades. It maps out both a personal journey and a disciplinary trajectory, for my own career as a dancer and a scholar traces many of the intellectual shifts that have taken place in dance studies over this time. What follows is neither a thorough nor an encyclopedic documentation of these developments, however, but rather an individual (and admittedly quixotic) investigation of the ways in which phenomenology has helped dance scholars to think about dancing bodies beyond the walls of the studio or the arch of the proscenium stage. The structure of my analysis follows my journey from philosophy through feminist theory to performance studies and back to philosophy, albeit with a critical distance. This intellectual pathway intersected with my dance training as I moved from a BA in philosophy to an MFA in choreography to a PhD in performance studies, and then began to teach in a dance department at a liberalarts college where, for the first time in my academic life, I could combine intellectual analysis and physical training in the space of one class session. Engaging students across the traditional mind/body divides of dance studio and academic classroom has, surprisingly, brought me back to philosophy, specifically phenomenology.

Over the course of the last thirty years, phenomenology has replaced aesthetics as the philosophical discourse of choice for dance studies, prodding scholars to think about a broad continuum of moving bodies within the cultures they inhabit. Generally speaking, phenomenology is the study of how the world is perceived, rather than the study of the essence of things as objects or images of our consciousness. It is a way of describing the world as we live in it—a philosophical approach that positions the body as a central aspect of that lived experience. Flipping Descartes's "cogito" ("I think, therefore I am") on its (in)famous head, phenomenology, as developed by Edmund Husserl, Martin Heidegger, and Maurice Merleau-Ponty, seeks to account for the structures of our situated "being-in-the-world."[1] This approach focuses on the body-based somatic and perceptual senses (including space and touch), as well as the more verbal and conscious aspects of our existence. I am deeply appreciative of phenomenology's multifaceted analysis—from discussions of posture to issues of ethical behavior—of the ways our bodies both shape and are shaped by our life experiences. Paying attention to how our corporeal engagement with the world creates meaning in our lives, phenomenology revises classical notions of the self as subject and the world as object of our reflections. Of course, now when I teach first-year students Merleau-Ponty's *The Phenomenology of Perception,* I realize that my approach to this seminal work is enriched by the interpretations and critical interventions provided by scholars whose interests cross many disciplines. Feminist philosophers such as Simone de Beauvoir, Iris Marion Young, Elizabeth Grosz, and Judith Butler, have critiqued the universalist approach of these early phenomenologists, stretching that philosophical discourse to include a consideration of cultural differences, all the while conserving the original focus on the corporeal as a key element in the constitution of subjectivity.[2]

Merleau-Ponty wrote *The Phenomenology of Perception* in four parts.[3] The first is an introduction that argues against figuring existence as pure consciousness (Descartes's "cogito"), and proposes instead that we try to understand the reality of our existence by recognizing that our perception is interactive with the world. Thus, the table around which my family gathers is not just an inert object made of wood—it means something and calls those meanings forth when I sit down at it. For Merleau-Ponty, it is our bodily experiences that provide the ground for our thoughts and not vice versa. Part 1 of the book, "The Body," is dedicated to refuting conceptions of the body as an object or a machine directed by our higher consciousness. Here, Merleau-Ponty analyzes in detail how our perceptions—moving through space, touching another person, etc.—create meaning. The next section, "The World as Perceived," includes an intriguing discussion of intersubjectivity ("Self and Other"). His final section, "Being-for-Itself and Being-in-the-World," upends traditional Western ideas of freedom as an exercise of individual will.

Throughout his project, Merleau-Ponty grounds human consciousness in everyday experiences of the world. His language, replete with gerunds, emphasizes the verbs—it is the acting (not the action), the perceiving (not the perception), the sensing (not the sensation)—that can provide us with insights into the nature of our existence. In addition to the great pleasure of discovering a subgenre of philosophy that takes bodily knowledge seriously, I was particularly interested in the ways in which Merleau-Ponty contradicts many earlier philosophers' pronouncements on selfhood, individual will, and freedom. For instance, in the last chapter of *The Phenomenology of Perception,* Merleau-Ponty discusses freedom not in terms of having abundant choices (of career, say), but rather as a kind of urgency—a necessity that ironically gives one the freedom to claim a career that does not always fit within culturally sanctioned expectations. I certainly experienced this rush of liberation when, as a twenty-year-old, I decided that my life would have to include dancing as my main focus and not just as an extracurricular activity or a hobby.

My entry into dance was unusual for a young woman of my generation in that I had no previous technical foundation in dance when I came to college. In fact, the first dance course I signed up for was dance composition. Due to the fortuitous combination of small classes (dance was offered for physical education credit back then), my own ebullient enthusiasm, and the deeply generous spirit of my early teachers, I was allowed to continue with the course, provided I joined the advanced technique class held right before. So there I was, an oddly energized but spastic presence in the back row, trying desperately to figure out which limb to move where. The majority of the other students (with some memorable exceptions) were high-school ballerinas who were having just as hard a time undoing the technical rigidity of their training as I was having trying to instill some in my body. In college, I was engaged in making dances, taking technique classes, reading my way through the GV 1700s, and writing about the dances I was witnessing in theaters and on video. Thus, I came to dance as a holistic enterprise—an intellectual, as well as a physical, discipline. I quickly recognized, however, that dance (unlike the visual arts) was not considered a legitimate academic major at Bryn Mawr College. The dance classes at my college were taught by women, many of whom had graduate degrees, but who nonetheless still held adjunct status. During my second year, I took a course on French women writers (from Mme. de Staël to Hélène Cixous) and one on political theory, all the while making connections with my dance experiences. My growing feminist consciousness made me realize the cultural urgency of bringing marginalized experiences and bodies into the academy.

The early 1980s were a formative time, not just for me personally, but also for gender and women's studies, as well as dance studies. These areas were not yet generally regarded as legitimate disciplines, but they were increasingly the sites of my intellectual curiosity. I read Simone de Beauvoir's *The Second Sex* (1953), whose famous line, "One is not born a woman, but rather becomes one," inspired so many early feminist analyses of the socialization of women's bodies.[4] Because phenomenology focuses attention on the circumstances of this active "becoming," it serves as a model for many studies on the complicated dynamics of bodies conforming to and resisting cultural norms. In 1990, feminist philosopher Iris Marion Young analyzed women's embodiment in her groundbreaking essay, "Throwing Like a Girl: A Phenomenology of Feminine Body Comportment, Motility, and Spatiality." This seminal piece of feminist scholarship is a brilliant example of a phenomenological movement analysis that articulates how women incorporate their social positioning. By describing how girls are taught not to take up space, not to use their whole bodies, and not to believe they can accomplish challenging physical tasks, Young provides a new framework for thinking about the interconnections between women's bodies and their sense of selfhood and social power.

Thirty years after its initial publication, "Throwing Like a Girl" is still extremely relevant for anyone exploring issues of gender in movement. Writing for a collection of essays dedicated to Young after her untimely death in 2006, dance scholar Susan Leigh Foster comments on Young's contributions not only to feminist philosophy, but also to dance studies. "In that essay, Young offers an innovative approach to the analysis of bodily motion, one that integrates movement patterns with psychological orientations and social roles."[5] Young grounds her insights with references to her own physical upbringing, acknowledging that while her observations are situated in a particular experience, they will likely resonate with many other women. Although general physical styles have changed for women and more girls are playing sports these days, the "inhibited intentionality" that Young identified is still very present in the adolescent female bodies I work with.

For the past seven years, I have directed an after-school program in the local middle school called *Girls in Motion*. This program, which uses college students as mentors, seeks to address on an embodied level what Peggy Orenstein and others have described as "the confidence gap."[6] By teaching movement forms—including capoeira, yoga, hip-hop, and some contact-based skills—that give girls an experience of mobilizing their own weight, not to mention taking up space, the mentors and I hope to guide them into a heightened sense of their own physical power. Young's classic essay is required reading for all the college women who work with *Girls in Motion*. If contact improvisation provided me with the physical foundation for this program, it is the work of feminist phenomenologists like Young that gave me the critical framework to articulate what I have always felt in my bones—that how we move in the world can make a difference.

During my second year of college, I was struggling with my own issues surrounding the socialization of female bodies, for I had recently hit the wall with the gender ideologies embedded in modern dance and I was finding it difficult to fit my punk body into the flowing skirts of our Graham-inspired dance-club recitals. Indeed, I might have left dance altogether if I had not stumbled across a contact improvisation class. It was the summer of 1980, I was twenty years old, and I knew immediately that I had found a dance form that fed my rambunctious physicality and my intellectual energy. Contact's task-based focus relieved my self-consciousness, and I liked that this improvisational form provided the space for an individual expressivity as well as my need for group interaction. I treasured the possibilities that contact improvisation offered of moving from fiercely combative to luxuriously sensuous in a split second. Over the next thirty years, contact improvisation would become a movement form that continuously nurtured both my intellectual and physical curiosities.

It was also the summer I was rereading *The Phenomenology of Perception* in preparation for writing my senior thesis. In retrospect, I realize that the movement form I was beginning to incorporate as an essential part of my physical identity helped me make sense of Merleau-Ponty's analysis of spatiality, motility, and intersubjectivity. For instance, in a section in the book called "The Phenomenal Field," Merleau-Ponty describes the experience of running through the woods and having one's body automatically move between the trees. Our bodies know that the tree is solid (not a figment of our imagination), not because they deduced it, or we remember a time when we hit the tree and thought, "let's not do that again," but because our bodies can perceive and react to things faster than our conscious thought can. Similarly, contact classes often begin with an exercise where everyone starts walking through the space, shifting directions and moving into the spaces between other people. It is always a fascinating experience because, just like navigating midtown Manhattan at rush hour, if you second-guess yourself or someone else, you tend to bump into people. But if you trust your instincts and keeping moving, nine times out of ten, you will slide through just as the hole disappears. One of the keys to "getting" contact improvisation is learning to dial down your conscious verbal commentary in order to let your kinesthetic intelligence take over. I began to see the experience of meeting someone else at the point of contact as a physical metaphor for the way Merleau-Ponty describes the interconnected relationship of self and the environment he calls "being-in-the-world."

Having graduated with a degree in philosophy (there was no dance major), I was keen to make up for lost time and dance all day, every day. Eventually, I ended up pursuing an MFA in choreography at Temple University. While there, I felt my body gradually incorporating a deep physical responsiveness, as I took lots of technique, improvisation, and somatic classes, along with the rigorous composition sequence. I was inspired by my modern-based teachers, and learned how to see and create choreographic structures and subtle variations in qualities of movement. I felt strong, but not smart, for there was little room in the program for much theoretical engagement with dance. This was an era when much dance writing was focused on descriptive criticism. As an alternative to the power toting, make-it-or-break-it kind of evaluative dance coverage, descriptive criticism set an important precedent in dance studies. Critics such as Deborah Jowitt and Marcia Siegel were instrumental in schooling a whole generation of dance writers in how to see and describe the movement priorities in modern and postmodern dance.[7] This was also the time when Michael Kirby proposed the possibility of an "objective" criticism that focused on recording events without any critical interpretation.[8] With a nod to ethnography, some dance writers were attempting to document the total dance-making process—from rehearsal to performance and its aftermath—but there seemed to be little interest at the time in a sustained analysis that probed the existing structures of cultural power, or investigated how dance reflected social identities or aesthetic ideologies.

In school, the influence of a Laban-based movement analysis combined with a focus on structural alignment in our technique classes stripped much of the dancing we did of its cultural moorings and kept us in a haze of the eternal present. We were training, rehearsing, and performing without much discussion of what it all meant or where we were going. Bodies were treated as neutral forms to be organized (sometimes manipulated) by the choreographer's vision. It was a moment when the Cunningham ethos ranked supreme and everyone seemed satisfied with a universal relativism that let each person find his or her own meaning in the material. I remember sitting in composition class and hearing elaborate analyses of the uses of lateral space, change in level, and rhythmic variation. When I pointed out the fact that the dance we were discussing included nine women dressed in black slips and red stiletto heels, and that those choices might carry a certain amount of cultural capital, I was politely told that that was my own interpretation, which I was welcome to, but that I should not assume anyone else would notice!

My frustration with this situation paralleled that of many feminist phenomenologists who were questioning the generic undercurrents of earlier discussions of the (presumably neutral) body in their field. Given what Elizabeth Grosz (1994) describes as the prevailing somatophobia of the Western philosophical tradition, bringing the body into this rarified discourse was an important first step (for which phenomenology deserves much of the credit), but it also clearly mattered whose bodies were being discussed. Although I did not articulate it in precisely these terms at the time, I began to feel uneasy with a rigidly composition-based approach to choreography. The language about dance that I encountered felt very insular. I found myself wanting to talk about dance and the cultural meaning embedded in the bodies that were dancing, but I knew I needed more analytic tools to work with. Thus I emerged from the stagnant air and florescent lights of the dance studios where I had spent the last three years sweating profusely, and began to train in a different kind of technique—feminist theory.

Eventually (each "eventually" in this text is a code for "nine months of waiting tables and teaching hundreds of aerobics classes to fund my next step"), I moved to New York City to dance and study. My movement curiosities took me to studios and lofts all over the city. My more scholarly endeavors were located at Movement Research, Inc., where I worked briefly as director of the Studies Project (a series of roundtable discussions between choreographers and critics), and at New York University, where I took classes in the Performance Studies department. There, I was fortunate enough to be part of a cohort of graduate students who were also intrigued by the insights that academic theory had to offer dance studies. At first, we eagerly embraced these new critical theories, particularly feminist film theory. It was exciting to trace the interconnections between moving images and moving bodies. Nonetheless, I was frustrated by the lack of awareness that the female body could be both a site of resistance as well as a site of cultural disempowerment.

I remember reading works like Teresa de Lauretis's *Alice Doesn't: Feminism, Semiotics, Cinema* (1984). In this work, de Lauretis tries to build a bridge from her discussions of narrative and desire in representation over to experience and subjectivity. Leading off with the famous passage from Virginia Woolf's *A Room of One's Own,* in which Woolf's female character is chided by a male academic for walking across the lawn where women are not allowed, de Lauretis redefines Woolf's use of instinct as cultural knowledge or habit. Instinct, for de Lauretis, has "too strong a connotation of automatic, brute, mindless response."[9] She prefers experience: "The notion of experience seems to me to be crucially important to feminist theory in that it bears directly on the major issues that have emerged from the women's movement—subjectivity, sexuality, the body, and feminist political practice."[10] However, once de Lauretis evokes the political relevancy of experience, she steers clear of the theoretical murkiness of material lived bodies. Yet it was precisely the messiness of bodies and ideas that I found so compelling in both the choreography and improvisational performances I was seeing all around me.

For instance, while I appreciated de Lauretis's articulation of experience as interactive process, I found her too quick to dismiss aspects of experience, particularly physical experience, that are not so easily categorized. Sure, this experience of Woolf's character—the "I" of the story—is a prime example of the social positioning of women. But suppose, for a moment, that de Lauretis had started to quote Woolf earlier in her essay:

> Thought . . . had let its line down into the stream. It swayed, minute after minute, hither and thither among the reflections and the weeds, letting the water lift it and sink it, until—you know the little tug—the sudden conglomeration of an idea at the end of one's line . . . But however small it was, it had, nevertheless, the mysterious property of its kind—put back into the mind, it became at once very exciting, and important; and as it darted and sank, and flashed hither and thither, set up such a wash and tumult of ideas that *it was impossible to sit still.* It was thus that I found myself walking with extreme rapidity across a grass plot.[11]

This wonderful stream-of-consciousness description by Woolf evokes a certain affective quality of physical experience that gets dropped out of many scholarly discussions of embodiment. It is the energizing engagement with her thoughts that brings Woolf's character to her feet, propelling her across the grass and smack into that black-robed keeper of those awesome patriarchal lawns. Mediated through a series of lived events in which the narrator follows the thread of an idea right up to the threshold of a (male) academic institution, this section of *A Room of One's Own* represented for me the interaction between somatic experience and social definitions, which constitutes the ongoing process of subjectivity. I would argue that the "I" of this passage does not evaporate as she confronts the robed male professor who puts her back in her place. Indeed, it was not the thoughts per se, but the somatic attitude of her body that was transgressive, not simply the geographic fact of her (mis)placement, but its energized concentration. At the same time that Woolf's character gets put in her place as a woman, she still has the experience of refusing that place—the experience of not being able to "sit still."

I am elaborating on this example because it is indicative of what I considered at the time as a prevalent myopia in feminist theory about what constituted meaningful experiences. Too often, these theorists addressed the body only in terms of its cultural constructions. This constructed body is seen as a sort of material blank page onto which society etches its own image. But dance, especially the contemporary dance I was surrounded by in New York City in the late 1980s and early 1990s, was increasingly political, and focused on the (sometimes contradictory) identities of the dancers' bodies, demanding different ways of seeing from the audience. My peers and I all began to realize that the more didactic theories of representation based on two-dimensional images could not do justice to the complex experience of watching live bodies move onstage. The critical essays we were reading were often brilliant and erudite, yet I often left my graduate seminars feeling rather depressed and strangely claustrophobic. I started to wonder if academic theory was not just as repressive at times as the cultural ideologies it was deconstructing. Whether pegged by academic theory or portrayed by artists, at the end of the day women's bodies were often represented as overly determined, and always already written over.

Interestingly enough, while dance scholars were investigating the theoretical usefulness of feminist theory, feminist and cultural studies were beginning to engage with performance theory. The result was an interesting hybrid of performance studies and phenomenology. One of the most influential examples of this was Judith Butler's work in *Gender Trouble* (1990). This short book offers a stunning analysis of the interdependent constructions of sex, gender, and identity. In it, Butler conjures performance (via Simone de Beauvoir's notion of "becoming" a woman) as a process or a "becoming, a constructing that cannot rightfully be said to originate or to end."[12] The "becoming" of women then, is an enactment, and as such resists both a biological teleology and a cultural ontology. Although Butler first defines gender as "the repeated stylization of the body, a set of repeated acts within a highly rigid regulating frame that congeal over time to produce the appearance of substance, of a natural sort of being," she recognizes the existential limits of performance and the ways in which "repeated acts" undermine the stability of the very gender they are said to express.[13] Performances (whether theatrical events or framed moments in everyday life) are physicalized within a specific time and space, often (although not always) with a live audience and therefore can never be exactly repeated.

This ephemeral nature of performance makes for a very intriguing slippage of identity in which the "natural" habits are recognized as "performed." Once the ideological "naturalness" of those conventions is deconstructed, however, their physical remnants are not so automatically displaced. Pulled away from its overdetermined psychic (and psychoanalytic) relationship to the body, gender is often figured by Butler as a place of resistance without accounting for the bodily echoes of those physically ingrained cultural patterns. Reading *Gender Trouble*, I kept wondering what this destabilized body actually looked like? A lot of feminist theory becomes pretty confusing when one insists on keeping the physical reality of material bodies within the conceptual framework. Butler's theory of gender as performance marks gender and sexual identity as a shifting category (one that is consciously "played" out), but it never accounts for how the body receives, produces and interacts with that very potent psychic instability. Fortunately, while in graduate school I was still dancing, and the kinetic experience of making work and seeing work refreshed my spirits and made me realize that contemporary dance could reinvigorate feminist discussions of bodily experience. I was inspired to try and articulate the particular phenomenology of late twentieth-century dance. My desire was not to dismiss critical theory per se, but to try and uncover the theories implicit in the work I was witnessing.

The result, many years later, was *Choreographing Difference: The Body and Identity in Contemporary Dance* (1997). This book—and the various articles that led up to it—is situated at the intersection of theory and practice, dancing and writing. It was equally informed by my academic graduate studies and by my years training in contemporary dance—attending rehearsals and watching performances. The arguments I make about the double moment of dancing in front of an audience in which the dancer negotiates between seeing and being seen, as well as my discussion of the slippage between somatic identity (the experience of one's physicality) and cultural identity (how one's body—skin, gender, ability, age, etc.—renders meaning in society) came out of my willingness to be corporeally saturated by the dancing I was analyzing. At the time, I encountered some resistance to this kind of scholarly engagement. I sensed a fear that this bodily connectedness would somehow sully my critical distance. I was told (more than once) that I could either write about someone's work, or dance with someone, but I could not effectively do both. In retrospect, I realize that many of the insights in that book came from a desire to engage with kinesthetic, visual, somatic, and aesthetic experiences, and to put those insights in dialogue with textual theories. As a dancer, as well as an emerging scholar, I was unwilling to treat the dancing I witnessed as simply the "raw material" for my academic pontificating. I wanted to give the experience of dancing its own intellectual credibility.

I was not alone. Dance scholars throughout the mid-1980s and 1990s were producing interesting hybrids of feminist theory, cultural and performance studies. Many of these works were influenced by a phenomenological approach to the study of moving bodies. For instance, Deidre Sklar worked on a movement ethnography of a religious fiesta in Las Cruces, New Mexico. In articulating her particular methodology for this study, Sklar developed a series of "essential theoretical parameters for considering movement or dance in cultural context."[14] Premise number five reads: "movement is always an immediate corporeal experience."[15] In her explanation, Sklar argues against treating the body as a text to be read. Instead, she suggests that the physical knowing in movement must be explored through the body, as well as observation and interviews. Sklar proposes a process of "empathic kinesthetic perception":

Emphatic kinesthetic perception suggests a combination of mimesis and empathy. Paradoxically, it implies that one has to close one's eyes to look at movement, ignoring its visual effects and concentrating instead on feeling oneself to be in the other's body moving. Whereas visual perception implies an "object" to be perceived from a distance with the eyes alone, empathic kinesthetic perception implies a bridging between subjectivities. This kind of "connected knowing" produces a very intimate kind of knowledge, a taste of those ineffable movement experiences that can't be easily put into words. Paradoxically, as feminist psychologist Judith Jordan points out, the kind of temporary joining that occurs in empathy produces not a blurry merger but an articulated perception of differences.[16]

What Sklar describes as "emphatic kinesthetic perception" underlies a number of dance studies that mix ethnography and cultural studies with a decidedly phenomenological twist, such as Barbara Browning's *Samba: Resistance in Motion* (1995), and Cynthia Novack's *Sharing the Dance: Contact Improvisation and American Culture* (1990).

For most of the 1990s, I participated in an interdisciplinary feminist study group called the Flaming Bitches (ah, yes, that punk sensibility strikes again). On one occasion, I invited the group to meet in the dance studio, where we did some bodywork and a few beginning contact exercises. Initially, I was amused to see my smart and capable academic colleagues freak out in an open space with no desks to hide behind. Once we started writing, someone asked me why I did not write about contact improvisation, since it so clearly informed my thinking in many ways. It was true—I had not engaged with contact improvisation much in my scholarly work. This was odd, I realized, since I was always arguing about the importance of bodily knowing within this group, and yet I had not articulated much about a dance form that arguably defined much of my social, aesthetic, and political sensibilities, not to mention my physical body. As Janet O'Shea suggests in her introduction to the second edition of *The Routledge Dance Studies Reader,* "[Methodological] approaches accrue strategic force at different historical moments and in different social and political contexts."[17] It took the experience and aftermath of 9/11, which brought with it its own political urgency, to pull me into addressing my practice of teaching and dancing contact improvisation. I wrote "Dwelling in Possibility" as an epilogue for *Taken by Surprise* (2003): a collection of essays on improvisation that I coedited with David Gere. This piece uses the improvisational score I created for the Oberlin community the day after 9/11 as a stepping-off point for a meditation on the ways in which improvisation can help us to imagine a personal and communal response to a global crisis. I began to think about contact improvisation not only as a movement form, but also as methodology—an approach to dance studies that used my body as a way of knowing.

Invigorated by new graduate programs across the United States and abroad, dance studies gained a clear theoretical momentum by the end of the twentieth century. Indeed, the July 2000 conference, "Dancing in the Millennium" (cofacilitated by Dance Critics Association, Congress on Research in Dance, Society of Dance History Scholars, and the National Dance Alliance), presented a rich array of approaches to dance, not the least of which was a growing interest in "embodied research." This (admittedly slippery) term has gained considerable currency in the first decade of the twenty-first century, particularly in the areas of the cognitive sciences (which are now, interestingly enough, taking embodiment seriously), as well as performance and dance studies. Loosely defined, embodied research is a blend of phenomenology, anthropology (with its long tradition of field studies and participant/observer dynamic), ethnography, and cultural studies. In dance programs, particularly in England and Europe, embodied research is one way to gain institutional recognition for choreographic production. For instance, at the 2004 Ethics and Politics conference at the Theater Academy in Helsinki, Finland, the dance department was celebrating a new PhD program whose goal was to give dancers and choreographers the scholarly foundations (with a strong emphasis on phenomenology) to reflect on their own artistic work. This program has produced some of the best examples of embodied research that I have had the opportunity to read.

In the United States, embodied research has started to gain currency as more dancers are involved in writing about their own kinesthetic practices. This is much harder than it sounds. More than just taking dance classes while doing scholarly work, embodied research (to my mind, at least) requires that one engage seriously with the ambiguity that results from trying to conceptualize bodily experiences that can be quite elusive. It requires patience with the partiality of physical knowing, as well as a curiosity about how theoretical paradigms will shift in the midst of that bodily experience. My next scholarly project intentionally positioned my dancing as a central aspect of the historical research on an early twentieth-century dancer.

Traces of Light: Absence and Presence in the Work of Loïe Fuller (2007) started with a somatic hunch. After reading one critic and historian after another dismiss Fuller's dancing prowess, I rebelled. A series of black-and-white images of Fuller shot in natural light by Eugène Druet convinced me, in a deeply physical manner, that there was something else going on. These images spoke to me with a force that spilled over the traditional boundaries of historical research and inspired me to engage my somatic, as well as my analytic, faculties. I decided to make a dance with every chapter I was writing—to explore through my body the ideas I was working with theoretically. This was not historical reconstruction, but rather creative interpretation with an awareness that I might touch some truths about her work that were not immediately visible at first.

Drawing on the possibility of a "connected knowing" through my dancing, I thought of my approach to historical research as a kind of contact improvisation duet, focusing on the artistic and intellectual reciprocity of touching and being touched. Ironically, it was through the writings of another French philosopher, Jean-Luc Nancy, that I conceptualized this relationship between moving and writing, contact and text. In his essay "Corpus," Nancy writes:

> In all writing, a body is traced, is the tracing and the trace—is the letter, yet never the letter, a literality or rather a lettericity that is no longer legible. A body is what cannot be read in a writing. (Or one has to understand reading as something other than decipherment.) Rather, as touching, as being touched. Writing, reading: matters of tact."[18]

Following Nancy's move from traces to tracing, allowed me to incorporate the tactile, and thereby refuse the traditional separation of object from subject. Reaching across time and space to touch Fuller's dancing meant that I allow myself, in turn, to be touched, for it is impossible to touch anything in a way that does not also implicate one's own body. (Interestingly, a similar point is made by Merleau-Ponty in his discussion of intersubjectivity in *The Phenomenology of Perception*.) Given the focus of the present essay, I might recharacterize my approach in that earlier project as phenomenological with a dash of creative license. Recently, literary and cultural studies (with their renewed focus on "affect") have begun to consider the experience of embodiment as more central to interpretation. In these disciplinary fields as well, phenomenology is receiving renewed interest as a methodology.

Sarah Ahmed begins her book *Queer Phenomenology* with a question: "What does it mean to be oriented?"[19] Playing across the phenomenological fields of spatial orientation and its implications for thinking about sexual orientation, Ahmed follows Merleau-Ponty's analysis of spatiality and sedimented habits to argue that spatial orientations are not simply a matter of choice. Rather, they are called forth by the world around us. We learn to turn towards certain things and directions, and away from others. Over time and with repetition, the act of turning becomes habitual and elided. We end up seeing simply what is in front of us. As Iris Marion Young and others have pointed out, the social positioning of gender, class, race, age, and ability affects how we inhabit space. For Ahmed, we make sense of space by following certain pathways—often those that are well trodden by others coming before us. These paths constitute lines of direction that point us towards certain ways of thinking and being in the world. Directions, Ahmed points out, are not only about the where we are going, but also tell us how we are to get there. She writes:

It is not, then, that bodies simply have a direction, or that they follow directions, in moving this way or that. Rather, in moving this way rather than that, and moving in this way again and again, the surfaces of bodies *in turn* acquire their shape. Bodies are "directed" and they take the shape of this direction.[20]

In her book, Ahmed wants to think about life experiences that disorient us, that teach us to turn around and reorient toward what may have been part of a background or what initially felt out of our reach. "By bringing what is 'behind' to the front, we might queer phenomenology by creating a new angle . . . To queer phenomenology is to offer a different 'slant' to the conception of orientation itself."[21] Ahmed claims that these moments of disorientation, while frequently disturbing at first, can also become "vital." Indeed, being lost can open up new directions and sensibilities that otherwise would escape our attention.

I too am interested in spatial disorientation, in experiences that "slant" our habitual perceptions and therefore open up other experiences of proximity and exchange. In this sense, my current project shares many of Ahmed's concerns, and I find myself pulled toward her discussions of moments that "throw" the body from its perceptual ground. As both Merleau-Ponty and Ahmed point out, we only begin to understand our orientations when we experience disorientation. Contact improvisation embraces moments of disorientation—both the physical experiences of being off-balance and the psychic experience of not knowing what comes next. I find the experience of teaching people to explore new directions can teach us a lot about our habitual orientations. As we all know too well, American culture focuses almost exclusively on what is ahead of us. Politicians, governments, and various other institutions claim to be forward thinking, and we are encouraged to leave the past (with its mounds of garbage and last year's fashions) behind us. When my college students enter the studio, I can see the strain in their eyes from spending so much time in front of the various screens that rule their lives. Often I send them moving briskly through the space, shifting directions and facings to try and shake up their habitual orientations. Another way to do this is to replace the sense of sight with attention to other tactile and proprioceptive sensations. Sometimes I ask people to fall backwards, or move in a direction where they can no longer rely on their sight to navigate their descent to the floor.

One of the fundamental skills in contact improvisation is learning how to give and support weight through one's back. This fairly simple task requires that we first cultivate an awareness of our backs, including the back of our skulls. Attending to what we cannot see, but can only feel, is not a "natural" or even comfortable situation for many people. Twenty-first-century post-industrial Western culture has so prioritized the visual and fetishized the textual, that other ways of being now take considerably longer to develop than they did when I first started teaching twenty years ago. On the other hand, the slightest shift in attention from front to back can lead to extraordinary results. When I ask a group of people—be they adolescent girls, college students, or teachers at a public institution for special-needs kids (all of whom I taught this past semester)—to lie down on the floor and feel their backs release into gravity, their experiences can border on the euphoric. Awaking layers of sensation with touch and weight can be remarkably reassuring. Moving through our back space—that is, moving without seeing where we are going—however, can be scary, especially at first. There is a certain satisfaction in becoming aware of one's "backspace," not only because it opens up new experiences of perception, but also because attending to the presence of what we feel behind us can produce a useful perspective on what is in front. The clarity of our future directions depends a lot on recognizing the footprints of our past. In fact, this essay, with its focus on the evolution of dance studies and its relationship with the development of phenomenology over the past thirty years, has done just that for me.

This is a particularly salient moment for me to reflect on that relationship. Thirty years after my first brush with Merleau-Ponty, I find myself looking at contemporary embodiment through a lens much indebted to his work. My interest in backspace is part of *Gravity Matters*—a new project that looks at contemporary embodiment in the twenty-first century, focusing on the corporeal dynamic embedded in a pervasive cultural rhetoric of falling at the beginning of the twenty-first century. Over the past several years, I have been thinking more deeply about gravity—both the phenomenological experience of one's weight because of the earth's pull, and the theoretical implications of being grounded in the midst of all the physical and psychic turmoil at the beginning of the twenty-first century. I am intrigued by how gravity is connected to falling, disability, and even death (having the same etymological root as grave), as well as a sense of profundity, rootedness, and an inherent connection to the earth. I am also aware of how many younger people (who grew up in the wake of 9/11) feel a bizarre sense of dislocation as their lives become increasingly implicated in the weightless exchanges on the Internet.

Influenced by my thirty years in contact with phenomenology, this new work is based on a conviction that there is a connection between how we think about the world and how we move through it. I draw from my experiences teaching and training bodies across many identity categories (including race, gender, age, class, and ability) and my sense that something is going on in these bodies (in a way that crosses over differences but does not homogenize them) that I want to explore. My research began with the following questions: (1) How are our bodies affected by images of falling buildings, falling bodies, falling economies, and falling governments; and (2) What are the physical implications of repeated evocations of stock markets "diving" or in "free fall," businesses "failing," or the housing market "plunging"? I ask these questions both in order to underline the importance of embodied experience in constructing theories of cultural meaning and because I want to think seriously about the somatic practices that might help us survive and revise these cultural metaphors of failure and doom. *Gravity Matters* is situated in a field of inquiry that I would call "engaged corporeal phenomenology," for it is both grounded in the interconnections between individual responsiveness and communal resonance, and mobilized by thinking deeply about other people's bodies through the intermediary of my own.

NOTES

1. See Martin Heidegger's writings, especially *Being and Time;* as well as his essays in *Poetry, Language, Thought* (New York: Harper and Row, 1971). See Edmund Husserl's *Phenomenology and the Crisis of Philosophy* (New York: Harper and Row, 1965), as well as the collection *Husserl at the Limits of Phenomenology,* ed. Leonard Lawlor and Bettina Bergo (Evanston, IL: Northwestern University Press, 2002).

2. See Simone de Beauvoir, *The Second Sex;* Elizabeth Grosz, *Volatile Bodies: Towards a Corporeal Feminisim;* Judith Butler, *Bodies that Matter;* and Iris Marion Young, "Throwing Like a Girl and Other Essays," in *Feminist Philosophy and Social Theory.*

3. Maurice Merleau-Ponty, *The Phenomenology of Perception,* trans. Colin Smith (London: Routledge, 1962).

4. Simone de Beauvoir, *The Second Sex* (New York: Vintage, 1973), 301.

5. Susan Leigh Foster, "Throwing Like a Girl, Dancing Like a Feminist Philosopher," in *Dancing with Iris,* ed. Ann Ferguson and Mechthild Nagel (New York: Oxford University Press, 2009), 69.

6. See Peggy Orenstein, *Schoolgirls: Young Women, Self-Esteem, and the Confidence Gap* (New York: Doubleday, 1994).

7. See for instance, Marcia Siegel's collection, *At the Vanishing Point: A Critic Looks at Dance* (New York: Saturday Review Press, 1973); Deborah Jowitt's *Dance Beat: Selected Views and Reviews, 1967–1976* (New York: M. Dekker, 1977); and Jowitt's *The Dance in Mind: Profiles and Reviews 1977–83* (Boston: D. R. Godine, 1985).

8. Michael Kirby, *New Theatre: Performance Documentation 1974* (New York: New York University Press, 1974).

9. Theresa de Lauretis, *Alice Doesn't: Feminism, Semiotics, Cinema* (Bloomington: Indiana University Press, 1984), 158.

10. Ibid., 159.

11. Virginia Woolf, *A Room of One's Own* (London: Hogarth Press, 1931), 7.

12. Judith Butler, *Gender Trouble: Feminism and the Subversion of Identity* (New York: Routledge, 1990), 33.

13. Ibid., 33.

14. Deidre Sklar, "Five Premises for a Culturally Sensitive Approach to Dance," in *Moving History/Dancing Cultures,* ed. Ann Cooper Albright and Ann Dils (Middletown, CT: Wesleyan University Press, 2001) 30.

15. Ibid., 31.

16. Ibid., 32.

17. Janet O'Shea and Alexandra Carter, *The Routledge Dance Studies Reader* (London and New York: Routledge, 2010) 3.

18. Jean-Luc Nancy, "Corpus," in *Thinking Bodies,* ed. Juliet Flower MacConnell and Laura Zakarin (Stanford, CA: Stanford University Press, 1994), 24.

19. Sara Ahmed, *Queer Phenomenology: Orientations, Objects, Others* (Durham, NC: Duke University Press, 2006), 1.

20. Ibid., 15–16.

21. Ibid., 14.

I

PERFORMANCE WRITINGS

I first started to write dance reviews for a small community newspaper in Philadelphia. Later, as an MFA student at Temple University, I persuaded the chair to let me launch a departmental newsletter called "Dance Dialogues," which included interviews with guest artists and short reviews of local performances. When I moved to New York City in the mid-1980s, I took classes and workshops all over the city and eventually became involved with Movement Research, Inc., coordinating their "Studies Project" for a while. Curious about experimental dance, I followed the emerging work of young choreographers and master improvisers at venues like St. Marks Dancespace, and Dance Theater Workshop (once fondly referred to as DTW, now known as New York Live Arts). At the same time that I was inspired by the movement community and kinesthetic energy in this downtown dance scene, I also began to realize that there was a dearth of thoughtful writing about this work. I felt that many of these performances, especially the amazing improvisational works that I regularly witnessed, were not receiving the critical attention they deserved. Fortunately, I had the extraordinary opportunity to study with dance critics Marcia Siegel and Deborah Jowitt. I was further inspired by reading the writing of Burt Supree, Elizabeth Zimmer, Wendy Perron, Sally Banes, and Anna Kisselgoff as well. Although I still wanted to perform and make dances, as time went on I became increasingly committed to thinking about the work I was seeing.

Because I came to dance at the same time that I was studying philosophy, French literature, and later, feminist theory, I have always been intrigued by the intersection of language and the body. How does the body "speak" its truth nonverbally? How do we craft words to capture the slippery experiences of dance? What are the implications of the mind/body split in academia, and what are the ways in which the knowledge of the body gets excluded or included in contemporary intellectual discourses?

At that time in my life, I often saw the same performance several times. After each show, I would write about it in my journal, beginning with a list of words inspired by the performance. Then I would draft short phrases, writing and rewriting them until I felt that they evoked something essential about the dance I saw. I tried to understand the difference between a visual picture produced by a pose such as an arabesque or a lift, and the ineffable quality of following something that disappears into the next movement phrase. Over time, I learned to use my corporeal memory and not just my visual memory to articulate the implications of the performance I was describing. I wanted to address not simply what was happening onstage, but also that dance's reverberations—how it could help us think differently about bodies in the world. It pleased me that fellow dancers and choreographers read my writing and felt that it spoke effectively about their work.

The majority of the dance reviews included here were written in the late 1980s and early to mid-1990s when I was living in New York City, and later in Ohio, when I moved there to teach at Oberlin College. They represent my desire to think seriously about the societal implications of the dancing I was seeing around me. I want to acknowledge my editors at *Women and Performance* (Marianne Goldberg) and at *Dialogue Magazine for the Arts* (Lorrie Dirske) for giving me the wonderful opportunity to write editorials and longer reviews that blended descriptions of performances with my fledgling forays into cultural theory. I realize now that many of these short pieces carry the seeds of my later, more theoretical work.

For instance, the first review included here takes up the issue of "play" in the early work of Pooh Kaye. There was something very intriguing to me about the feisty and rambunctious energy of her choreography and although it looked chaotic on the surface, I knew from taking a movement workshop with her that there was an internal kinetic synchrony that connected dancers across space and disparate actions. This idea that there was in fact a "mesh in this mess" led to a longer piece published later in *Contact Quarterly*, which is included in the final Occasional Pieces section of this book. Pooh Kaye also shows up in this Performance Writings section in a review of an evening of improvisation with her mentor, Simone Forti. By the time I reviewed *Active Graphics* three years after seeing her work for the first time, I had been thinking about the dance stage as a framing device, and I later expanded the discussion of the way frames get disrupted in this dance in an essay entitled "Mining the Dance Field," which is included in the Feminist Theories section.

Many of the discussions in these reviews, especially those written for *Dialogue Magazine for the Arts* in the early to mid-1990s, focus on the relationship between the physical body and cultural identity at stake in the choreography I was seeing on stages in New York City and Ohio. At the time, I found an interesting confluence of themes in many contemporary dances where American history, geography, African-American identity, and individual artistic practices were woven into what I identified as "The New Epic Dance." Several of these short reviews focus on work by Blondell Cummings, Jawole Willa Jo Zollar, Bill T. Jones, and Garth Fagan, as well as that of larger repertory companies such as Dance Theater of Harlem and Joseph Holmes Chicago Dance Theater. Ideas that were briefly sketched out in a paragraph or two here, later became developed in a longer essay entitled "Embodying History," which focused on an in-depth comparative analysis of Bill T. Jones's *Last Supper at Uncle Tom's Cabin/The Promised Land* and Urban Bush Women's *Bones and Ash*. That piece can be found in the Dancing Histories section.

I have chosen to include these early dance reviews because I believe they are a powerful example of how something that begins as a simple observation can grow into the central theme of an essay that incorporates multiple layers of historical or sociological research, not to mention somatic contemplation. Oftentimes I do not know which ideas are going to take root until much later in the process. Thus, rather than jumping right to the mature arguments of my later writing, I have decided to keep these fledgling efforts at writing about performance intact so that younger dancers and scholars can trace the threads of ideas as they weave their way through the various political and poetic strands in this collection.

1

Pooh Kaye and Eccentric Motions

Dance Theatre Workshop, New York City, October 1984.
Women and Performance 2, no. 2, 1985.

Pooh Kaye uses "play" in her performances with conscious intent. In a recent interview, she stated, "Play creates an emotional and immediate response which requires a different way of looking at dance. If the critics were to deal with it seriously, they would realize it is a radical, political notion—a challenge to traditional ways of structuring art." In the evening of dance and film at Dance Theatre Workshop's studio space, Pooh Kaye and the women who dance with her—Claire Bernard, Amy Finkel, Ginger Gillespie, Jennifer Monson, and Sanghi Wagner—smiled and laughed in response to one another while catapulting into each other, rolling together, or mutually supporting each other's weight.

The program began with "an almost finished film by Pooh Kaye." Shot with the endearing quality of a home movie, the film, *Inside the House of Floating Paper,* mixes the animated movements of human beings with those of objects, creating a kind of funhouse where chairs, people, paper, and typewriters roll, hop, and skitter interchangeably. The first image is of a woman dressed in a winter coat, sitting in a chair on rollers. This chair has a mind of its own. It moves, she slides off, and the next few minutes involve a mutual struggle for the top. It is no longer clear here who has control, the woman or the chair, nor does it seem to matter—it's play.

The camera's focus shifts to the middle of a condemned building with gutted, graffiti-lined rooms. A follow-the-leader lineup of people, chairs, and a typewriter is joined by big, animated sheets of colored paper as it tumbles its way out of the building and disperses onto the street. Driving away in mimed, invisible cars, a man and a woman leave the crowd and take refuge in one another's arms, on a boat tranquilly floating down the river.

In *Swept-up,* movement and film are layered to make what is described in the program notes as a "chaotic texture." The dancers play with a new prop—lightweight aluminum garbage cans—that can be carried on the head, used as weapons or hiding places, or simply as playmates. The film is similar in its animated, fun-loving quality, but it speaks a more potent message. Outrageously dressed characters with colored objects, paper, party

hats, chairs, and zebra-striped mattresses are defined as garbage by an unknown voice. Collection teams of Mr. Cleans in spotless white sanitation
trucks chase after this "garbage," dumping people head first into trash bins.
Again and again there are shots of the happy "trash" playing in the streets,
while unidentified work boots are shot menacingly pushing huge brooms
that slowly enclose the people/object garbage.

Unfortunately, we cannot play with colorful paper and garbage cans all
our lives—little girls grow up and their imaginations and bodies are re-
cruited for the real world of urban offices. The program notes that the next
piece, *Bring Home the Bacon,* is an assault on this urban work coercion.
Pooh Kaye explains: "This piece is about the economy and its effects on
small-income people. It is consciously feminist. I chose to work with office
machinery because we were all women, and office work is a woman's job."
The lights brighten to reveal six old-fashioned typewriters meticulously
lined across the back wall. Sparse at first, then rising like a submarine, the
sound surfaces into the disturbing monotony of a computerized typewriter.
This appropriate barrage of sounds is composed by John Kilgore. A dancer
in a rolling desk chair is flung onstage from the wings, followed by a fellow
speeder on a rolling typewriter. There is a mass rush of dancers in black
work pants and uniformly white tops, all on typewriters, enthusiastically
involved in an office game of bumper cars. Agility is at play here, as smash
encounters blend imaginatively into acrobatically coordinated resolutions.
The pace is driven, interrupted only when the dancers are caught in neat
asymmetric poses.

Soon, order prevails as dancers crawl and collect one by one in a unison
sequence that nudges them all over to the far wall. Six rear ends face out,
subdued. But only momentarily; as a shift to handstands frees these office
workers to bang their feet (not their heads) noisily against the wall. Spring-
ing back to their feet, the dancers scatter and bound into the air, landing
indiscriminately on their hands, feet, chests, or backs.

Yet Big Brother is watching, and a censoring force seems to bind these
free movements. Antagonism sets in as three standing women face three
squatting women. The squatters furiously beat their fists against the others'
thighs, but to no avail. The standers hold fast until the subjugated realize
their best offense: blow them away. They puff up their cheeks and noisily
spout gusts of air that send the couples sprawling across the space.

Later, a circle is formed with each woman seated at a typewriter. Fingers
tap frantically at the imaginary machines before them. Elbows are pinned
to the sides, bodies are restrained; even the breathing is bound. Nonetheless,
this circle provides a safe community in which each woman can leave her
imposed office role to swirl, twist, shake, and rebound in an individualized
statement against temporary employment agencies and their suppression of

women's physical and emotional energy. Pooh Kaye explained, "It was as though you could just walk in or out of the office as your anarchistic self. There was definitely an element of shelter in this circle of women."

Pooh Kaye and the dancers of Eccentric Motions are fearless. Although there is little sense of traditional technique, the dancers are skilled in their sheer physicality. Flinging themselves and each other through space, they have mastered the coordination of unexpected interactions: if someone is in the way, cartwheel over them. Visibly enjoying themselves, these dancers have rediscovered the possible affinity we humans could have for the floor, if only we wore more playclothes and sat in fewer desk chairs. Whether Pooh Kaye is framing sheer physicality, chaos, urban offices, or symbolic collection teams, her work carries a joy in the sheer pleasure of the activity, but also a seriousness of conception. The films are funny, the moving is fun, but the messages about society and artistic anarchy are clear.

2

Johanna Boyce

Dance Theatre Workshop, New York City, April 11–22, 1985.
Women and Performance 3, no. 2, 1986.

Johanna Boyce's *Raising Voice,* a brilliant revisionist version of Handel's Hallelujah Chorus, opens with a "family portrait" of a group of diverse women: construction worker, preppy businesswoman, East European peasant, East Village New Yorker. Although their body sizes, hair styles, and clothing preferences differ markedly, these twelve women are joined in a common song. Hailing the "queen of queens," the "lady of ladies," and declaring that "she shall reign forever and ever," the performers unravel their tableau into a joyful skipping procession.

Singing while moving, the women weave through a series of lines, loops, circles, and polkas, forming human mountains and bridges for one another to climb over or step across. Smiling, acknowledging a partner, or greeting someone at the other end of the stage, they encourage a support where a woman can dare anything—even a final, running, leaping nosedive into the arms of others. This Hallelujah Chorus speaks not to "the kingdom of the world," but to the "queendom of her might."

Raising Voice is the first section of a series of narrative vignettes that bring women's lives, sensibilities, and concerns onto the stage. In the dim lights that separate the first section from the second, four women help two others undress. Calmly, purposefully, shirts and pants are folded and placed on an attending arm; socks and shoes are gently arranged. The lights break the strange peace of this interlude and Annuel Dowdell and Cydney Wilkes, dressed in undershirts and pants, present part 1 of *Ties That Bind.* This dance centers on Annuel's and Cydney's emotional histories with their sisters, and perhaps with each other.

Climbing one another like trees, they recite episodes from their early family life. Stories about trips to the dentist, the day-care center, and piano lessons spill out with a raw youthfulness that fluctuates, as do their movements—from timid and gentle to headstrong and rough. Cydney's helpful hand becomes too helpful as it jerks Annuel up and flying in the opposite direction. A teasing scramble ensues, then a wrestling match, until they finally collapse—exhausted. As the two are racing around in a circle, Annuel complains of her sister: "I always felt like I could never catch up to her," while

Cydney declares, "I always felt like she was on my heels." Moments later, the playful competition melts into a friendly embrace. They walk off the stage, hand in hand.

In the middle of *Ties That Bind* part 2, Jennifer Miller stands on Susan Seizer's shoulder and declares, "I see no reason why I should bow down to what Nelson Rockefeller says is beautiful." Jennifer has a beard that grows naturally on her face. Jennifer and Susan are lovers. Shuffling a soft shoe, they introduce one another to the audience as a Taurus and a Gemini. We learn that they met in a contact improvisation class; that they both have exceptional grandmothers. Bit by bit, facts emerge that color in the unique lives of these two women.

Jennifer and Susan are comfortable with their own bodies. Flexible, grounded, and trained in the casual art of giving and carrying each other's weight, they move like young bears—nudging, rolling, and pouncing all over each other as they wind their way across the stage and through the story of their lives and their relationship.

As Jennifer executes a precarious balance on Susan, she tells us (quite naively) that she comes from the insurance capital of the world. Later, when the two are rolling together, arms and legs intertwined, they mention that people often wonder what two women do in bed. The duet becomes intensely personal at times. During a humorous dialogue with Jennifer, Susan details her early friendships and the response of her parents to her coming out. She shrugs her shoulders as she impersonates her father's sleepy "did you wake me up for this?" response to her mother's declaration that "Dear, your daughter has something to say . . ."

In a more serious mood, Jennifer speaks of her mother's illness and relates her experience of spending a year back with her family. Kneeling, she caresses the space in front of her. Her voice softens as she remembers the beard that grew, unencumbered by the usual cosmetic treatments, on her mother's chin while she was ill. Her mother had previously gone to great lengths to rid herself of the beard.

Boyce's work deals with women's expectations and desires. Never treated abstractly, these concerns are explored in the day-to-day personal stories that come from the lives of her performers. The narratives portray experiences of female identity, friendship, and choice. The intimate duets engender a sense of community in the mixed audience, even when they introduce a variety of "hot coals," such as traditional conceptions of female beauty or a direct expression of lesbianism onstage. When Boyce presents an image of community, it is with full preservation of individual differences. Twelve voices in her Hallelujah Chorus create a harmonious sound, yet the ensemble is achieved without homogenizing the women. Presented as individuals, they have an unusual freedom of expression. The open possibility of choice only strengthens the larger identity and connection of the group.

3

Improvisations by Simone Forti and Pooh Kaye

Second Annual Festival of Women Improvisers, Kraine Gallery, New York City, October 10, 1987.

Blood on the Saddle. Choreographed by Jennifer Monson in collaboration with Zeena Parkins. Danspace, New York City, November 7, 1987.

Active Graphics II and Tangled Graphics. Choreographed by Pooh Kaye. Performed by Eccentric Motions. The Kitchen, New York City, December 5, 1987.

Women and Performance 4, no. 1, 1988/1989.

There is a finish on most dancing these days. Highly aerobic, polished, and preened, bodies flash across the stage and then are gone—finished. Watching this kind of spectacle may be visually exciting to some, but it rarely moves me. What did move me last fall and winter was a handful of performances by a three-generation lineage of dancer/choreographers.

There is something powerful and sensuous about the open, raw physicality of Simone Forti, Pooh Kaye, and Jennifer Monson. Historically, these women share a branch on the family tree of postmodern dance. Pooh Kaye studied with Simone Forti from 1973 to 1978, and Jennifer Monson danced with Pooh Kaye for two years. While they now work separately as soloists, or in collaboration with others, these women's work continues to be linked by a commitment to improvisation as a movement source. By allowing for non-technique-oriented movement, improvisation celebrates an idiosyncratic investigation of dancing possibilities. Although their movement personalities are radically distinct, Kaye, Forti, and Monson are all skilled at the wit, risk taking, and playfulness that are central to improvising.

Recently, Simone Forti has been performing a series of solo improvisations called *News Animations*. Forti is known for her movement studies of animals in the zoo, as well as for her devotion to exploring the forms and structures that appear in nature: plants, rocks, the weather. Her teaching seeks to develop an awareness of individual bodily sensations within the changing landscape of movement. This internal attention often gives her dancing an absorbing deliberateness. Usually when I watch Forti, I feel as if I am right next to her, listening to the physical forces that guide her dancing.

On the evening she shared with Kaye and Deidre Murray (a musician) during the second annual Festival of Women Improvisers, Forti's approach seemed a little less holy, less Eastern. She entered the performing space in darkness, her pathway erratically lit by the flashlight dangling from her waist. As the lights brightened, she stood among piles of newspapers, engaged in a slightly sardonic verbal monologue about the news. She used her body as a topographical map on which to act out the Persian Gulf crisis (the subtext of which was ironically sexual), as she accumulated a momentum of language and gesture that hinted at the crazed underside of world events: "Cause they suck the oil out. They suck the oil out of the ground. They suck it out and then they make it into fertilizers and into pesticides and they just spread it back over the top . . . Pump it and pump it up and pump it up."

It is a fine line that Forti balances; reaching out to the edge to find the place where behavior becomes manic, and then recycling that source. Whether she is dealing with personal or political material, Forti is interested in evolving a relationship between dancing and the culture as a whole. And who knows, maybe it will catch on—maybe one day we will turn on the news and find her there.

During the second half of this evening of women improvisers, Kaye joined Forti and Peter van Riper (a musician). The fact that they have rarely worked together since 1978 seemed to color Kaye's and Forti's dancing with a peculiar mixture of wariness and curiosity. Tentative about renewing this dancing relationship, they retreated into their own private games for a while. But soon their fingers and noses became antennae that they used to sniff and prod one another. As they pushed and pulled their movements into frank expressions of affection and combativeness, Forti and Kaye rekindled a connectedness that led their dance to an exhilarating end.

Jennifer Monson's concert—a collaboration with Zeena Parkins at St. Mark's Danspace—was provocatively titled *Blood on the Saddle*. The audience entered through the performing space, in which a line of nine people, shrouded in white sheets, slowly turned from facing backward to forward. "Who are they?" I asked, trying to connect their draped costumes to the Arabic music playing over the loudspeakers. This was the first of several tableaux whose juxtaposition of imagery and events were charged with strange, often unconnected, meanings. The evening was segmented by such divergent performances as the unison, upbeat Jackson Five dancing of the ensemble, or the *entr'actes* performed by Jackie Shue and Jennifer Miller.

Miller juggled vaudevillian wit; she seemed to conspire with the audience. Shue's *entr'acte* was stark and compelling: she was rolled into the center of the space on a neon surrealistic door. Framed by this glittering mosaic of lights and trash, dressed in a makeshift white ball gown and white gloves, she calmly opened a pomegranate and, with increasing ferocity, devoured it. As she ate, her face, dress, and gloves became smeared with the blood-red juice of the fruit. A second before the lights surrounding her blacked out, she looked up with an astonished expression as if she did not know what had just come over her.

Softening the effect of these disturbing tableaux was the very human physicality of Monson's dancing. Engaged and enlivened by the experience of dancing with one another, she and her partners swept through a staggering display of hungry lunges, diving chest rolls, and floor spins, surfacing from this deluge of movement to acknowledge each other's presence before dropping back into its current. While their body types and dancing styles differed drastically, the performers stayed connected through a sympathetic physical synchrony. Even when Monson was the only dancer, weaving her furious bull-like head thrusts and lyrical back arches into a probing, poetic solo that vacillated between willfulness and vulnerability, Monson partnered the music, drifting in and out of the musician's space and the rhythm of her playing.

Pooh Kaye's recent choreography for her company, Eccentric Motions, is characterized by an avalanche of backbends, handsprings, and tumbling floor work, which are fast becoming the company's trademark. In *Active Graphics II* and its sequel, *Tangled Graphics,* although the movement is set and perfected in rehearsals, there is a raw edge to this dancing that harkens back to some of Simone Forti's structured improvisations of the 1970s. In those, the movement task was so difficult to accomplish that all of the performer's energy was concentrated on getting it done.

Active Graphics II opens with a solo within a slender rectangle of light. Slipping her body in and out of the lighted space, a dancer wavers at first, but then dives into the lighted arena. She could be plunged in another substance—water, for instance—for her movements seem to defy earthly rules in their rolling, tumbling procession. Framed—but not contained—by the lit rectangle, she slips in and out of its edges, spreading her energy out beyond its boundaries. Joined by another dancer, and then another like her, she darts through a hopscotch of changing lights that are never quite able to catch up with her.

As I watch the dances of Forti, Kaye, and Monson, I feel as if am watching women move in a manner that escapes traditional representations of dancing women. Working close to and with the floor, using any part of their bodies (arms, shoulders, chests) to hold weight, moving at times with a great deal of momentum, these dancer-choreographers rarely use typically inscribed dance gestures such as an arabesque. Like the soloist in *Active Graphics II,* they slip out of conventional frames. Perfecting a gesture, finding out the effect of momentum in a leg whip, or what it is like to fall while running, Forti, Kaye and Monson discover who they are as dancers. Their performing, then, allows them to exult in movements that most fully represent their desires and experiences. Hovering on the edge of conventional dancing, they whisper to the audience, beckoning us to follow them outside the frame, letting us see what goes on beyond the spotlight.

4

Song of Lawino

Directed by Valeria Vasilevski and choreographed by Jawole Willa Jo Zollar. Aaron Davis Hall, City University of New York, New York, January 5–8, 1989. *Women and Performance* 4, no. 2, 1989.

There is an intriguing, almost eerie mesh of self and other, community and dissent in the dance/theatre piece *Song of Lawino*. As I walked from the lobby, which was filled with people greeting, hugging, and chattering away, into the darkened theater, the flood of community feeling dissipated as I stared at the laundry line hung with brown braids and various hair pieces. What was the meaning of these disembodied remnants of some woman's vanity, some woman's life? It wasn't until I read the short biographies of the performers included in the program that I realized that a few of these hair pieces were actually physical bits of the performers' own life stories. While chopping her childhood braids off gave Connie Chin a sense of liberation from the traditional values of her parents, for Ching Valdes-Aran, cutting her hair was simply a way of earning money to support her fledgling acting career. Strung up among other, more anonymous hair pieces, these braids also served as visual symbols of the difficulty many nonwhite, non-European women have conforming to Eurocentric stereotypes of beauty.

Directed by Valeria Vasilevski, and choreographed by Jawole Willa Jo Zollar with the performers' participation, *Song of Lawino* was inspired by the writing of Okot p'Bitek—a Ugandan poet who died recently in political exile. In his epic poem, also called "Song of Lawino," p'Bitek speaks out against Western political, economic, and social colonialism. Taking on the voice of an Acoli woman, he confronts the reductions of modernization—most poignantly symbolized by the husband's attraction to Westernized "modern" women—by reaffirming the spiritual meanings of traditional Acoli culture. Realizing a dream of p'Bitek's in bringing his message to the stage, the ten women performers weave music, dance, and song into a texture of community and resistance.

The performance of *Song of Lawino* begins with an extraordinary solo by Pat Hall-Smith. Moving cautiously, tentatively onto the stage at first, her back rippling to the sparse melodic sounds of Edwina Lee Tyler playing the thumb piano, Hall-Smith approaches a school lectern with an increasing ferocity of movement. The mythical creatures, ghosts, and ancestral power, which had momentarily swelled her body in a wave of dancing, subside as she begins to read "Let Them Prepare the Malakwang Dish." But her body cannot stand still and separate itself from the anger and purpose of the words she recites. Soon hand gestures, indignant thrusts of the head, and impatient shifts of weight punctuate her speaking until finally her verbal and physical protestations join in a moment of deep, rich song.

Aroused by the powerful authority of her rich voice and the drums that accompany it, other performers begin to sing and dance, setting the whole stage in motion. Later in the performance, the women line up with their arms interlaced, their backs facing the audience. One by one, they turn around to spit back the insults their husbands have showered on them. Phrases like "He called my mother witch" and "He says I am stupid" give testimony to how these absent men have tried to belittle their wives' "old-fashioned" identities and beliefs. This ritual of talking out—of verbally exorcising these insults—serves both to confirm the women's community with one another and also to pull the audience into their emotional struggle. Because they have experienced the kind of double oppression of being both ethnic and female, these ten women from different cultural and ethnic backgrounds can make the bitter, sarcastic language in p'Bitek's writing express their own anger too.

The celebration of anger as well as the ecstasy of a communal release of pain through the lively physical rejoicing of dance and song makes *Song of Lawino* both politically alive and a pleasure to watch. This mix of brilliant, defiant energy and entertainment was particularly evident in a drum solo by Edwina Lee Tyler. Coming after the upbeat, chatty chorus-line style of numbers like "I Do Not Know the Dances of White People," Tyler's testimony is potently nonverbal. Her drumming begins offstage with cadences of soft-mulling rhythms. As she makes her way across the stage, her body takes on the emotions sculpted by the sounds of her hands. Raised eyebrows, winces, furtive glances, knowing smiles, and compassionate nods flash across her infinitely expressive face as she retraces the personal and archetypal stories we have just witnessed. Slowly building a foundation of resistant beats into the melody of her drumming, Tyler inspires both the performers and the audience with a triumphant sense of the creativity and power of community that can emerge out of the shared articulation of oppression and pain.

5

Joseph Holmes, Sizzle and Heat

The *Cleveland Reader*, April/May 1992.

I went to the Joseph Holmes Chicago Dance Theater's January 24 performance at the Ohio Theater in Cleveland with two goals: I wanted to enjoy some high-powered dancing, and I wanted to start to think about the connections between the genre of modern jazz and the politics of a marketing strategy that focuses on the "sheer sizzle" and "heat" of this "multiracial" company. Two and a half hours later, I left the theater filled with a palpable kinesthetic excitement and a heightened curiosity about what the tag "multicultural" might really mean.

The program—which was choreographed, with one exception, by the artistic director, Randy Duncan—opened with *Bittersweet Av* (1987), a dance that portrays the raucous and raunchy milieu of nighttime urban life. This setting was, of course, a perfect backdrop for the kind of physical display that plays such a key role in jazz dancing. Embedded within the theatrical convention of a dance about strutting your stuff on the city sidewalk is a very frank exchange of seeing and being seen between the dancers and the audience.

The dance began with the company exploding onstage in an all-out bump and grind. Enlivened by the sheer satisfaction of outdoing one another, the dancers sauntered downstage and then abruptly launched into a series of energetic movements that frequently ended with a signature toss of the head or swoosh of the hips. Like the tag on a break-dancer's routine, this final flourish left the dancers' individual marks in the air as they turned to swagger offstage with a "Top that if you can!" attitude. Patrick Mullaney emerged from the crowd to perform a marvelously witty and extraordinarily virtuosic solo. A genial and compact Irishman, Mullaney moved with a sly smile that hinted at a delightful ability to parody himself. Roaming all around the stage, he wove in and out of the beat of the popular tunes in the background, lingering over a hip roll in one place, only to dive double-time into the next phrase of spectacular dancing. With a sideways glance and a wiggle in his walk, Mullaney eased into a slower section, acknowledging, with a wink, both his own healthy appetite for daredevil dancing and the audience's desire to watch him move.

The dancers' knowing nods to the audience—these physical references to the theatrical frame of the stage space—were surprisingly empowering. In the section that came after Mullaney's solo, for instance, four men—Arturo Alvarez, Cuitlahuac Suarez, Roger Turner, and Rodni Williams—filled the stage with bold unison movements that rocked pelvises on both sides of the curtain line. Yet the frank sexuality of their dancing did not reduce them to mere objects of the audience's adoring gaze. Rather, the groundedness and power of their movements revealed an individuality that made me feel as if these dancing men were still in control of their own self-representations. The decisiveness with which they all swung into the downbeat coupled with the leisurely pace allowed these dancers the extra split second to insert their own interpretation—to finish with their own movement signature.

Unfortunately, I did not get the same feeling from the duet by two women (Ariane Dolan and Kimberley McNamara) that followed this section. While the men's dancing mostly stayed within a jazz idiom, the women's dancing drew much of its style from classical ballet technique. The abundance of arabesques and pirouettes stifled a certain spirit in the dancing for me, mostly because ballet movements tend to end in a formal pose, rather than an idiosyncratic, signature gesture. Not only did this classical aesthetic have a ridiculous effect when juxtaposed to the blues vocals in the soundtrack, but it served to reestablish many of the typical theatrical conventions of the stage. Along with the ballet style came what one famous dance critic once called a "visionary" gaze—a dry spatial focus that pretends that the stage is a separate world and the audience is not really on the other side of the footlights. By not clearly meeting or acknowledging the audience's own gaze, the two dancers missed the opportunity to subvert the power dynamic implicit in being seen, but not seeing. No matter how high they kicked their legs, these women seemed unable to claim their dancing as their own subjective experience.

The next three dances on the program, *He and She* (choreographed by Joseph Holmes, the founder of the company, in 1983), *Delta* (choreographed by Duncan in 1986), and *Turning Tides* (choreographed in 1986 by Duncan as a tribute to Holmes's legacy) blended the jazzy movements of *Bittersweet Av* with modern and African-American dance styles. Sometimes this combination created a slightly weird effect that made the dancing look cautious or tentative; but at other times, this fusion of styles seemed appropriately mysterious. In *Delta,* for instance, a beautiful blue fabric awning framed the dancers' movements, evoking a surreal landscape where mythic half-animal, half-human beings drifted across the space to a dissonant score by Andreas Vollenweider. The slow-moving angular shapes and deep central contractions of the dancers' bodies created an otherworldly atmosphere that seemed to distill their movements into liquid crystal. Out of this stillness arose a very touching duet between two men that resonated with images of a timeless and enduring companionship.

Dedicated to Holmes, *Turning Tides* most fully incorporated the company's African-American heritage. Set against a solo by Cuitlahuac Suarez, the larger group section brought the individual dancers together with a real sense of dramatic purpose. For the first time all evening, the ensemble danced together as one group (not simply a collection of men and women), and the joy of this communal physicality seemed to both mourn the death of a leader and celebrate the continuity of his vision.

Placed against a backdrop of skyscrapers at night, the final dance was set to a medley of songs by Aretha Franklin. Choreographed jointly by Holmes and Duncan in 1983, *Aretha* brought the audience back to the vernacular styles of city life, milking the high-stepping, leg-kicking routines that characterize much of contemporary jazz dancing. Interspersed throughout the dancing was an occasional short vignette that simultaneously presented and parodied contemporary African-American culture. Much of this hip-swinging, finger-snapping theatrical business came from a small, feisty dancer named Robyn Davis. While I was watching her dance a solo set to Aretha's "Dr. Feelgood," I thought of Josephine Baker and the subtle ways in which Baker could both please a crowd and please herself by dancing. Like Baker, Davis would momentarily step out of the choreography to reference her own sexuality, using Aretha's lyrics to punctuate her own desire.

Significantly, it is through presenting herself within specific cultural frames that Davis was able to extend her own individuality. As the sassy black woman bossing her man around in the trio she danced with Roger Turner and Ariane Dolan, Davis seemed to delight in the eye-rolling, self-parodying archetype that Josephine Baker made famous. Playing back and forth over the stereotype as she crossed the very edge of the stage, Davis acknowledged at once the significance of the image as well as the sheer fun of mocking it. Unfortunately, this kind of complex cultural reference was rare overall, and when it did occur, it often took place as a comic interlude set aside from the dancing. Nonetheless, these brief moments in *Aretha* point to the possibility of creating a jazz style that could incorporate every dancer's cultural icons into the movement itself. This would allow the company individual movement signatures that would truly be multicultural.

6

Performing across Identity

Dialogue Magazine for the Arts, November/December 1991.

"Performance gave me a vocabulary and a syntax to express the processes of rupture and deterritorialization I was undergoing."
—GUILLERMO GÓMEZ-PEÑA

Who am I? is a complex question for minority performance artists working amid the cultural rubble of the late twentieth century. Splayed between different communities, these artists must negotiate a minefield of strategic allegiances and shifting identities. Although "ethnic" forms of artistic and performative expression are finally being supported by many arts foundations, too often the emphasis of these programs is on preserving a static notion of a traditional cultural identity that can remain safely marginalized within American society. I know a classical Indian dancer, for instance, who can readily get a grant for a performance if she applies under a "traditional" arts category, but has difficulty getting funding if she wants to incorporate her experience of living in America for the past twenty years into her dancing and chooses to wear jeans instead of an appropriately colorful sari.

Currently, there is little ideological space within arts organizations for artists whose work threatens to explode tidy assumptions about the role of minority artists in contemporary American society. Ironically, it is precisely these artists who are creating performances which I feel can significantly contribute to one of the most interesting discussions in contemporary cultural theory—that of identity politics. Refusing the categorization of "other" by refusing to limit themselves to a single "authentic" heritage, these artists circle around the hyphen that marks the ambiguous nature of their identity. Artists like Blondell Cummings, an African-American choreographer working out of New York City, and Guillermo Gómez-Peña, a Mexican-American performer and writer, are creating work that attempts to represent the fluid space of their multicultural experience.

Basic Strategies V is the last section of a cycle of dances by Cummings that explore how people grapple with the intersecting political and social webs of work, money, and power. In what she terms her process of "collage," Cummings layers texts by the Caribbean writer Jamaica Kincaid and music by composer Michael Riesman with her own choreography to create a series of connections between individual identity and communal legacies. A remarkable text by Kincaid focuses the dancing in the first section. The flowing, abstract movements of the group's dancing are juxtaposed with a story that braids the history of an indigenous people with that of a colonial Anglican cathedral. Smooth and liquid, the taped narrator's voice loops back on itself repeatedly:

> My history before it was interrupted does not include cathedrals. What my history before it was interrupted includes is no longer absolutely clear to me. The cathedral is now a part of my history. The cathedral is now a part of me. The cathedral is now mine.

During a brief interlude, another text by Kincaid begins to describe with encyclopedic detail the habitat, production and reproduction of the silkworm. Read like an article from *National Geographic,* the information seems tame enough, at first. As the interlude finishes and Cummings's solo begins, however, the context changes and this scientific discourse transforms into a series of metacomments on the politics of colonial enterprise, cheap Third World labor, and the production of Western luxuries.

At the beginning of her solo, the lights fade up very slowly to reveal a statuesque Cummings, wearing a shimmering black evening gown and cape. Slowly raising and lowering a champagne bottle and fluted glass, she turns in a vague, disembodied manner, as if she were a revolving decoration in the middle of the ballroom floor. Her impassive face and glittering dress are reflected in the large mirrors that fan out to either side of her. Functioning as a kind of *Huis Clos,* these mirrors confine her movements, meeting each change of direction with multiple reflections of her own body. Sometimes Cummings moves with proud, grandiose strides, covering the space with a confident territoriality. Other times, she seems frantic and possessed, pacing the floor in this prison of mirrors where she can neither confront nor escape the reflections of the woman she wants—was intended—to become.

In the midst of a luxurious, waltzy section where she is swirling around the stage, Cummings abruptly drops to her knees and, drawing her skirt over her face, begs for money. The spilt-second transformation of her body from ease to despair reminds the viewer of the fragility of that seductive, glamorous world. While the early fracture is quickly smoothed over by the romantic music and Cummings's lyrical dancing, this crack in the illusion widens as photographic slides are projected on a screen above her head. Alternating images of Third World famine refugees with Western signs of wealth and power depicted in Ralph Lauren-like advertisements, these slides throw Cummings's whole intention into question. Is she trying to insert herself into these white, patriarchal images? Or is this whole scenario a conscious attempt to point out the problems inherent in such assimilation?

Cummings's solo forces the audience not only to confront the issues at stake in being a black woman in a white man's world, but also to see the difficulty with representing that experience. No one image, sentence, or gesture can describe an identity that must always shift between cultural icons. With each movement, Cummings introduces an image of herself that is simultaneously vanishing and reappearing in another direction. Her physical presence—the constant turning and turning again—compounds the vertigo of watching both a live body and its multiple refractions. Confronted by their own inability to follow just one image, the audience must shift their attention to the spaces between the mirrors—the space of her dancing. Because the impact of her performance is located in neither her "real" physical body nor its surreal reflections, but rather in the transient movement between these poles of representation, Cummings can fashion a self that insistently exceeds the visible. Turning, and turning again, she is always in the process of re-creating herself; at once suggesting and refusing the boundaries of her own identity.

This crossing and recrossing of boundaries and identities also creates the existential vibration of Guillermo Gómez-Peña's multilingual monologues. Traveling between San Diego and Tijuana, Gómez-Peña works in what he describes as "the fissure between two worlds." In biting, spitfire performances like the one he gave at the Wexner Center for the Arts in April 1991, Gómez-Peña elaborates a network of visual and textual references to his cultural moorings, while simultaneously cutting himself loose from any "ethnic" ties that might bind him too closely to one fixed identity.

Seated at a table overflowing with artifacts of both the pop and sacred cultures of his intercultural existence, Gómez-Peña launches into a monologue that continues to shift relentlessly between languages and cultures. The "Border Brujo" character suggested by the visual effects of his "Chicano" costume or his "Latin" looks is quickly disrupted as Gómez-Peña switches from English to Spanish; from the talk of a streetwise macho hood into postmodern artist-speak; from the rhythmic incantations of a priest to the thick, slurred tempo of a drunk's rantings; and from the breathy accent of a transvestite to the repetitive sloganism of a politician. Although this linguistic smorgasbord evokes typical border characters, the superbly performed dialects that conjure up these talking heads also expose them as simplistic stereotypes.

Like Cummings's mirrored images, Gómez-Peña's many voices echo back upon themselves to create an aural texture that is always in the process of appearing and receding. Over the course of a performance, this cacophonous sound mixture becomes a wonderfully elusive representation of multiple locations of his self. The rapid onslaught of his multilingual text underlines Gómez-Peña's inability to identify with one, fixed "ethnicity." This intense sonal whirlpool of languages and dialects can easily disorient those not immersed in the same reality. Yet it is precisely in the midst of this disorientation that the audience can begin to appreciate Gómez-Peña's ability to situate himself within this turbulent border lifestyle.

Hopefully, the work of increasingly visible performance artists like Blondell Cummings and Guillermo Gómez-Peña will begin to have an impact on the structures of institutions that support the arts, forcing them to reevaluate the inherent racism in their funding criteria. Refusing to be limited to either one category or another—to either here or there—these artists are exploring ways in which to express a cultural experience that is itself always in flux. Watching their performances, we must admire their willingness to risk the terms of their own representation and confront the ambiguity of these cross-cultural identities.

7

In Dialogue with *Firebird*

Dialogue Magazine for the Arts, May/June 1992.

With its powerful combination of visual and romantic subtexts, the pas de deux is the cornerstone of classical ballet. Traditionally, this duet sequence is marked by an elaborate attention to the ballerina. The male dancer partners the female dancer so as to display her technique; his steady hand helps her extend into an arabesque and his lifts help sustain the illusion of her ephemerality. His presence frames the ballerina in three critical ways: physically, with his partnering; visually, with his gaze; and narratively, with the story of his desire for her. One consequence of this structure is that the danseur's sight becomes a lens which directs the audience's own way of looking. We see not only what he sees, but how he sees her as well. In addition to being eroticized in this fashion, the classical ballerina is also frequently framed as an enticingly elusive creature from another world and thus becomes exoticized as well. When an African-American ballet company stages these classical pas de deux in the 1990s, the implications of this doubly—erotically and exotically—objectifying gaze are foregrounded in important ways.

In their recent Cleveland season (State Theater, March 11–15), Dance Theater of Harlem presented two ballets: *Dialogues,* a contemporary choreography by Glen Tetley, and *Firebird,* a reconstruction of the famous 1910 collaboration between Igor Stravinsky and Michel Fokine for Diaghilev's Ballets Russes. *Firebird* is a fairy tale about the triumphs of good over evil that begins with an elaborate pas de deux between a magical half-woman, half-bird creature and her captor. While Fokine's movement vocabulary infused the classical idiom with expressive gesture, his choreography maintains, for the most part, the double gaze embedded in the classical duet form. Staged by Dance Theater of Harlem in a mythic jungle environment, this version of *Firebird* reflects back on itself, highlighting the cultural situatedness of its own representation. In other words, by watching a black ballerina dance the role of Firebird, I become aware of the ways in which classical ballet has traditionally both eroticized female bodies and exoticized black bodies. In Dance Theater of Harlem's production, this history of the gaze is made obvious and subverted in interesting ways.

Even though it is based on a series of four pas de deux, *Dialogues* manages to shift the dynamic of the gaze in order to physically articulate a mutually interactive pas de deux based on the equal exchange of seeing and being seen, moving and being moved. The ease with which the dancers in these duets respond to one another also suggests the possibility for a different viewing relationship between the performers and the audience. The juxtaposition of these two ballets within one program both allows for a critique of the hegemonic structure of the pas de deux, and offers an alternative vision of this particular form in classical ballet.

Dance Theater of Harlem was founded in 1969 by Arthur Mitchell, an African-American classical ballet dancer who had trained with Balanchine and danced in the New York City Ballet, and Karel Shook, his ballet teacher. Mitchell's original goal was to form an all-black dance company in order to prove to the rarefied and Eurocentric world of ballet that African Americans could successfully dance the classical idiom. In addition, he set up a school and a series of public outreach programs to attract and train young black dancers. Mitchell believes that art is a realm that can speak to many cultural traditions and that ballet provides a sort of universal language with which to speak one's own experience. Yet the specific context of that experience, especially of an African-American dancer, suggests the possibility of making that universal language speak in a different way.

The range of Dance Theater of Harlem's repertory, which includes jazz-inspired and Afrocentric dances, as well as several neoclassical works by Balanchine, and traditional narrative ballets such as *Giselle, Swan Lake,* and *Firebird,* reflects this breadth of experience. When he produces traditional ballets, Mitchell strategically alters the settings and costumes in order to incorporate the company's cultural heritage. Thus, Dance Theater of Harlem's version of *Giselle* is set in a southern creole community, and their version of *Firebird* is staged in a mythic jungle environment.

Their production of *Firebird* begins with a young man walking stealthily across the stage. He is a hunter, stalking unseen prey. As the music speeds up, a bright red light swirls around his head. Startled by this elusive light, he moves to the side and watches (unseen) from a distance as the Firebird dances onstage. She is dressed in a fiery red costume that shimmers as she crisscrosses the stage in a series of exuberant leaps and turns. The Firebird holds a pose momentarily, and in these moments the fascinated hunter draws closer to get a better look. Eventually, he captures her unawares. Suddenly entrapped in his arms, the Firebird freezes. The vitality of her previous dancing immediately drains away and she appears delicate and fragile in his arms. What follows is an elaborate negotiation in the form of a pas de deux. Bit by bit, she regains her strength and gradually convinces the hunter to release her. Enlivened by the preciousness of her refound freedom, the Firebird repeatedly breaks away from and returns to the hunter in a series of increasingly daring leaps.

Although the Firebird's beginning solo is characterized by brilliantly fast and expansive dancing, conveying her voracious appetite for the freedom of soaring through space, it is also ironically contained by the hunter's scopic presence. Visually in awe of such a fascinating creature, the hunter becomes wrapped up in the desire for her elusive image, and he physically enwraps her in his arms. This double intertwining—at once physical and psychic—is, of course, the basis for many duets in traditional ballets. Yet the potency of this mutual connection is diluted here by the ever-present gaze of the hunter. Although she leaves the stage in a glorious leap, the Firebird's presence is still framed by the hunter, who watches transfixed until the lights fade.

Because the Firebird's subjectivity is ultimately dependent not only on escaping the physical grasp of the hunter, but also on eluding the overpowering dynamic of his gaze, it is in the second scene of the ballet—when the hunter's eye is transferred to the Princess of Unreal Beauty, another figure of exotic femininity—that her real empowerment occurs. In this climactic scene, the quiet pastoral atmosphere of this enchanted jungle is thrown into chaos as the Princess of Evil and her creatures swarm around the stage. Leaping onstage in the midst of this bedlam, the Firebird propels the evil creatures with the energy from her fast, tight spins, all the while helping the young man subdue the Princess of Evil. Once the battle is won and the stage is clear, the Firebird reappears to dance a triumphant solo marked by a serene powerfulness. Her dance ends with an extraordinary cascade of small bourrée steps that set her whole body vibrating, and seem to release her spirit into the air. As a figure whose body and spirit refuses containment, the Firebird can be interpreted here as an important symbol of the struggles of Dance Theater of Harlem—a company which was born out of its founder's refusal to be contained by the overwhelming elitism and racism of American ballet.

Dialogues, which received its company premiere in 1991, is based on physical conversations between men and women. The four pas de deux in this modern ballet are choreographed to four movements of Alberto Ginastera's Concerto for Piano and Orchestra, Opus 28. One of the reasons that the duets in *Dialogues* felt like the physical meeting of two equal partners was that, unlike the pas de deux in the first scene of *Firebird*, these duets were based on a mutual exchange of looking. Indeed, this visual give and take constituted an integral part of the dancing and displaced the traditional voyeuristic frame of the male gaze.

Watching this piece, I was amazed at how inventively Tetley had used ballet vocabulary to make a dance about relationships between men and women that allowed each dancer his or her own physical integrity. Although the classical lines of the body were present throughout the dancing, the ballet vocabulary had been expanded to include rich successive movements initiated by the central body. The focus of this dance was on the flow of two bodies' movement together and apart from one another. Like a couple ice-skating together, the dancers often stayed in close contact with one another, basing their interaction on a tangible sense of physical synchrony and movement dynamic, rather than the more dramatic relationships staged in many narrative ballets. It was kinesthetically satisfying for me to see these couples dancing with an acceptance of their bodies' weight and a real physical enjoyment of the resulting momentum. That sense of satisfaction was a result of a very different visual dynamic between the dancers themselves and, by extension, between the performers and the audience. The physical meeting of the two dancers allowed me to enter the dance as well, constructing a representational frame in which both the dancers and the audience could meet as mutually empowered participants.

8

Dancing Bodies and the Stories They Tell

Dialogue Magazine for the Arts, March/April 1993.

The one, overwhelming image I have of La La La Human Steps' multi-media extravaganza is of Louise Lecavalier flying through the air like a human torpedo. She gets caught by another dancer, thrashes around with him for a while, then vaults right out of his arms and halfway across the stage, only to rebound back into his face. Two minutes and who knows how many heartbeats later, she rears up from the floor one last time, shakes her mane of bleached-blonde hair and struts off the stage with an attitude that would make the most vicious heavy-metal rocker look like Pete Seeger by comparison.

Louise Lecavalier is the star of Édouard Lock's dance and rock creation *Infante c'est destroy,* which I witnessed during the Festival International de Nouvelle Danse in Montreal this fall. Throughout this nonstop, seventy-five-minute spectacle, Lecavalier's body—both its hardened aerobic energy and its filmed image—is continuously on display. Pitted against the pounding sounds of Skinny Puppy, Janitors Animated, David Van Tiegham, and Einsturzende Neubauten, her dancing uses the driving beat of the music to stretch dance movements to the outer limits of physical possibility and endurance. At one point, Lecavalier grabs one of the various mikes littered around the stage and panting, discusses the metaphysical dimensions of music, heartbeats, and physical energy. She then produces a mini mike, which she solemnly attaches to percussionist Jackie Gallant's chest. With the kind of cosmic, synergistic intensity that makes heavy metal so seductive to teenagers, Gallant begins to pound away at her drum. The harder Gallant drums, the faster her heartbeat. The faster her heartbeat, the faster she drums to keep up. As Gallant builds quickly to the orgasmic peak of her auto-aerobic union with the drum, Lecavalier comes crashing back to center stage, riding the musical tidal wave just as Gallant finishes.

The first ten minutes of Lecavalier's dancing is absolutely awe-inspiring. Within a few minutes, her well-defined muscles are pumped up and her body is practically pulsating with untapped energy. The way she launches her body across the floor and at various partners is phenomenal. Physically, she is powerful. But, unfortunately, much of that power gets stripped away by the relentless repetitions of the same old stunts, as well as by the sexist frames of Lock's stage design. Most of the time, Lecavalier and her two female backups, Pim Boonprakob and Sarah Williams, dance around in various stages of undress, frequently throwing themselves at the male dancers who are unusually dressed in suits. By contrast, Lecavalier is usually totally naked, topless, or dressed in a black bustier and tight short-shorts. Occasionally, she will sport a black leather jacket, but usually that is when she is wearing nothing else on top. My point, of course, is not that the women get naked onstage; it is that they are the only ones who do so. And although their bodies are all superbly delineated, the physical power in their dancing gets subdued by the context of Lock's choreographic presentation.

Édouard Lock is a filmmaker, a photographer, as well as a director of mega pop spectacles. Critics frequently call Lecavalier his muse, likening her role in *Infante c'est destroy* to a blend of Madonna and Joan of Arc. Visually, they have a point, but spiritually, Lecavalier—in spite of her bulging muscles and daredevil feats—usurps none of the power or male prerogative in the way that Joan of Arc and Madonna did. Whether she is framed by the camera as in the huge blown-up films of her falling slowly through space, or by the men onstage, Lecavalier's physicality never seems to be able to break out of Lock's own vision of her body.

Donna Uchizono's body takes on a frail, rag-doll quality in *Désirée*, especially in the moments in her dancing when her head is flopping from side to side and her arms are held stiffly out in front of her. But there are other moments, as when her whole body is lashing out at some unknown force; when the intensity and clarity of her rapid-fire movement creates its own sense of purpose. The juxtaposition of these moments of claiming control over her body versus being controlled by some outside force create the drama in this solo, which I first saw as part of the Yard's annual choreographer's showcase in New York City this fall.

The piece begins as Uchizono, dressed in black, drops a huge bunch of red flowers over her head all the while facing away from the audience. The spotlight fades and she retreats upstage to begin a journey towards the flowers. This time she is facing the audience—her arms bent and fists clenched in furious movements that are alternately self-directed, as when she hits her torso, and directed outward, as when she randomly punches the space around her. As she approaches the pile of strewn flowers, her feet break out in a stamping pattern, crushing and scattering the flowers around her. The deluge of pain and passion is over for the time being and she is still, listening for a while before she nosedives into the flowers and back into the fury of her earlier dancing. Later, in one of the most beautiful moments of the dance, she takes off her top to reveal a long-stemmed red rose running up her spine. The stark contrast of her black pants, naked back, and red rose creates a powerful image of strength and vulnerability. She turns to touch it and ends up spinning faster and faster, like a cat trying to catch its own tail. Uchizono finally grabs the flower and holds it in front of her, allowing it to lead her dizzy stumbling back and forth across the stage as if it were a divining rod.

It is not clear to me exactly what the flowers mean to Uchizono, but I find them to be a potent metaphor for a certain feminine beauty and physicality that Uchizono seems to be struggling with. The image of the rose on her back reminds me of a story by Maxine Hong Kingston called "White Tigers," in which the heroine's back is carved with the names of her family. Applied painfully and indelibly on her skin, these names give her the strength to go forth into the world, but they also insist on her eventual reincorporation into a structure that confines her. Similarly in *Désirée,* the flowers provide both the visual space and narrative impulse for Uchizono's dancing, but they also imply an image of "woman" that her body is unwilling to accept.

While *Désirée* alludes to the issues of body image only very obliquely, Marta Renzi's excerpted solo *I'm Not Very Pretty,* which was shown in her Lincoln Center Out-of-Doors program in August and the solo which David Dorfman presented in December at the Danspace Benefit to support artist fees, both explicitly tackled issues surrounding their own changing perceptions of their bodies.

A full-bodied yet casual dancer, Marta Renzi has a luscious movement style that emphasizes the pleasure of moving through off-balance tilts, as well as the precision of bold leg gestures and intricate footwork. Her solo adds another layer as she works her way through a monologue about her self-image as a girl in dance class. The taped text is actually a conversation between Renzi and her husband, Daniel Wolff. Renzi's voice often sounds doubtful and hesitant, causing her husband to reassure her that he thinks she is beautiful. But she slips through a maze of sensuous movement phrases, which tumble almost effortlessly out of her body. Eventually, the reality of this dancing overcomes the memory of her vulnerability and the piece ends as she realizes that she does not need to be beautiful in order to dance, but rather that it is when she is dancing that she feels most beautiful.

Out of Season or Eating Pizza While Watching 'Raging Bull' was David Dorfman's contribution to Danspace's benefit, "Amazing Grace." Billed as a work-in-progress, *Out of Season* starts as an autobiographical monologue about Dorfman's mother's death and his subsequent weight gain, and quickly unravels into a series of free associations that intersperse pop images with the more jagged-edge truths of interracial romance, death, and human suffering. While some of his text smacks of sentimental clichés (including his final litany of "I care about x, I care about y, I care about you"), his physical presence nevertheless conveys a certain noble concern about the world.

Dorfman first appears walking nosily over to the off-center mike onstage. He is dressed in sports shorts and a T-shirt, with a plastic crash helmet on his head and football shoulder pads, kneepads, and odd-looking protection gear attached to his hips. This weird outfit makes his large frame look even bulkier and as he stares unprepossessingly out to the audience, he looks like he has wandered into the wrong place. He launches into his monologue anyway, interrupting the text at key moments to step away from the mike and into a battery of drill-like movements that often slam his body into the floor. Arising almost apologetically from the ground, Dorfman adjusts his padding and continues with his monologue.

I was profoundly intrigued by this fragment of a dance because of Dorfman's willingness to address his body image on stage. With few exceptions, this issue has been confined to the province of "hysterical" female performance artists like Karen Finley, and it is gratifying to see men begin to grapple with the implications of the "dancer equals thin" mentality too.

All varieties of male bodies have appeared in the work of Bill T. Jones/Arnie Zane Dance Company. Indeed, the focus of some of the early duets between Jones, a tall black man, and Zane, a short, compact white man, was on the ways that two men with such different physical builds could partner one another. It is not unusual to see all sizes and all races of male bodies dancing in their choreography, including the heavyset frame of Lawrence Goldhuber and the emaciated, AIDS-debilitated body of Demian Acquavella. Watching the company's New York season at the Joyce this October, I was again struck by the incredible diversity of these male bodies. (I was also struck by the absence too—Zane died in 1988; Aquavella, in 1990.)

Continuous Replay was originally a solo, then a duet, and now it is a group work for seventeen people, all of whom appear nude at sometime or other during the piece. This dance is based on a series of hand and arm motions—gestures that accumulate as more and more dancers come onstage. Often the choreography juxtaposes the unison movement of the group with a solo variation, and it is interesting to watch how different bodies perform the same motions. But what struck me most in this dance was the rigidity of female body types in the midst of such flexibility concerning male ones. While the women's heights and skin colors may vary, all the female dancers in Bill T. Jones/Arnie Zane Dance Company were thin, sleek, and muscular. Even though their dancing was uniformly extraordinary, it tended to fade into the background of several dances, and none of the women's personalities shone through the choreography in quite the same way as the men's did. Watching, I realized that although Goldhuber could move his graceful 250-pound body across the stage without a stitch of clothing on, we were still a long way from seeing the same size women dance in this company.

Laurie Carlos is a big woman who makes strong theater pieces about heavy subjects. I saw her *White Chocolate for My Father* the same weekend that I saw the Bill T. Jones/Arnie Zane Dance Company, and the contrast was remarkable. While the male dancers were the stars in that company, women clearly owned the show in Carlos's work. Based on the intersecting life stories of six African-American women, *White Chocolate* combines Carlos's text and stage direction, with music composed by Don Meissner, choreographed dance sequences by Jawole Willa Jo Zollar, the director of Urban Bush Women, and a stage design by Seitu Ken Jones.

The piece opens with a blitz of five women crisscrossing the stage from every direction, talking, gesticulating, hollering, and pounding on the floor with big sticks that looked like crosses between maize pounders and giant phalluses. They are all dressed in eccentric versions of 1950s clothes, and as the dust begins to settle after the first onslaught of talk, talk, talk, their characters take on the personalities implied by their costumes. There is the uppity, churchgoing grandmother, complete with fussy shoes and an even fussier hat. There is the trying very hard to stay young mother who is glamorous and overly dependent on male approval, and the three sisters who have grown up in body, but not necessarily in attitude. The fragmented story of equally fragmented lives is told from "Lore's" (played by Laurie Carlos) point of view, and it is her physicality that generates the constant vibration and much of the energy onstage. Every time Lore speaks, her body is right there with her, shaking, prodding, and sometimes even twitching in agreement with what her mouth is saying.

Moving in the shadows of this hysterical commotion are two figures who represent the wisdom and integrity of generational survival. White Light Spirit (Cynthia Oliver) is the African spine of the piece—a kind of core physical identity whose silent presence and low, serpentine movements flow almost unseen among the other characters. Emilyn is the mother slave (played, ironically, by a white woman, Evangeline Johns), whose mantra of "I have never had no white man's child'in" foregrounds the network of racism, misogyny, and abuse, which slowly emerges over the course of the performance. These two mythic figures act as shepherds, physically weaving in and among the extended family of women whose interpersonal relationships become increasingly troubled as the stories of mothers who allow their men to abuse their daughters surface in each generation.

One of the most powerful moments for me was a unison group dance that temporarily interrupted the emotional narratives. This section began with all the women pointing on a diagonal, stamping and gesturing as they marched towards the audience. The mix of African movements with fifties dance steps, and the wonderfully diverse manner in which their different bodies approached the movement (for instance, some women leaning over to touch the ground and others simply gesturing towards it), seemed to acknowledge the physical connectedness that these women experienced even in the midst of their often abusive relationships. Knowing the kinds of contradictions we all must live with in order to forge communities across differences, I was moved by how this double bind of pain and love, of separation and continuity, was captured in *White Chocolate* through the potent juxtaposition of these women's dancing bodies and the stories they tell.

9

Embodying History

The New Epic Dance

Dialogue Magazine for the Arts, March/April 1994.

Garth Fagan and Bill T. Jones are both African-American choreographers working within a genre of contemporary performance that I think of as the "New Epic Dance." Garth Fagan's *Griot New York* and Bill T. Jones's *Last Supper at Uncle Tom's Cabin/The Promised Land* are two evening-length works that explore various facets of their own cultural heritages, refiguring written history in order to embody a tale of their own making. Using dance as a kind of metaphor for the physically inexplicable, the suffering, and glory of a people so long denied the right to speak their own histories, these two choreographers and their collaborators have created theatrical spectacles that evoke the elegiac as well as celebratory spirit of a people wedged in between the past and the future. In many ways, these works remind me of the term that Audre Lorde used to describe her autobiographical work *Zami: A New Spelling of my Name.* Grounded in, but not limited to the historical facts of a people's existence, these dances weave what Lorde calls a "biomythography," elaborating a complex texture of sound and motion into a visionary saga of social and personal survival.

Although Bill T. Jones and Garth Fagan share similar cultural projects and identity categories, their dances are, in fact, strikingly dissimilar, separated both by a historical generation and a world of aesthetic difference. While these differences are manifested in multiple ways, I think that they are rooted in these men's divergent conceptions of the place of the performing body in their choreography. For Garth Fagan, the dancing body is framed as his artistic medium, a technical life force with which he creates his choreographies. For Bill T. Jones, the performing body first locates itself onstage as a human body, and then proceeds to wow the audience with some fantastic dancing.

Garth Fagan was born in Jamaica fifty-three years ago. During his youth, Fagan performed with the Jamaican National Dance Company. Although he originally moved to the United States to study psychology, he was soon haunting New York City dance studios, absorbing the various influences of the seminal figures of American dance. In 1970, Fagan moved to Rochester, New York, to teach dance at the State University of New York, Brockport.

There, he launched a fledgling dance company, wittily called Bottom of the Bucket, but . . . Later, as the company developed and became increasingly professional and technical, the name was changed to Bucket Dance Theater, and subsequently became Garth Fagan Dance. It was on this final incarnation, a company of technically superb dancers, that Fagan choreographed his evening-length dance *Griot New York*.

Commissioned by the Brooklyn Academy of Music (BAM) for the Next Wave Festival (with additional support from the Vienna Festival-Tanz '92, the Houston International Festival, the University of the Arts, and the University of Kansas concert series), *Griot New York* is an extraordinary artistic collaboration between choreographer Garth Fagan, jazz composer and musician Wynton Marsalis, and sculptor Martin Puryear. When it was staged last fall at the Wexner Center in Columbus on October 14, 1993, Marsalis's band accompanied the dancing, lending an exciting improvisational quality to the performance event. Based on a short poem by Fagan that evokes the energy of New York City, as well as the spiritual center of his Afro-Caribbean heritage ("Rife ancestors ritual/Ritual skyscraper riffs"), *Griot New York* is a movement epic in eight sections that weaves different historical vignettes together with joyous moments of spectacular dancing. A *griot*, the program notes informs us, is a West African storyteller: a cultural custodian who preserves and transmits a people's history and traditions. Here Fagan is figured as an invisible griot, weaving his commitment to dancing into a parable about a people's survival.

The dance begins with a section aptly entitled *City Court Dance*. At first there are only two dancers onstage, executing a stylized pas de deux that splices jazzy moments of off-balance pelvic tilts into a classically based duet. Soon, they are joined by the rest of the company, as the original "courting" couple is multiplied into an ensemble court dance of social stalking and being stalked. Throughout this section, the dancers maintain the "cool," slightly distanced presentation of the self that marks much contemporary classicism.

In the next section, *Bayou Baroque,* the long elegant arms and legs of the dancers shift context to become insect-like appendages, intertwining with one another in an abstract mating ritual. Facing each other, but most often not looking at one another, these dancers seem like otherworldly creatures evolving through an elaborate series of entanglements, like cosmic three-dimensional puzzles. Eventually, these creatures leave the stage to two lovers in *Spring Yaounde*. Recasting the same entwining gestures into a slower pas de deux, Fagan softens the edges of his choreography for the first time here, allowing for a broader range of emotional qualities in the supporting and embracing of their interconnected dancing.

During his career, Garth Fagan has sought to digest the multiple influences of modern, ballet, and Afro-Caribbean dance in order to create his unique movement style appropriately dubbed "Fagan" technique. His dancers are virtuosic, combining the fast feet and high legs of ballet, the weight and floor work of modern, and the rhythmic energy and torso isolations of Afro-Caribbean dance. Yet this technique is based on a certain formal presentation of the body that continually frames it as dance, creating an odd dynamic within the more naturalistic sections of *Griot New York*.

For instance, in a later section of the work called The Disenfranchised, the movement is based on gestures of reaching up toward the sky—a staircase to (heaven?) placed stage right gives a sense of religious overtones to these movements—and then falling in despair and rolling on the floor. The weight, effort, and repetition of these gestures seems to drag the dancers down even further. As they become increasingly isolated, they are unable to find solace in one another or the messenger figure who moves through the masses, encouraging them not to lose faith. For me, this section paradoxically evoked a powerful sense of pathos, and yet at the same time, produced an oddly melodramatic effect. Even with the torn costumes that symbolized their destitution, it was hard to read these perfectly defined dancers' bodies as "homeless," perhaps because their pleading, grasping gestures were laid on top of a physical attitude in the torso that still bespoke a certain grandeur of classical presentation.

Even in his most theatrically self-conscious works like the evening-length epic *Uncle Tom's Cabin/The Promised Land* (which Midwestern audiences saw two years ago in Columbus and Chicago), Bill T. Jones's choreography evokes for me the sense that I am watching a group of people who happen to prefer the language of movement to express their situation, rather than dancers who are "performing" choreography. There is a certain ease with which his dancers approach even the most strenuous and difficult movement combinations that makes me feel the interconnectedness of aesthetic and human expression in his work. This was especially true of the group of dances that the Bill T. Jones and Arnie Zane Dance Company presented recently in Cleveland at the Ohio Theatre on January 21 and 22, 1994.

The story of Bill T. Jones's and Arnie Zane's artistic and personal relationship is a story of a love affair—a love affair not only of a short and a tall man, of a black and a white one, but also of dance and pictures, bodily motion and visual imagery. When they met at the State University of New York at Binghamton in 1971, Jones was an athlete working his way into becoming a dancer and Zane was a budding photographer. Dance quickly became the common language through which their lives, hopes, dreams, attitudes, and eventually Zane's death (in 1988), would acquire both a deep personal meaning and a means of public expression. During their performances together, this immediate reality of their relationship always seemed to dwell just outside our view in the wings of the theater. Now that Zane is gone, what Burt Supree has called "the daily fact of absence" shades the physical states of Bill T.'s own dancing, as well as that of the company. This is most evident in pieces like Jones's solo *Red Room,* the dance that opened the Cleveland concert.

Although it was originally commissioned in 1987 as part of Robert Longo's performance epic *Killing Angels,* it is difficult not to see this dance as a powerful evocation of a survivor's existential suspension. Why God? Why Arnie? Why me? Why now? The piece begins with Jones onstage, splayed in a Christ-like position against a rich blood-red curtain. The material is gathered at the center, so that it looks like a beautiful giant angel hovering over Jones's body. Accompanied by a musical score that sounds at first like a heartbeat, Jones leaves the security of the angel's shadow, coming forward in measured steps. Still powerful and intricately sculpted, his naked torso looks thicker now, and his movement seems more weighted, less flighty, and quick. In this solo, Jones's dancing seems fragmented, as if it is inspired by the memories of his collaborative dances with Zane. There are the gestural tidbits which I associate with their mid-1980s style (in pieces like *Secret Pastures*), as well as the moments of full-bodied, almost exhibitionist dancing that Jones has always executed with breathtaking spontaneity. But mostly, I remember the poignancy of his supplicant gestures towards the sky, questioning, always questioning . . . why?

If *Red Room* evokes the elegiac quality of memory, *Soon,* a duet choreographed by Jones in the late 1980s, seems to recapture the joyful, youthful exuberance and ironic wit of Zane's and Jones's earlier collaborations. Set to music by Kurt Weill and Bessie Smith, this duet begins with a soft-shoe routine that at first camps the romanticized dancing of figures like Fred Astaire and Ginger Rogers, and then proceeds to embrace the sheer pleasure of moving side by side with someone you love. Performed by Arthur Aviles and Eric Geiger, *Soon* plays contemporary gay contexts against the backdrop of heterosexual romantic conventions. As Lotte Leyau sings in her husky voice of those "young men who woo you with words," Aviles shimmies up to Geiger while seductively and yet somewhat humorously rubbing his own belly. Here, the audience grasps at once the celebration of passion in the music, the queer commentary on a heterosexual norm, as well as the very potent physical exchanges between the two dancers.

Later in the dance, in the midst of vaudevillian show-upmanship and the bluesy sounds of Bessie Smith, these two men exchange short solos, interchanging the roles and the pleasures of performing for one another. At one point near the end of the duet, Aviles sits on the floor, providing with his legs a diamond-shaped shelter into which Geiger repeatedly dives. This image of giving a partner the security and space of one's own body seemed an apt physical metaphor for the caring, intersubjective relationship that marked Jones's and Zane's artistic collaborations. The directness and frank sexuality of the dancing in *Soon* was rendered even more potent during the final curtain calls, when Bill T. announced to the Cleveland audience that the Ohio Theatre was the last place that Arnie performed before he got sick. Almost six years after Arnie's final dance, his spirit still vividly informs much of the company's work, as Bill T. and the others continue to dance their lives.

While I situate both Fagan's and Jones's full-evening length works in what I call the "New Epic Dance," I believe that these two choreographers approach the notion of "epic" differently. In works like *Griot New York,* Fagan uses the genre of epic to create a heroic saga of a people's history. Destitution, love, and celebration are some of the themes that document that struggle. As metamorphosed through a dance technique that draws on a classical presentation of the body, these themes recall those of earlier epics of Western civilization. In contrast, Jones reworks the genre of epic, refusing many of its elitist assumptions by emphasizing the contradictions of heroism and the ambivalence of survival. His choreography continues to maintain a dialogue between the person performing and the specific nature of the part performed. This creates a kind of self-reflective communication that makes me feel both as if the dancers are truly embodying the movements, and likewise that the choreographic choices really seek to embody the dancers' own physical presences. Jones's revisioning of epic is particularly potent given the contexts of much of his recent focus on the issues of life and death. In fact, his next full-evening-length work is entitled *Still/Here,* and deals with the ageless and yet vitally contemporary issues of hope and survival in the face of loss. Based on survival workshops that Jones has been doing all around the country, this new epic will no doubt push the genre even further, refusing the classical model in order to ask: what is the use of a heroic death?

10

Desire and Control

Performing Bodies in the Age of AIDS

Dialogue Magazine for the Arts, March/April 1996.

At the post-performance discussion of choreographer Elizabeth Streb and her company Ringside's recent performance in Cleveland on January 19 and 20 at the Ohio Theater, an audience member asked the dancers what their physical training regimes consisted of. Actually, the question went something like this: how did you get so built-up? Now, Elizabeth Streb and her seven young company members are pretty awesome dancers-cum-gymnasts. They have cultivated tight, muscular bodies that maximize their movement potential. Streb began making dances in 1979, and formed her company Ringside (a tongue-in-cheek reference to both circus and boxing rings) in 1985. Streb's dances are built on mastering the very real physical challenges of moving across, with, through, and in various pieces of physical equipment, including a twelve-foot wall, a twenty-two-foot pole, a coffin-like box suspended sideways in the air, a bouncing mat, two 4 x 8 plywood panels, and a trampoline complete with adult jungle gym. Sometimes when I watch Streb's work, I get the feeling that I am at a circus and all I can do is to marvel at the sheer spectacle of her dancers launching their bodies through the space. Other times, my attention is drawn away from the mere fact of what they are doing to the how of it, as I notice the physical coincidences between the dancers, and their spatial, kinesthetic, or rhythmic interactions.

Streb/Ringside's recent program was entitled POPACTION. Over the course of the evening's six pieces, the performers flung themselves at walls, catapulted one another into the air, and dive-bombed through the space, just barely missing one another as they landed on a mat. In the first piece of this concert, *Wall* (1991), five dancers in bright blue Lycra unitards throw themselves against a red wall. During this short piece (Streb's work often has a slightly clipped feel to it, as if to say "Let's do it and move on."), these dancers climb up one another in their efforts to reach the top of the wall, and then they slide down it, bash against it, and hang from various body parts on it.

Streb's choreography highlights a hyper-athletic physicality. She is interested in movement for movement's sake; not in order to tell a story or to express an emotional state. Her dances are about the raw physics of bodies in motion. Ironically, however, her audience seemed much more interested in the shape of the dancers' bodies—their defined musculature and sleek look—than in their dancing. The people sitting around me during the performance (the lengthy equipment setups gave me good opportunities to eavesdrop on my neighbors) kept commenting on various dancers' bodies, wondering how often and how much they worked out. This reaction made me realize how the fit body has become, now more than ever, a privileged icon in American culture.

Over the past decade, bodies on display—in advertising, the media, MTV, and dance—have become increasingly muscular and delineated. This is particularly striking in women's bodies. Thirty years ago, it would have been unheard of for most middle-class women to have desired clearly defined arm muscles. Today, not only are delineated biceps de rigeur, the fashion industry has even provided women with the perfect apparel with which to display their upper-body muscles in the varieties of racing-back dresses, jogging bras, and the newly feminized version of the muscle shirt. For the first time in Western history, women are entering athletic clubs (traditionally bastions of homosocial bonding) in droves to work out. Given the ways that women's bodies have been physically constrained and historically represented as "naturally" passive and "weak," there can be no denying that sensing the rush of adrenaline and the aliveness of one's body after exercising can be an incredibly powerful experience.

But this physical liberation comes with its own form of enslavement, for a muscular body requires constant working out and considerable financial resources. Exercise has become a commodity, as the various technologies of contemporary fitness—nautilus machines, universal gyms, free-weights, StairMasters, and stationary bikes—can attest. Of course, this new look is not only about changing fashions of a bodily aesthetic. As Susan Bordo quite rightly points out in her book *Unbearable Weight: Feminism, Western Culture, and the Body,* "the firm, developed body has become a symbol of correct attitude; it means that one 'cares' about oneself and how one appears to others, suggesting will power, energy, control over infantile impulse, the ability to 'shape your life.'"[1]

Bodies, however, tend to elude control (both physically and politically). Inherently unstable, the body is always in a paradoxical process of becoming—and becoming undone. As any dancer or athlete will readily admit, the body never reaches a stable location, no matter how disciplined and rigorous the training. The daily practice required to keep a body in shape exposes the body's instability; its annoying tendency to spill over its appropriate boundaries. The obsessiveness with which American culture approaches body management (exercise and weight training, etc.) always makes me wonder if we are not trying desperately to refuse what I see as a fundamental experience of our bodies—that of continual loss. Thus, I see Streb's relentlessly pumped-up movement style as embodying a deep cultural anxiety about the inevitable fragility of human bodies. For me, her company's dancing is one possible response to the chaotic loss of control—over the environment, our health, the neighborhood—that we are experiencing at the end of this millennium. There is something reassuring each time the dancers mount an obstacle or complete a difficult task—a sense of satisfaction in how they take charge of the physical situation. Fit and strong, young and daring, they embody the possibility of success, the productive harnessing of physical energy. Watching them move, we can participate vicariously in their extraordinary physicality.

Our desire to control the body is connected to the need to control desire. The desire to control bodies, natural resources, national destiny (others' as well as our own), has historically been one of the (mis)guiding forces of Western civilization. Many of the great advances in our culture are seen in terms of control: the widespread use of antibiotics to "control" infections, the damming of rivers to "control" flooding, the establishment of economic sanctions to "control" commerce. Oddly enough, as the century of advancement draws to a close, we are forced to realize our own impotence as disease and malnutrition, the environment, international trade, even our livelihood, continually slip out of our control.

It should come as no surprise to anyone forced to read Nathaniel Hawthorne's *The Scarlet Letter* in the sixth grade, that American society has a long tradition of trying to regulate its citizens' bodily desires. Nowhere is this more visible than the fierce battles currently being waged over homosexuality. If the disciplined, fit body has become, as Bordo suggests, a symbol of the "correct attitude," then cultural logic has it that the undisciplined, "weak" body reveals a "wrong attitude." Caught in a self-perpetuating binary of good and evil, the religious right has been trying to represent the AIDS crisis as a result of undisciplined, loose, immoral bodies, whose physical extravagances have brought on their own (well-deserved) destruction. Fortunately, however, performers, artists, and activists have responded by creating a new body-centered theater that flaunts and affirms those desires in the face of censorship.

Bodies, boundaries, fluids, joyful, messy desires—this is the stuff of Tim Miller's *My Queer Body,* his 1992 coming out/coming-of-age saga. Miller's recent revival of *My Queer Body* at the Cleveland Public Theater was part of the Performing AIDS conference held at the Omni Hotel in Cleveland. The conference was hosted by Northeastern Ohio Universities College of Medicine (NEOUCOM) and organized by Teresa Jones (a postdoctoral fellow in the Human Values in Medicine program and editor of *Sharing the Delirium: Second Generation AIDS Plays and Performances*). The conference sought to bring various populations concerned with AIDS issues together to explore how AIDS is being represented in the mainstream media and contested through the performative energies of activists and artists. The night I saw it, Miller's performance was an enthusiastic, fantastical, autobiographical journey into the terrain of his body's memories, his body's desires, as well as his own mortality. In describing the piece's origins, Miller says, "I am listening to the places on my body and speaking their tales, the places of hurt and the places of pleasure. I do this as a way of knowing who I am and to reclaim my flesh and blood from those who try to control it."

Unlike Streb's dancers, who are dressed uniformly in Lycra bodysuits and whose focused physicality and high-risk movement tasks create a veil of anonymity—rarely giving them the chance to look up and connect to their audience—Miller begins his show by waltzing through the audience, trying to get a feel for his viewers. Part master of ceremonies, part show-off, part flirt, Miller cruises around in a cocky, conversational manner before he takes his place onstage to begin the story of his life with the story of one queer sperm fighting all the others to impregnate a "dyke ovum."

Over the course of the evening, Miller chronicles his first gay date in high school, his involvement with ACT UP/LA anti-homophobic protests, and his frantic search for "truth" among the lost lives of his friends and lovers. This latter section is a classic quest journey framed in the mythopoetic language of the men's movement. The climactic moment of revelation takes place in a volcano in the desert into which Miller, now stripped naked, has descended to meet the demons of his present reality. Grieving over the dead bodies that surround him, Miller rages against a society and government that does so little to stem the loss of lives. Exhausted, he eventually leaves this theatrical no-man's-land to return, dick in hand, to the reality of his own desire.

What follows is an extended incantation to his penis. "Get hard because it still feels good to be touched . . . get hard because I want those boners before I am a bag of bones, get hard because I know only one thing: This is my body and these are my times so get hard, get hard, get hard." I wish Miller's performance had lingered in that emotional space for a moment, so that the failure of his penis to get hard and the difficulty of representing desire in these times of conflicting bodily experiences would give us pause—so that we might reimagine this very traditional scenario of the phallus as life force, and look for other ways for bodies and desires to manifest themselves. Instead, Miller shakes off any trace of mourning or hesitancy and, imagining himself the performance art laureate of the nation, triumphantly marches into a final utopian fantasy of phallic presence and productivity.

Seeing Streb's and Miller's performances within a month of each other compelled me to question the hidden ideologies behind the various systems of "body management" that are so popular today. Is the current fitness craze somehow connected to our refusal to deal with the ailing bodies in our culture? Looking at the legacies of fit and frail bodies as we near the end of the twentieth century, I cannot help but think that despite our extensive technological know-how, we have yet to truly understand the importance of every body in our world. Frankly, I believe that we need a new ethos of the body—one committed to controlling disease without trying to control desire.

NOTE

1. Susan Bordo, *Unbearable Weight: Feminism, Western Culture, and the Body* (Berkeley and Los Angeles: University of California Press, 1993), 195.

II

FEMINIST THEORIES

This section contains some of my earliest theoretical writings in which I read late twentieth-century dancing through the lenses of feminist film theory and feminist literary criticism. These critical perspectives on language and image taught my generation of dance scholars to move beyond traditional analyses of movement style or compositional strategy in order to think not only about the "what" but also about the "how" of a performance event. Feminist theory insisted on a fuller examination of the social dynamics of dance training, as well as the cultural ideologies embedded in various modes of dance production. Rather than focusing on dance as the presentation of a shared kinesthetic experience, we set off to explore the gendered moorings of dance as a form of representation. Influenced by feminist analyses of the camera as a framing device that positions a woman's body within a male gaze, we began to regard the proscenium stage as another kind of visual apparatus, producing a similar frame for viewing bodies. Feminist theory provided many useful critical tools with which dance scholars could dismantle the assumptions about dance as primarily a form of aesthetic and expressive movement, providing a much-needed critical distance and introducing important discussions of cultural meaning into our evaluations of line and shape, technique and phrasing. In addition, feminist theory helped us navigate the complex relationships between bodies and subjectivities, movers and viewers within dance performances.

The first essay, "Mining the Dancefield: Spectacle, Moving Subjects, and Feminist Theory," addresses questions that I was grappling with at the time about how staged dance creates the conditions of its own representation and how certain performances can consciously disrupt those viewing structures. This essay uses Yvonne Rainer's film *The Man Who Envied Women* as a springboard into a discussion of subjectivity, mobility, and visuality in contemporary dance. Rainer's experimental strategy in this film was to try and preserve the protagonist's subjectivity by making her an invisible, disembodied voice. Recognizing the limits of this strategy and noticing that there is, in fact, one shot of Trisha Brown's slippery and evocative dancing in the background, I propose in this essay that we look to experimental dance for other options. Through a comparative analysis of the work of Pooh Kaye, Jennifer Monson, Ann Carlson, and Marie Chouinard, I argue that these contemporary performances can disrupt conventional structures of representation without erasing the material presence of the female dancing body.

The next essay, "Writing the Moving Body," takes up the question of authorial signatures in feminist literary criticism. I was interested in tackling the central question of how we can write the female body into language without erasing its gendered specificity by way of an exploration of how we can write the moving body. How can we translate motion and gesture into a textual form without losing its embodied presence? In this piece, I situate Nancy Stark Smith's hieroglyphs—improvisational movement figures that are written quickly after dancing in an attempt to directly capture that movement experience—as a midway point between dancing and writing. Rereading the work of French feminist theorists Hélène Cixous and Julia Kristeva through the lens of improvisational dance helps to loosen the essentialist notion that women's bodies can only be scripted in a certain way. Interestingly, I end this essay with the example of Gertrude Stein's prose portrait of Isadora Duncan, unaware, of course, that I would write a book two decades later on Duncan that foregrounds Stein's use of language to write the moving body.

The next essay continues the interconnected themes of language and movement, body and voice, writing and dancing. "Auto-Body Stories" uses Isadora Duncan's autobiography to frame a discussion of the autobiographical subject in contemporary dance. I look at the theatrical work of Blondell Cummings as an example of a destabilized (postmodern) subject that is nonetheless materially present and grounded in a black female body. Written five to seven years after the first two pieces, "Auto-Body Stories" articulates the tensions between a somatic identity (the internal experience of one's physicality) and a cultural one (how one's body is read by society), but in a way that draws its theoretical argument from inside the choreography itself.

I decided to include "Femininity with a Vengeance" because it contains what I consider to be a paradigmatic feminist analysis of Loïe Fuller's performances of Salome. This excerpted chapter from my book on Fuller, *Traces of Light: Absence and Presence in the Work of Loïe Fuller,* looks at the trope of veiling and the role of the femme fatale in nineteenth-century Orientalist fantasies within a discussion of the feminist possibilities of what Mary Russo calls "making a spectacle of oneself." Toward the end of the essay, I leap forward a century to make an intriguing comparison between Fuller's over-the-top performances of Salome and those of the (in)famous Ethyl Eichelberger: a late twentieth-century drag queen. At turns serious and ludic, this essay was enormously fun to write, and it is my hope that the reader might enjoy a similar pleasure in its reading.

Mining the Dancefield

Spectacle, Moving Subjects, and Feminist Theory

Contact Quarterly, Spring/Summer 1990.

I

In her film *The Man Who Envied Women,* Yvonne Rainer steers clear of
a troublesome pothole in feminist film theory—that of imaging a female
body—by simply removing the visual presence of her main female character.
Trisha appears to the audience through another kind of presence—that of
her voice. Sometimes her voice is the film's conscience—a sort of distant
everywoman's voice. Sometimes her voice is like that of a close friend, whispering a story to you at a crowded party. The human voice has a paradoxical quality. It comes from inside a person and its textured cadences bespeak
individuality, yet the voice flows beyond the person, spreading out into the
space around her.

As a voice, Trisha cannot be caught on the screen by the conventional
gaze of an audience. This is, of course, precisely Rainer's strategy. It affords
Rainer a much greater mobility for her character. Without a visual body,
the character cannot be objectified in the usual manner; that is, glamorized
or idealized in the camera's and the audience's eyes. This slipping out of
the filmic framing also gives Trisha a subjectivity rarely found in female
characters—she is a speaking subject. It seems, then, that by removing the
screen image of Trisha, Rainer has evaded the problem of representing female characters in film. Hers is, perhaps, the ultimate feminist film coup.

I wonder, however, about the limits of this maneuver. Are we to assume
that the only way to present the subject-ness of a female character is by
erasing her object-to-be-looked-at-ness? And does this feminist strategy really
confront the issues of spectacle that surround the representation of the female body? Of course, Rainer's film is much more complex than I have suggested so far, and its multiple layerings address several theoretical issues—
political, aesthetic, psychoanalytic, and feminist—at once. As a phantom
presence who floods the film yet is nowhere to be seen, Trisha inhabits a
different kind of space—one which lies just outside the frame, influencing

how we see the images inside it. This space of possibility Teresa de Lauretis calls the "space-off." In her latest book, *Technologies of Gender,* de Lauretis discusses this space as a vital place of feminist revisioning—the place of "the ongoing effort to create new spaces of discourse, to re-write cultural narratives, and to define the terms of another perspective—a view from 'elsewhere.'" By using Trisha's disembodied voice to fracture the conventions of the filmic gaze, Rainer envelops her audience in this "elsewhere."

Interestingly enough, Rainer hints at another "elsewhere" in her film. Projected above the head of Jack Deller, Trisha's husband in the film, is a fleeting glimpse of a film by Trisha Brown, the choreographer, dancing *Water Motor* (1978). The dance is a series of quirky energetic movements, where flung limbs and off-balance suspensions hang briefly in the air before sliding back into movement. The dancer's body is never still and her head is as loose as her arms are, tailing behind the movement like the last person in a game of "crack the whip." Seen for less than a minute, this film clip is enough to give the viewer a lasting visual impression of strong, personable aliveness in a female moving body. It is ambiguous whether this dancer is, in fact, a representation of the film character of Trisha, her alter ego, or merely a figment of Jack's imagination. Yet the dancer's spectral presence shares, in my mind, a certain ubiquity with Trisha's voice. For in this moment Rainer has targeted a visual experience that breaks through the traditional syntax of looking at the female body. As elusive as Trisha's voice, this dancing body cannot be controlled by the camera's image of her. Her movements seem to pour out of the frame to engulf the whole space of the theater, locating the physicality of the female body both in the film and in the space just outside of it—the "space-off."

It is this visual flash of dancing footage, or rather the possibilities it suggests, that I want to explore here. For it seems to me that contemporary dancing (like that in Trisha Brown's *Water Motor*) finds ways to rupture the traditional representations that objectify the female body by alluding to, including, or focusing the audience's attention on, the "elsewhere" in which de Lauretis put so much hope. Slipping in and out of their culturally determined frames, the ebullient bodies in these dances elude a traditional gaze and defy the powerful pleasure of spectacle—that of looking at some thing to be looked at. Surprised by a disruption of their gaze, the audience, in turn, can be pushed out of its conventional consumption of these bodies. Thus jolted, the spectators will (ideally) begin to look elsewhere; to find a new focus; to look at the physical experience of the dancer—her moving, her motion, her movement—her subjectivity.

And then if I spoke about a person whom I met and who shook me up, herself being moved and I moved to see her moved, and she, feeling me moved, being

moved in turn, and whether this person is a she and a he and a he and a she and a shehe and a heshe, I want to be able not to lie, I don't want to stop her if she trances, I want him want her, I will follow her.
—HÉLÈNE CIXOUS

Images of women abound in dance. While dance performances are not the imaging machines in quite the literal way that cameras are, they often manifest a politics of imagery that raises questions concerning the presentation of "woman": woman as a spectacle, as an object to be admired, as a vision of beauty, and as a site of pleasure. The stereotypical dancer-cum-seductress of Western dance forms like ballet, or Broadway musicals, tends to embody some kind of eternal or essential woman. Framed by the proscenium stage and courted by one or more male partners, the female dancer is raised up to iconic heights. However idealized, this image serves to represent not the experience of the particular woman who is dancing on stage, but rather her role in the lives and fantasies of the male directors, choreographers, and audience members.

The arrival of modern, postmodern, and post-postmodern dance has brought alternative images of women to dance. But although many of the pointe shoes and frilly tutus are gone, there remains a conventional framing in representations of the female body—they simply have a more sleek and updated look to them. Molissa Fenley, for example, makes fast dances that require that she and her dancers train rigorously for stamina and strength. Their bodies look quite muscular. One would think that this kind of physical strength would give the dancers an aura of confidence and self-possessiveness. Within the possibility of making the audience aware of this power, this physical selfhood is usurped, however, by the conventional context that presents these bodies as objects to be looked at. They may be riding on top of a constant cycle of motion, but one gets the feeling from the presentational address of their vertical, pumped-up bodies that they are more involved in showing off their dancing bodies than in doing the movement. One of Fenley's most famous publicity photos shows her standing still, displaying (as she has done for *Vogue* magazine) her muscular torso. The sense I have is that her choreography is merely an elaborate way to accomplish the same thing.

Fenley's dances fail to challenge a traditionally static male gaze because they continue to accept the classic split between the audience and performer— placing the dancer (the object) on stage for the admiring audience (the subject). Seen within this context, Fenley's movement cannot make the audience aware of the physical experience of those moving bodies, thereby presenting them as active subjects, no matter how many calories they burn.

II

The driving, percussive music begins in darkness. In the midst of banging rhythms, a narrow block of light becomes visible. First a leg, an arm, then a head enters this rectangle of white suspended in a sea of blackness. A body teeters on its edge. Is she unsure whether to continue, to enter the spotlight? Is she teasing us; playing with the power she has to engage our pleasure with her presence? Or is she simply enjoying those moments of wavering— of suspension and being off-balance—as she surfs in and out of the spot-light? Luxuriating in the fall, she dives toward the mat, landing chest first. The impact of her body sponsors a rebound—actually a series of rebounds. Each jump intensifies the previous one by adding an arm, a twist. Finally, a thrown head propels her into a back arch. She lands like a lizard and stays there for a moment, but I can see the energy coursing through her limbs.

Choreographed by Pooh Kaye with help from the dancers, *Active Graphics II* subverts, in several different ways, the traditional frames I have been discussing. For instance, the most literal frame—the proscenium arch—is obliterated by the dance's intriguing lighting effects. Beginning and ending in complete darkness that merges the stage space with that of rest of the theater, the lighting is tailored to illuminate only specific areas on the stage floor. These rectangular shapes almost seem to float in midair. As the only lights on stage, they frame the dancing, but they do not box in or contain the movements of the performers. In fact, because the dancers play with slip-ping in and out of the light, those lit areas heighten the sense of the dancers' power. The blackness surrounding them suggests de Lauretis's "elsewhere" of female subjectivity and influences the way we see these performers. It is as if the dancers choose when to go into the light, when to allow the audience to see their dancing. In a later section, the dancers even seem to motivate the changes in lighting, calling the cues by their movement. In a game of follow-the-leader, they lunge beyond a lit area with a broad stamping motion and a few seconds later, the lighting appears, barely catching an arm or a leg gesture before they move on. One dancer's movement becomes the next's as she trails along in her footsteps. Sometimes they dance in unison; often they seem to pass movement to one another, smoothly braiding and adjusting the space—sometimes coming together, other times spreading apart.

When it is fully lit, the movement style of *Active Graphics II* flaunts a looping explosive energy that rarely addresses the audience in a frontal, pre-sentational manner. Rebounding from the floor to spring back into it, this dancing does not place the dancers on the stage only for the spectator's view. While it is certainly true that they are performing for us, they also seem to be performing for themselves and for one another. Whirling, tumbling, and swooping in and out of the lights, the dancers affirm a physical aliveness that claims subjectivity from within the context of their roles as performers for an audience. The costumes—black bicycle outfits with white stripes running down the front and across the back—also reinforce this new possibility, accenting not the curves of the dancers' bodies, but rather the movement of those lines as the dancers roll and dive onto the floor.

Like Trisha's voice in Rainer's film, Kaye's *Active Graphics II* goes beyond the frames of conventional representation and brings the spaces and experiences hovering just outside that frame into the audience's awareness, providing an alternative viewing consciousness. The lit rectangles of *Active Graphics II* could be a frame of film where the images of the women are allowed to scamper in and out of the frame at will, foiling at long last an ideology of imagery. Of course, for some members of the audience, these dancers will always be objects. Some people will continue to look at the dancing in much the same way they ogle the front lineup at the Moulin Rouge—but it is not easy. Too often the dancers elude their gaze. The dancers move on their own desire, unbuttoning this girdling gaze by slipping out of the light to reappear in some other place, concentrating less on being seen than on the lived experience of dancing. Negotiating between the positions of object and subject—between being inside the frame and moving on the other side—the dancers in *Active Graphics II* underscore the contradictions in the representation of women on the stage.

III

One by one, three dancers enter the stage with a lazy, looping elephant walk. Just as the group stretches across the stage in a diagonal line, another dancer walks behind a scrim and the three dancers explode into separate movements. Thrashing their limbs and hurling their bodies through space in a curiously frenetic yet nonchalant manner, they first orbit individually and then cluster to the side. Separate movements connect in a single suspension and they all shoot to the floor, each one finding a different path downward. Two more dancers vault onto the stage, just in time to pick up the speed and energy of the others, who now rest subdued on the floor. They dance in unison for a while and then split off into two tangents. Their action spawns another reaction that sends all five dancers reeling and tumbling through the space in individual explosions of wild vigor. Everyone is doing everything, every which way. And then almost magically, like a blurry picture brought into focus, this chaotic field etches itself out across the stage in a single, long diagonal line. The dancers squat and pause, crystallizing a moment of stillness and visual simplicity.

Jennifer Monson's concert, *Blood on the Saddle,* was a collaboration with composer Zeena Parkins. Performed in New York City at St. Mark's Danspace—a non-proscenium setting—this evening-length work juxtaposes visual tableaux and a self-consciously presentational performance style with sequences of dancing which eschewed these elements. Several times during the piece, the ensemble of nine very different-looking people establish a tableau by lining up a few feet from the audience and, smiling gleefully, sing and dance in an upbeat, unison Motownesque manner. Finished with their "number," the group holds the final pose for a moment and then shuffles off, completely shattering the effect of their earnest, if awkward, entertainment. The *entr'actes* also flaunt this showy Broadway performance quality. In one of the most compelling moments of the evening, Jackie Shue is rolled in to the center of the space on a neon surrealistic doorway, which is framed by a glittering mosaic of Christmas lights and tinsel. She is dressed in a white ball gown and sits demurely, first peeling and then eating a pomegranate. The bright-red juice of the fruit runs down her chin, stains her mouth, gloves, dress, and, by extension, her reputation. Moments before the lights fade out, she looks straight out of the audience, slightly dazed by the whole experience.

The images in these tableaux are familiar and easy to digest: the line of chorus dancers, the juggling side act, the display of the beautiful woman in white. Yet they are made strange and ironic in the context of Monson's work. The dancers look awkward; they are a little too close to the audience. We can see how hard they are working. The juggler is a bearded woman in an evening dress, and the lovely woman in white is too hungry for comfort.

Softening the effect of these disturbing tableaux, however, is the very human physicality of Monson's own style of dancing. Engaged and enlivened by the experience of dancing with others, she and her partners sweep through an engaging romp of lunges, diving chest rolls, and floor spins, surfacing from this deluge to acknowledge one another before slipping back into the current of movement. The dance floor stretches out like a field, with the dancers roaming from one end to another. Catching up with one another, they blend their diverse rhythms into a physical synchrony. They face each other (not the audience) as they push, spin, or guide one another through the bumpy texture of the dance.

In its tableaux and chorus line numbers, *Blood on the Saddle* draws on the familiar pleasures of spectacle only to subvert them into uncomfortable and strange juxtapositions. Shaken by this somewhat alienating wrenching of convention, the audience embraces the friendly, rambunctious dancing of the duets and trios. There is no irony posed in these wide open sequences of playful dancing, no narrative; only a spread of dancers merging in and out of each other's spaces and rhythms. This dancing is virtuosic, not unlike that of Pooh Kaye's *Active Graphics II,* but what strikes me most about it is the sense of connection among the dancers. Contrasting the two-dimensional—almost cardboard—quality of the chorus line (whose attention is projected solely out to the audience), these dancers seem to be fuller beings, engaging both the audience and one another in their movement.

IV

The theater is dark. From underneath blackness, a strange, muffled sort of uneven humming starts. Gradually, there is a crescendo as a spotlight reveals a woman squatting comfortably in a corner, her head immersed in a basin of water, blowing bubbles. The closer her mouth is to the surface, the louder and more percussive the sound is. By blowing bubbles in different depths, she can shape a song. Songs shape her performance: visual songs, vocal songs, movement songs, even silent songs. Short moments of poetry, they may be soft or harsh, strong or fleeting, but they are always personal. The sounds, like her movements, originate deep inside her body, and in her performing she lets the audience see the beginnings of these songs.

Marie Chouinard can be very quiet at times. Out of those still, silent moments—moments of resting, of waiting for a call—comes a trickle of movement, a song. Fluid and supple, Chouinard swirls and glides across the floor with ease; at other times, her movement is as slippery as her long, soft hair. She can be convulsive and terribly fierce as when a series of small, jerky vibratos explode into a violent demonic passion that sweeps and pounds her body into the floor. Throughout her dancing, there is a sense that Chouinard is choosing between being in control of her body and releasing that control, enjoying the results. Changing the rhythm and quality throughout her dance, Chouinard's songs call forth the immediate rawness of her physicality.

She takes her place next to the skeleton, on a piece of grass sod, and looks out to the audience for the first time. Shaping her hand like a swan shadow puppet, she luxuriously extends her arm in a full arc, raising her face to greet the hand bird that glides down to her mouth and deeper into her throat. A collective shudder darts through the audience as her abdomen contracts convulsively. She does this again, standing with her profile to the audience. This time there is something amazing in the moment when her body responds. The deep contraction spawns a series of ripples that spread out through her body. What at first seemed like a reaction to an almost cruel gesture, now seems to be a healthful, awakening release. Her next gesture leads her to her hands and knees and she begins to crawl back and forth across the space with a soft, yet steady, attentive sensuality.

In some sense, Chouinard's performances are like rituals. The mythic, earthy quality of her performance environments—a tub of water, a skeleton, a piece of grass sod—as well as the spiritual inner attentiveness of her moving can evoke a myriad of personal and archetypal associations for the audience. Her role is like that of a shaman, insisting that the spectators witness and thus share in the creation of a communal event. As she sticks her hand down her throat, as the saliva oozes out of her mouth, as she masturbates, as she sings, Chouinard's experience—her inner space—loops out into the open for all (including herself) to see. Not only does she pull the viewer's focus into her world, she pulls the inner space of her body out into the performance space, making the audience attentive to the passages through and around her body. Performed in a space with no proscenium arch or even a stage, she merges her space with the audience's, melting an important distinction between performer and spectator.

By crossing over into the audience's physical and psychic space, Chouinard's dancing suggests the possibility of a different relationship between the spectators and performer. Her body is too close, too disturbing, too inquisitive, too demanding to be positioned as an object of their desire. When she draws the viewers' focus into her experience and space by making them aware of her breathing, her shifts in weight, a quiver in her fingers, she meets them on equal terms, confronting the spectator's desire with her own.

She begins to walk. Light, yet sure on her feet, she circles the stage, swooping down to the ground intermittently. She is dancing to an inner song; at times stepping high on her toes with her face and arms lifted upwards; at times curled and inching low toward the ground. Then, very simply, she walks over to a corner and sits on one leg. Looking out to the audience, she slips one and then the other sleeve of her shift off her shoulder and with the same open comfortableness that pervades her movement, she slides one hand down her pants. There is stillness, then a deep, light tremor in her breathing. Breaths become more audible, as her undertones cadence into an antiphonal vibrato. She sings. And as she sings, stories, chants, and myths are called up from deep inside her throat and brought out into the space by the husky archaic sound of her voice.

In her essay, "A Desire of One's Own: Psychoanalytic Feminism and Intersubjective Space," Jessica Benjamin introduces her concept of "intersubjective space" as a feminist re-visioning of female desire. Rather than predicating desire on an opposition between the desiring subject and a desired object, Benjamin outlines the possibility of an "intersubjective" model of desire, where the act of desiring erases neither your own nor another person's position as subjects. "The intersubjective mode assumes the paradox that in being with the other, I may experience the most profound sense of self." Benjamin's intersubjective space is a kind of cosmic slide rule that stretches between people. It is a place where one can move closer or further away from another without either losing intimacy or risking incorporation. In other words, it provides a connectedness with another without short circuiting a connection with oneself.

Although Benjamin uses the dynamic of mother/child relations as a base for her essay, we could easily insert the performance situation into her paradigm, for the concept of intersubjective space is similar to the spatial experience of audience and performer. The physical distance of the seating to the stage (if there is one), or the spatial design and pathway of the dancers in the space (are they close to the audience, facing them or not) as well as the psychological identifications, sympathy or kinesthetic empathy can all affect this interaction. However, as it is while performing that dancers often experience the most profound sense of themselves, it seems to me that an audience could be made aware of that experience, could be trained to see it. The first step in this education of the audience must come from the performance itself—from the ability of the spectacle to disrupt the traditional measures of the spectator, forcing them to look elsewhere.

V

An ominous music fills the dusky twilight onstage. Wrapped in a blue gray, strapless evening dress and perched upon high-heeled shoes, she stands center stage. She seems at first glance to embody all the traits of a cultured seductress. Mostly her movement is confined to her face and upper body—a white expanse of flesh framed by the sheen of her gown's satiny texture. Her arms and mouth are magnificent, stretching open in a luxuriously beckoning gesture. Then the image shatters as a low, guttural sound rises up from her throat and floods out into the audience. Instantly, she is a whale. Large, strong, and impressive, she rears gracefully out of the ocean and then plunges back into its depths. Enigmatically evoking and mixing the embodiment of a whale and a lady vamp—the literal and metaphorical images of a man-eater—she leads the audience into seeing a woman, a whale, a whale woman, a woman whale; moving with her, being moved by her.

In February 1988, Ann Carlson premiered a suite of dances entitled *Animals*. This concert effectively included faces, movements, and experiences that normally lie outside of a performance event. Carlson adeptly altered our perception of a performer as spectacle by including in her dance work performers who were unfamiliar and unconcerned with how the audience saw them. This extraordinary cast included two goats, a dog, a goldfish, a kitten, and a Down's syndrome child. Her program note attunes the audience to the fact that the usual conventions of presentation and address are particularly fragile in this situation. "The involvement of animals in this performance has been an intrinsic part of the development of the works. They are well loved and cared for. Please refrain from any calls, whistles or gestures of distraction to the animals. If any animal or human performer should become disoriented, the performance will be immediately altered to accommodate or offer support. Thank you." Before the performance actually begins, while the stage crew is setting up the corral for the goats in the first piece and as we read the program note, Carlson's own approach to her performers has edged into our consciousness, making us aware of their experience.

The Dog Inside the Man is a duet with Brunelleschi, a golden retriever. Dressed in a shirt and tie, boxer shorts (did she forget her pants?), and shoes and socks, Ann Carlson briskly walks out with the dog, talking to it and the audience through a microphone that amplifies her breathing and walking. The text she recites is interspersed with comments about her health, the dog's behavior, and the immediate situation. At one point the dog becomes frantic, and Carlson excuses herself for a moment as she takes the dog away. Returning to the performance space alone, Carlson continues her duet, accumulating a sequence of movements that are punctuated by erratic fits and starts, and an increasingly desperate, "Down girl, down, down." The audience sees both the dog that used to be beside her and the one acting up inside her, and follows her efforts to control first the one and then the other.

Duck Baby is performed by a Down's syndrome child, a young woman, and a young man. Their movements are athletic, but none of the performers have the technical prowess or refined physical shapes which a contemporary dance audience is used to seeing. These performers do not apologize for their awkwardness, but move with a frankness that is curiously disconcerting. The unpredictability of seeing a young child dancing about—one time bending over to look at the audience from the ripe perspective of upside down, or running to one side to plop down and fastidiously rip sheets of paper apart—is a strangely involving experience for the spectator. In watching her perform, the audience is forced to follow her desires, seeing her choose what to do, which activities give her pleasure (being caught and thrown by the other two performers), and which ones make her quiet. Tired of a sequence of movement or a certain activity, she looks out into the audience and around the space, hesitating and then deciding (or remembering) which way to go next.

Carlson's work is filled with the contradictions inherent in revisioning the conventional relationship of spectator and performer. By directly addressing the audience in the program notes, or vocally during the performance, Carlson attempts to cross over the usual gulf, bringing an awareness of the performers' experiences to the spectator's attention. Because some of the performers she uses are rarely seen on a dance stage, the audience does not have a preformed image of them. Rather than being presented as circus sideshow attractions, they are treated as subjects whose experience we can all appreciate, and their presence is an integral part of each section. I think Carlson set the order of her program with an eye to training—or retraining—the spectators in how to see the performers. Watching animals and people dance with one another leads the spectator to look at all species of performers differently. Curious about how two goats will react to a woman falling between them, we watch their reactions with an attentiveness rarely given to the performer's experience. Attentive to the animal's experience, we learn to be aware of the human performer's experience as well. Perhaps this is why Carlson saved her two solo dances for the end of the evening.

In her final solo, *Visit Woman Move Story Cat Cat Cat,* Carlson lumbers around the space, tumbles on the floor, sits with her back to the audience, and mothers a kitten—naked. It is a shock, at first, to see her so exposed; to see her full, white flesh against the black floor. Galloping around the space in wide, uneven strides, some of her movements suggest those of primates. At other times she moves with the amazing grace of a feline, crouching low to the floor and easing into a long, elastic roll. The kitten onstage captures her attention and she befriends it, eager to love and care for a smaller creature. Unpretentious about the presentation of her naked body onstage, Carlson does not negate its human expressiveness by miming an animal. Slipping through movement images with the same ease with which Kaye's dancers slip through the light in *Active Graphics II,* she evokes a girl child, a mother, and an infant during the course of this intriguing duet. While watching the dance, the audience is absorbed by the intensity of her performance and her play with the kitten, but once it is over, we are left to ponder the awesome frankness of her naked body.

VI

The work of the four contemporary choreographers discussed in this essay rubs up against the wall of traditional representation; pressuring and splitting its facade, oozing through its cracks and gaps, perhaps creating enough friction to someday wear it down. By experimenting with the format of spectacle and playing with different kinds of presentations, Pooh Kaye, Jennifer Monson, Marie Chouinard, and Ann Carlson highlight and expose the problematical dynamic of a conventional performer/audience relationship. Dissatisfied with an equation that always identifies the audience with an active desiring subject and the performer with a passive, desired object, these women are trying out new forms of presentation that disturb or dismantle this formula.

When Pooh Kaye allows her dancers to move in and out of the light, reveling in the space just beyond the light's frame, or when Jennifer Monson brings her homespun chorus line so close to the audience that they are breathing down the spectator's necks, the audience is jarred by this disruption of their taken-for-granted pleasure. Once the performers have slipped outside of the frame of spectacle to move into the audience's physical and emotional space, as in Marie Chouinard's or Ann Carlson's performances, another kind of conversation is possible. De Lauretis's "elsewhere" becomes Benjamin's "intersubjective space" as the audience becomes aware of the performer as an active participant who can engage, comment on, and direct the audience's focus. For what lies just outside of the frame of representation in dance—the "space-off"—is precisely that space between the performers and the audience. And it is in this space—this new frontier—that women dancers can begin to claim their own subjectivity.

a person whom I met and who shook me up,
herself being moved and I moved to see her moved,
and she, feeling me moved, being moved in turn . . .
—HÉLÈNE CIXOUS

12

Writing the Moving Body

Nancy Stark Smith and the Hieroglyphs

Frontiers: A Journal of Women Studies 10, no. 3, 1989.

Now more aware of the empty space we are replacing with every splash of
ink on the page, [we find] yet another expression of the awkward movement
through a forest of words toward a clearing that might be found waiting in
the space between them.

—NANCY STARK SMITH

Estranged from language, women are visionaries, dancers who suffer as they
speak.

—LUCE IRIGARAY

In 1980, when I was taking dance classes in Paris at the Centre International de Danse, I remember we had two sorts of accompanists. One was a
wonderfully eclectic musician who would come in with all sorts of ethnic
and homemade instruments. He sat on a stool in the corner and arranged a
strange assortment of sound makers in a half-moon shape around him. The
other accompanist was not a musician; he was a painter. He would arrive
once the class had started and set up his working space next to the musician. Sitting with his legs loosely crossed underneath him, the painter would
dip his thick brush into a well of black paint and, with a series of darting
glances up at the dancers, begin to trace the lines of our movement onto
thick sheets of paper. We had a Limon technique teacher at the time, and the
painter's abstract drawings reflected the circular, spiraling spatial pathways
of the movement, as well as its rhythmic suspensions and releases. Each
drawing would take him less than a half-minute to do. By the end of the
class, the floor around him was covered with these figures. Although these
drawings had many more loops, sweeps, and swirls than Chinese characters,
it seemed that the artist was influenced by this form of script. I remember
being amazed at how lightly he held the brush, and how the movement of
his sketching arm originated at the bottom of his spine. His strokes, though
much more delicate, seemed related to the strokes of rowers who involve
their whole bodies in the motion of continuous cycling. Each movement of

his brush looped up through his back, out his arm, onto the paper, and back around again.

I never mustered the courage to ask this artist for one of his drawings; indeed, I had completely forgotten about his efforts to draw our dancing until, several years later, I encountered Nancy Stark Smith's movement hieroglyphs. Written in a grid-like pattern, often from right to left, Smith's hieroglyphs are unique little insignias of a moving body. Although they are informed by several writing traditions (Chinese characters, cursive writing, drawing), these whirls, loops, curves, slashes, dots, ovals, and tangents do not adhere to any one symbolic system. Each hieroglyph is a burst of ink—an eruption on the blank page. The thin lines of ink seem to be constantly in motion, playing on the page like a group of Calder's wire circus figurines. Though there is no one-to-one correspondence to specific movements in these hieroglyphs, there are indications of rhythm and motion in their shapes and lines. Even the words with which I can describe these designs—slash, loop, curve, whirl, chute, pretzel—suggest the qualities of movement in the ink. While the hieroglyphs are extraordinarily idiosyncratic, they can be read by others. An effort/shape analysis would reveal, for instance, the dynamics and spatial pathways of the movement. But most people, when handed a hieroglyph, usually have some sort of movement response.

These movement hieroglyphs position themselves at the intersection of the feminist analysis of how women's bodies are inscribed in cultural representation—how we "write the female body"—and that ever-present stumbling block in the dance field of how to "write the moving body." By analyzing Smith's hieroglyphs and contact improvisation, the movement form that inspires them, in a context provided by two very different French writers—Hélène Cixous and Julia Kristeva—I hope to show the significance of the hieroglyphs as a form that writes the female moving body.

In an essay concerning women's "Ceremonies of the Alphabet," Sandra Gilbert and Susan Gubar document the diverse and imaginative ways that women writers have subverted and inverted names, words, and the alphabet (which they refer to as alpha beth) in order to claim their own experiences in writing. "Women of letters have for centuries defended themselves against the intimacies of linguistic mortality conveyed to them by the nature and the culture of the alphabet through fantasies about names, letters, ideograms, hieroglyphs, characters and calligraphies."[1] These new signatures seek to include a corporeal experience in writing, claiming for their authors not only a voice but also a body. Like these women writers, dancers, and choreographers have also sought to rework the alphabet, moving beyond the confines of known letters and words in a desire to translate the physical immediacy of dancing. An endless array of idiosyncratic squiggles, stick figures, and arrows indicating directions place themselves next to the more formalized systems of movement scoring such as Labanotation, in which each aspect of dance movement is meticulously documented so that it can be accurately reproduced from the written score. Unlike Labanotation, Smith's hieroglyphs are somatic stream-of-consciousness movement reflections that are inspired not so much by the outside shape or appearance of the movement as by its internal motion and sensation. This alternative suggests a new vision—a signature that validates the body as a source for writing.

The hieroglyphs bring into one space two of Smith's interests: writing and contact improvisation. Since 1972, when she graduated from Oberlin College with a degree in creative writing and an ever-increasing involvement in the budding movement form of contact, Nancy Stark Smith has sought not so much to bridge the gap between writing and dancing as to probe this space itself: "my focus was not on the historical context nor the visual form of the written symbols, but on what happens between an experience and the telling of it, the translation from one medium to another."[2] As an exploration of the gap between writing and dancing, the hieroglyphs tell us much about both forms of experience and communication.

As elusive as the hieroglyphs, contact improvisation slips through most conventional definitions of either folk or theatrical dancing. Its casual style and informal presentation (dancers wear sweat pants and T-shirts, and feel free to talk with one another and to the audience during a performance) make contact improvisation seem at times like a "dance sport" in which nondancers can also participate. Contact improvisation is informed by the 1960s ethos of community and the cultural translation of Eastern ideas and movement practices like tai chi chuan and aikido. It began in New York City in the summer of 1972, when a group of students, including Nancy Stark Smith, joined Steve Paxton, then a member of the postmodern dance ensemble, Grand Union, to improvise with a dance form based on two bodies sharing their weights. Since then, the work has spread through formal workshops and training sessions and informal jams (sessions of leaderless dancing) to reach all over the world.

Contact improvisation trains dancers to move with a consciousness of dancing as physical communication. The dancers concentrate on internal sensations, rather than on the shapes or designs that their bodies are creating for the audience. Curt Siddall, an early exponent of contact improvisation, describes the form as a combination of physical forces: "Contact Improvisation is a new movement form, improvisational in nature, involving the two bodies in contact. Impulses, weight, and momentum are communicated through a point of physical contact that continually rolls across and around the bodies of the dancers."[3] But human bodies, especially bodies in physical contact with one another, are difficult to abstract, and part of the project of contact improvisation is allowing these stories of the body to evolve. Thus David Woodberry sums up contact improvisation another way: "Contact

Improvisation is a duet form, the deuce dance, faster than thought. It deals with the flows of gravity, your partner, and yourself. Somewhere between jitterbugging, wrestling and making love."[4]

In this space between social dancing, physical intimacy, and combat lies a dance form whose engagement with a physical way of knowing can inform the project of writing the body. A common exercise for a beginning contact improvisation class demonstrates one of the most fundamental concerns of contact improvisation—the messages of physical touch. Two people stand facing one another, eyes closed. Pressing their right forefingers together, they wait until they feel that point of contact begin to move in space. Following it anywhere and everywhere, the dancers concentrate on the qualities of that touch, allowing their bodies to move comfortably with little thought to the specific shapes of movements they are making. Soon this touch takes on a being of its own, speaking to the dancers and guiding their actions.

Touch, the point of contact, sets up the meeting ground for the duet. While there may be a shared compact of physical skills such as rolling, learning when and when not to give weight and how to receive weight, and learning how to fall softly, these skills are only bits. More than the physical techniques, it is the common choice to improvise—to explore an unforeseen moment, to give value to the potential stories of physical contact—that informs the dancers' engagement in the duet. Like a kaleidoscope, contact improvisation can arrange and rearrange whichever piece of the world it focuses on. Social relationships, physical hierarchy, gender roles, and personal interaction are constantly rolling, shifting, and sliding in and out of view.

In a description of dancing from the inside, John Gamble speaks of this touch as a process of exchanging somatic messages within the duet:

> Moving against my partner, the point of contact becomes a window through which I can see our common Gestalt. This window is more than a transmitter of mechanical information. Through it I can experience a "state of being" made up of fear, excitement, impulses, caution and hidden secrets. Different parts of my partner's body reveal different things. Some windows are transparent, some only translucent, and some opaque. I experience my own body as a surface covered with tiny frames of glass. Each frame is a window through which I can look out and a mirror against which I can reflect in. Each frame is activated by my partner's touch.[5]

In this dance form, the traditional focus on the space between the audience and the performer changes, as does the dancer's sense of a performance persona. Less aware of the physical space between herself and the audience (the theatrical concepts of downstage and upstage) and more focused on the space between her and her partner, the dancer is no longer concerned with the "window" or "mirror" looking out to the audience. (I once took a contact improvisation class in a studio that was normally a ballet studio. The entire atmosphere of the previous class's valiant last leaps was radically altered when the teacher pulled the forest green drapery over the enormous mirror—read audience—that spanned the length of the studio.) A whole system of theatrical presentation—the outward focus, the facing-front stance, the smiles—is bypassed as the dancer's focus and concentration are pulled inward to the point of contact. Visually, then, the space between the dancers becomes more important than either the dancers' individual movements or their spatial relationship to the audience.

Actively working against the flattening, two-dimensional effect of the proscenium stage or the mirrored studio, contact improvisation is often taught and performed with a spatial consciousness that includes not only front and back, but sides, diagonals, upside down—what Cynthia Novack calls "an orientation towards 360 degree space."[6] This sense of being "in the round" is often built into performance situations; audience and performers may create a circular enclosure within the box frame of the stage or studio. The dance area thus becomes a field rather than a picture—a space rather than a stage, with no front, no one best seat or royal box to which the performers must "play." Contact classes also work in the round, employing specific exercises to interrupt the dancer's more traditional relationship to the room and the people in it: rolling on the floor, moving in spiraling, curving pathways, dancing for a long period of time with eyes closed, or playing human bumper cars. Less concerned about what the audience sees, the dancers can concentrate on the space between them—the space of the duet.

The frames of glass that John Gamble describes reflect both a physical and a psychic space. Physical impulses of momentum and weight become more and more meaningful within the developing context of the ongoing duet. Friendly, curious bouts of push and shove quickly become combative when one partner remains insistent. A slow, testing and balancing section can suggest different things depending on whether it comes at the beginning of a duet or after a spectacular sequence of turns and lifts. As the dancers move with the evolving point of contact, their identities also move, merging and surfacing within the waves of the improvisation. In 1977, Christina Svane, a veteran contacter, wrote in her piece "In Praise of Bad Dancing": "I value this work not only for the rare glimpses of in-touch, in-time, in-tune, but for the companionship of the ever-present indications of what is possible. The form itself, if one exists beyond the instances of attempts to experience it, is none other than the existence of the possibility of a dance in which wills, instincts and verges merge. Emergency, emerge, merge."[7]

Svane's word *merge* seems particularly appropriate to describe a duet danced by Andrew Harwood and Nancy Stark Smith at the Ethnic Folk Arts Center, March 2, 1987. Merge gives a sense of blending together, as if the surface of the containers that separate one entity from another could just dissolve. Lovers and families merge, lanes of traffic merge, and, with acutely capitalistic wit, Tiffany's advertises expensive wedding rings for new "mergers." But merge can also mean to dive or plunge, and it is the gliding from one meaning of this word to another that marked Harwood's and Smith's dancing together.

Their duet began with a dialogue of quick solo vignettes. Winding their way through the space, they tested their own energy and each other's. They passed by one another, hesitated, and then moved along, until Smith catapulted into Harwood's arms. Catch. A moment of stillness. Gradually melting together, they began a rolling sequence on the floor. Like a pair of pebbles tumbling down a hill, they picked up a circular momentum, resting now and then in a suspension or a lift. Circling up from the floor, they revolved into their own orbits. When they next passed near one another, Harwood dived headfirst toward Smith, becoming a human mat to soften her fall—one he had initiated. Later, they separated, and Smith whirled into a rambunctious series of body bounces, joyously throwing herself around the space and at Harwood, who helped facilitate her landings but chose not to join in. Finally, he followed her lead, and several rolls later they ended up cradling one another in a moment so tender that it caused someone to ask if they were lovers.

What was particularly noticeable in this duet was the narrative flexibility that went along with the dancers' mutual rompings. Many stories of the body were picked up for a slide and a roll or two and then dropped. Humor and tenderness, struggle and bravado surfaced intermittently, usually unexpectedly. Certain images of the dancers' relationship flickered for a moment and then subsided, consumed by the demands of the ever-changing physical momentum. This flexibility to play, to deconstruct, or to reconstruct stories of power and love, is a direct result of a different relationship between bodies and space.

Implicit in the spatial experience of contact improvisation is a willingness, indeed a curiosity, to be disoriented. The contact point usually requires both partners to give up complete control over their own weight in exchange for some of the responsibility of another's weight. Radically diverging from a great many other dance techniques, contact improvisation embraces moments of being off-balance. In fact, one might say that being off-balance is the form's strongest motivating force. Subverting the most common responses to being off-balance—either trying to right oneself or tensing the body—contact improvisation teaches its dancers not only how to fall softly, but also how to enjoy those moments of falling. In the process of becoming comfortable with spatial disorientation and learning how to enjoy circling upside down/supporting one's partner's weight on one's knees/rolling onto her back and then spinning in the air, the contacter also becomes comfortable using peripheral vision.

Being at ease with spatial disorientation is a physical response that contacters feel has considerable psychic ramification. The movement training is only part of contact improvisation; there is also the improvising—the movement toward an opening. For Nancy Stark Smith, "improvisation is a practice in disorientation—training the reflexes to read confusion as a challenge not a threat; that a movement cut loose from its moorings has the advantage of being able to move in any direction, and further, that a temporary absence of reference points can clear the way for impulses from unexpected quarters."[8] This desire for disorientation helps contacters confront an open space, another body, or a messy physical situation with ease—indeed, eagerness. Consciously working to reroute old movement habits—not to dive where one always dives, not to lift in all the predictable situations—contacters stretch movement and improvisational possibilities, trying to see a moment anew, trying to find out what a pirouette feels like upside down.

> EXERCISE: Imagine a writing instrument is located at the top of your head, at the soft spot where the bones of the skull meet. Imagine you can draw with this instrument as a sky-writing plane draws in space. The space around you is a three dimensional canvas. Allow your writing instrument to draw pathways on the canvas, letting the rest of your body be loose and responsive. Adjust your body to accommodate your drawing pathways, always letting the top of your head lead. Explore different speeds, levels, and degrees of locomotion. Allow your eyes to scan, seeing all but focusing on nothing. Work to the point of disorientation and stop."[9]

If there really were a writing instrument on the top of that head, it would probably draw something like a hieroglyph. Visually, hieroglyphs can be disorienting—their meanings are elusive. Yet as representations (however abstracted and distilled) of a body or bodies, hieroglyphs parallel many of the desires at play in the dancing of contact improvisation. For, while hieroglyphs are a form of writing, they are also a form of improvisation. Spewed out in a moment of immediacy, inspired by an experience of dancing and enlivened continually by the physical act of tracing them on the paper, these movement drawings skip across the page with a freedom seldom seen in writing.

Smith constructs her hieroglyphs in a single spontaneous gesture. "I would sit down with a napkin, notebook or pad, a black ink pen, thick or thin, and make a series of 'first thought, best thought' pen movements across the page. I liked the way they looked, they satisfied me. They seemed to precisely capture the frequency of my mood, mind, and body rhythm."[10] Because there is no intention of capturing a specific movement or phrase of movements, any danced interpretation of the hieroglyphs is perfectly valid. A squiggly line could as well be a pathway on the floor as an S curving through the body. The openness of the "text," however, does not efface the subjectivity of the writing hand. When dancers in Smith's classes first work with moving in the space and then later write their own hieroglyphs, there is usually a recognizable connection between how a person moves and the "signature" of her hieroglyphs. The group can guess which hieroglyphs go with which dancer.

Interestingly enough, an early version of the hieroglyphs in Nancy Stark Smith's notebooks suggests how they originated in her handwriting as well as her signature. On a page that has a sprinkling of doodles (stars, cactus-like figures, clouds) are the words "other language" and "parts of speech." In a box on the center of the page is Smith's signature, written in bold, cursive style. Underneath it are increasingly stylized and illegible lines of ink that seem to capture a movement flow similar to her signature without being concerned about tracing specific letters. A later entry reveals the same fascination with letting go. Written on New Year's Eve 1977, its rambling train of thought invokes the ambivalence of this turning point—the seeing one year out and welcoming another one in. After several paragraphs she ends: "no predictions, no resolutions. Here it is." What follows are lines, large, bold, crawling lines that look as if her normal handwriting is wrestling with a teeming energy (desire?) that makes it illegible. A first impulse is to scan the writing (for it still resembles writing), looking for a familiar letter or word. But soon my eyes are content just to follow the movements of the lines on the page. In later hieroglyphs, where each figure is separated, I am less likely to see the lines of ink themselves; my attention is drawn instead to the spaces and shapes those lines create.

As written signs of individual bodies, the hieroglyphs make visual and accessible the place that women have long tried to open up—the place of the female body in language. By inscribing the experience of the writer in the very act of writing, the hieroglyphs subvert the uncomfortable, alienated relationship that many women have with the language of a culture that often denies or conceals the importance of their somatic experiences. These writhing, thriving lines of ink allow a kind of expression that includes the female body. In this sense, the hieroglyphs are analogous to *écriture féminine* (writing the feminine), the central impulse in the work of Hélène Cixous, who emerged from the theoretical and political aftermath of the 1968 uprisings in France to proclaim that "woman must write herself." Cixous believes that ideological and social structures are built into our language. Because these institutions of power have often negated or silenced women's voices (among others), the first step in challenging the power structure of dominant culture is to break down its hegemonic hold on language. Cixous's strategy is defined in the very first lines of her trademark manifesto, "The Laugh of the Medusa." "I shall speak about women's writing: about what it will do.

Woman must write herself: must write about women and bring women to writing . . . Woman must put herself into the text—as into the world and into history—by her own movement."[11]

Although Nancy Stark Smith's hieroglyphs are not by any means as self-consciously feminist as Cixous's vision, they do emphasize the creative physicality and imaginative movements of a female body. They place a physical communication inside written language. The hieroglyphs do not try to describe or talk about the moving body. They try, rather, to *speak* that experience directly. This is also Cixous's project. "In fact, she physically materializes what she is thinking; she signifies it with her body. In a certain way she *inscribes* what she's saying, because she doesn't deny her drives the intractable and impassioned part they have in speaking."[12] In an interview during the summer of 1987, Smith spoke about words and the dancing experience in terms that echo Cixous's desire to speak the female body. Smith sees writing as a way to "induce" a state of being similar to the experience of dancing. "Language can be used to experience the movement of ideas in the same way that I would experience the orientation of movement in a dance—you're moving through the space and things are coming at you, and you're working them."[13] Like a partner in a contact improvisation duet, language can mirror the dancing, giving the reader a "feel" of the movement.

Reading the euphoric passages of Cixous's writing is a little like dancing contact improvisation. Her images of fluidity and motion guide me through an experience in language that reminds me of the merging and emerging, the tumbling and flying of the duet described earlier.

> Text: my body-shot through with streams of songs; I don't mean the overbearing, clutchy "mother" but, rather, what touches you, the equivoice that affects you, fills your breast with an urge to come in language and launches your force; the rhythm that laughs you; the intimate recipient who makes all metaphors possible and desirable; body (body? bodies?), no more describable than god, the soul or the Other; that part of you that leaves a space between yourself and urges you to inscribe in language your woman's style.[14]

By calling forth the experience of the body via language and by attempting to break through representations of the female body that address its physicality only in a distanced, objectified manner, Cixous's writing changes the role of the reader. Physically caught up in the experience, the reader becomes a partner in a duet. Nancy Stark Smith describes this new attitude toward reading in terms that reflect a contact improvisation duet: "It's a level of involvement that sort of takes you in—where you trust the person (the writer) and you're willing to go for the ride with them. You trust that they won't drop you—it's like dancing in that sense."[15]

In contact improvisation, partners communicate when to give or take weight, when to lead or follow a pathway, and when to pursue or resist movement primarily through physical sensations. The requisite attentiveness is often referred to in contact improvisation as "listening with your body." A dancer's responsiveness, her readiness to "go for the ride," implies both a physical and an emotional willingness to merge with someone else. Dancing with a variety of partners, often ones with radically different body types and movement styles, forces contacters to adapt their own movement preferences in order to find a way of moving that will be comfortable for both partners. Implicit in this physical dialogue is, of course, a flexibility of social roles and an ease with multiple movement identities. Men and women interchange traditional roles of lifting or movement dynamics of strength and softness, and each dancer changes his or her own movement in relation to the particular energies in the duet. Cixous's description of woman's embodied language evokes not only the multiplicity of movement identities in contact improvisation, but also the freedom of written expression in the hieroglyphs.

> Her writing can only keep going without ever inscribing or discerning contours, daring to make these vertiginous crossings or the other(s) ephemeral and passionate sojourns in him, her, them whom she inhabits long enough to look at from the point closest to their unconscious . . . Her language does not contain, it carries; it does not hold back, it makes possible. When id is ambiguously uttered—the wonder of being several—she doesn't defend herself against these unknown women whom she's surprised at becoming but derives pleasure from this gift of alterability.[16]

The fantastic, euphoric quality of Cixous's writing and its insistence on certain "essential" metaphors for women's desires and sensibilities strike a number of feminists as coming very close to reinforcing traditional sexual differences. But Cixous does not hold onto a consistent theoretical stance. At times in her work women are closely identified with their bodies and with "writing the feminine"; at other times she insists that écriture féminine is a way of writing found in the work of both men and women—particularly avant-garde writers. It is not my aim in this discussion to pin down Cixous to a specific position. The difference that is crucial here is not that between men and women or masculine writing and feminine writing, but rather the difference between writing that takes its impulse from and includes the body and writing that negates it.

Which is not to say that this is not a feminist issue. As female bodies have historically been both overexposed and under-self-represented, the issue of writing the body in a way that allows the body's movements and rhythms to surface is particularly important to women. This writing not only brings to the surface of language what has traditionally been submerged in it but also inspires another kind of reading attentiveness—one that might alter how we look at and read about women's bodies.

Nevertheless, a fluid movement of the dancing body into abstract traces and into writing is not without historical precedent. Gertrude Stein's portrait of Isadora Duncan, "Orta, or One Dancing," requires that the reader engage with the movement of the words; that s/he enter the dance. Rolling like a wave, over and over again, Stein's language braids "even if she was one," "she was one being one," and "this one is one" into a rhythmic phrase not unlike a series of Duncan's dance movements:

> This one is the one being dancing. This one is one thinking in believing in dancing having meaning. This one is one believing in thinking. This one is one thinking in dancing having meaning. This one is one believing in dancing having meaning. This one is one dancing. This one is one being that one. This one is one being in being one being dancing. This one is one being in being one who is dancing. This one is one being one. This one is one being in being one.[17]

When spoken, Stein's portrait sounds the motion of a dance. Stepping out and then back again, cycling and recycling, Stein's words create not a description of the woman or of her dance, but an evocation of the woman dancing. I feel Duncan's movements when I read Stein's portrait. I become caught up in the rocking of a mature body; the sways and bends; the under curve of a woman rising up to greet the skies with open arms. Willing to be lullabied, I enjoy feeling the words cascade over me in a continuous wash of "one dancing."

Stein's written portrait has an analogue in Abraham Walkowitz's sketches, which trace the movement of Duncan's dancing body.[18] Some of his sketches of Duncan are dark and powerful, with black strokes of draping material arcing along her outstretched arms. These thick marks carry the flow of Duncan's body from the abundant weightiness of her wide stance to the breath and mobility of her upper body. Other drawings are lighter, their thin lines tracing the afterimages of a movement. Because Walkowitz's drawings emphasize the pathways of Duncan's dancing rather than her static (photographic) features, they bring forth the presence of her moving body. One page of Walkowitz's sketches is framed by a clipped series of totally abstract drawings that could easily be called hieroglyphs. Straight, angular lines intersect the space to form geometric figures. In the midst of the fragmented triangles is a circle, a head, suggesting that these forms are traces of a dancing body. I interpret these angular hieroglyphs as a radical experiment meant, perhaps, to inform Walkowitz's later, somewhat less harmonious drawings of Duncan. Because they defy conventional representations, these lines draw an experience of movement and force to the surface of the sketch, pulling the viewer into contact with the dancer's—and the sketcher's—energy.

In order to evoke Duncan's dancing body, Stein and Walkowitz had to invest their media with an involvement with the body—both Duncan's and their own. Before they could adequately represent her dancing, these artists had to let themselves ride along with her movement, risking the disorientation, the dizziness of following another's kinetic rhythms. This sense of merging and emerging in Stein's and Walkowitz's portraits of Isadora Duncan connects them to Cixous's call to write the body, as well as to Nancy Stark Smith's hieroglyphs. Keeping the body active and vital as it is articulated through words is half of the dialogue that the hieroglyphs engage between the dancing body and language. The other half of that dialogue has to do with what these written figures can tell us about the social mechanics of our language. What, in other words, is the theoretical space that the hieroglyphs inhabit?

Throughout her life, writing in many forms—letters, diaries, journals, notebooks—has been important to Smith. Once she became involved with contact improvisation, she used her writing as another vehicle with which to explore it. With the beginnings of the hieroglyphs in 1979, the dancing began to inform the writing as well. In each issue of *Contact Quarterly,* Nancy Stark Smith writes a page called the "Editor Note." In the 1987 Spring/Summer issue she writes:

> Maybe sitting here facing this blank page is the closest I'll be able to get in writing to the feeling of improvising. Because how can you describe something that isn't there yet? I want to be able to write from inside the movements of an improvisation and tell from there how things look, how they feel, how they're going. But I keep finding myself back here walking the line, on the page, trying to make pens pirouette, words walk and ideas bounce and split open, like dancing can do.
>
> I'm impressed and informed by all the efforts evident in this issue of people putting a finger on what isn't there. It's like talking about a hole. In this issue, we're trying to say what shapes the hole from within.[19]

A paragraph later, Smith is still circling around this absence of definition, but instead of calling it a hole, she now refers to it as the "Gap":

> Where you are when you don't know where you are is one of the most precious spots offered by improvisation. It is a place from which more directions are possible than anywhere else. I call this place the Gap. The more I improvise, the more I'm convinced that it is through the medium of these gaps—this momentary suspension of reference point—that comes the unexpected and much sought after "original" material.[20]

The space implied is not a negative space, but rather a freeing, creative space—an opening up in the absence of traditional reference points. Julia Kristeva, who has influenced contemporary feminist thought both on the

Continent and in the United States, is also interested in this "momentary suspension of reference point." Working at the point of intersection between current linguistic theories and psychoanalysis, Kristeva juxtaposes the formal acquisition of language and the social ordering implicit in that learning (what she calls the symbolic) with the primary psychic process of the nonverbal (what she calls the semiotic). Pulling on the etymological roots of *semiotic*, Kristeva plays with its meaning as a "distinct mark, trace, index . . . engraven or written sign, imprint."[21] Much like traditional hieroglyphs, Kristeva's semiotic has a mysterious edge, an undecipherable meaning that throws into question the safe, superb rationality of civilized languages. Kristeva imbues her notion of the semiotic with an energy and movement that are associated with the body—most often the female body. The semiotic is a process or a drive—a "pulsion" that is often described by Kristeva as a sort of "kinetic rhythm." Nesting in the "unnamable" currents that surround and seep through our language, but are normally glossed over, the semiotic pulls meaning away from its traditional moorings. Nancy Stark Smith records a process that also digs under and around the usual meanings of her words in a stream of writing that precedes a group of hieroglyphs in her 1981 notebook:

> Glyphs, symbols, figures, languages, we continue to discover (uncover) invent and communicate by means of our own. Do we say what we mean, mean what we say? Are we "saying" anything? Do we care? Is it enough to express and suggest (even and especially to ourselves) states of mind we inhabit. We are choosing to record. Landmarks. Do we try to return there by way of these markings we leave. A place. A state.
> State of affairs.
> State of the art.
> A statement.[22]

Kristeva's semiotic and Smith's hieroglyphs parallel one another in several ways. I can imagine that the hieroglyphs would represent, for Kristeva, a kind of fantasy moment when letters and words have been swept up and reshaped in a semiotic storm of physical rhythms. Kristeva writes of finding the holes in the linguistic fabric, of slipping through the cracks in the symbolic to find another world like some Alice in Wonderland figure. Building on the imagery of texture and textiles, Kristeva notes that art "weaves into language (or other 'signifying materials') the complex relations of a subject caught between 'nature' and 'culture.' . . . between *desire* and the *law*, the body, language and 'metalanguage.'"[23] Smith uses a similar metaphor in an "Editor Note" that talks about the choices of improvisation: "She's looking for the hole in the fabric, through which stories are told, magic carpet rides are taken, information is exchanged. But to find the holes, she has to first weave the fabric."[24] I would call Smith's hieroglyphs an attempt to weave a fabric that invites one to slip through its openings.

In both Kristeva's concept of the semiotic and Smith's hieroglyphs, there is an intriguing relationship between kinetic rhythms and the space that movement creates or inhabits. Suspended, as if in midair directly above the page, the hieroglyphs dwell in a nebulous space somewhere between dancing and writing, where the movements of the one influence the rhythm and figures of the other. As a visual representation of the new linguistic/kinetic texture that both Smith and Kristeva envision, the hieroglyphs contain within their form the gaps (those momentary suspensions of reference points) that Smith and Kristeva believe encourage a fluidity of perception—both visual and imaginative. The loops and swirls of each figure encircle a space, but usually there is a crack, a leakage through which the inner and outer spaces can merge. Although the written script stays on the page, there is a sense in the visual interplay of these lines in motion that encourages a flow of space around and through the hieroglyphs.

This attention to the spaces in between coincides with the spatial features of the semiotic and with Kristeva's notion of the *chora*. Explaining the *chora* in a section of "Revolution in Poetic Language," Kristeva notes, "We borrow the term *chora* from Plato's *Timaeus* to denote an essentially mobile and extremely provisional articulation constituted by movements and their ephemeral stases."[25] Like the hieroglyphs, which funnel movement into writing, the kinetic rhythm of the *chora* can shake up and disrupt the symbolic order. The ruptures that result from that movement create spaces in which the unexpected or unnamable can emerge. Ironically, it is in an essay entitled "Women's Time" that Kristeva describes the importance of these spaces for women. Playing with less linear, more spatial concepts of "cyclical" or "monumental" time while simultaneously analyzing the historical moments of feminism, Kristeva posits another space in the last section of the essay, "Another Generation in Another Space." Transferring the temporal into the spatial, she notes, "My usage of the word 'generation' implies less a chronology than a signifying space, a both corporeal and desiring mental space."[26] This imaginary space is not a separatist's feminist utopia, but rather the place where the semiotic meets the symbolic. Kristeva envisions this space as being elastic enough to encompass the mixed and multiple identities that contemporary women must affirm.

It is telling that both Kristeva and Smith want to slip through a hole in the symbolic and dive into the gap and then come right back up to the surface to reintegrate that experience. Nancy Stark Smith sees the hieroglyphs as a sort of boomerang that will take her beyond the traditional uses of language but will eventually return her to that form. "I keep wanting to get back to the English language. I'm curious to see how the spontaneity and individuality of the hieroglyph writing will inform our use of words; how we can keep the dance moving, through the hieroglyphs and into our mother tongue."[27] Kristeva's desire to reenter the symbolic realm is based on her belief that little effective political action comes from staying in a space that is too easily marginalized or dismissed by conventional attitudes. As Jacqueline Rose comments in an essay on Kristeva, "The question therefore becomes not how to disrupt language by leaving its recognizable forms completely *behind*, but how to articulate the psychic processes which language normally glosses over *on this side* of meaning or sense."[28]

Nancy Stark Smith's hieroglyphs work on two levels to stretch language and open up new possibilities in writing. On a visual, perhaps more literal level, hieroglyphs take the body's movements into script. Infused with the flowing improvisational movements of contact improvisation, these symbols represent the body not in a static position or pose, but rather in a fluid, variable state. While these figures may be "read" in many different ways—all equally valid—they involve the reader in an active, personal, physical manner. Situated in the intersection of Cixous's notion of *écriture féminine* and the dancing of contact improvisation, Smith's hieroglyphs also take their place in Kristeva's notion of the semiotic, moving in and out of socialized discourse and awakening its appetite for more gaps, more movement, more body.

It is, of course, no coincidence that a woman who moves between the physicality of dancing contact improvisation and the writer/editor's constraints of verbal articulation would produce a personalized signature that tries to combine these culturally distinct ways of being. Using writing to "speak" the dancing and using the dancing to infuse certain fluidity into the writing, Smith has crafted an alternative that takes an important place in the ongoing dialogue between women and words. Because female bodies have been written into language as objects (of male desire) for so long—the equivalent, in some sense, of being completely written out of language—it takes radical experiments like those of Cixous, Kristeva, Stein, Walkowitz, and Smith to puncture the linguistic strongholds of dominant Western culture and bring women to language as subjects. Working within these cracks, writers like Smith can begin to put the feeling, breathing, moving bodies of women back into language, opening more possibilities for including the knowledge of the body in the language of the mind.

NOTES

1. Sandra Gilbert and Susan Gubar, "Ceremonies of the Alphabet," in *The Female Autograph*, ed. Donna C. Stanton (Chicago: University of Chicago Press, 1987), 25–26.

2. Nancy Stark Smith, "Dance in Translation: The Hieroglyphs," *Contact Quar-*

terly 7, no. 2 (Winter 1982): 45. Nancy Stark Smith has edited *Contact Quarterly* since it began as the informal *Contact Newsletter* in 1972. Now a self-supporting journal, *Contact Quarterly* publishes articles and creative writings about contact-related dance forms and body-awareness techniques.

3. Curt Siddall, "Contact Improvisation," *East Bay Review,* September 1976, cited in John Gamble, "On Contact Improvisation," *Painted Bride Quarterly* 4, no. 1 (Spring 1977): 36.

4. David Woodberry, *Contact Newsletter* 1, no. 2 (November 1975). This material was originally printed on a publicity flier for Woodberry's contact class.

5. Gamble, "On Contact Improvisation," 41.

6. Cynthia Novack, "Sharing the Dance: An Ethnography of Contact Improvisation," PhD diss., Columbia University, 1986.

7. Christina Svane, "In Praise of Bad Dancing," *Contact Newsletter,* November 1977, cited in "Editor Note," *Contact Quarterly,* 10, no. 3 (Fall 1985): 3.

8. Nancy Stark Smith, "Editor Note," *Contact Quarterly* 10, no. 2 (Spring/Summer 1987): 3.

9. Gamble, 38.

10. Smith, "Dance in Translation," 45.

11. Hélène Cixous, "The Laugh of the Medusa," in *New French Feminisms,* ed. Elaine Marks and Isabelle deCourtivron (New York: Schocken Books, 1981), 245.

12. Ibid., 251.

13. Nancy Stark Smith, personal interview with the author, Northampton, Massachusetts, summer 1987.

14. Cixous, 252.

15. Smith interview.

16. Cixous, 259–60.

17. Gertrude Stein, "Orta or One Dancing," in *Two* (New York: Books for Libraries Press, 1969), 288.

18. Abraham Walkowitz, *Isadora Duncan in her Dances* (Girard, KS: Haldeman-Julius Publications, 1945).

19. Smith, "Editor Note," 3.

20. Ibid.

21. Julia Kristeva, "Revolution in Poetic Language," in *The Kristeva Reader,* ed. Toril Moi (New York: Columbia University Press, 1986), 93.

22. Nancy Stark Smith, collected notebooks (unpublished; courtesy of Nancy Stark Smith).

23. Julia Kristeva, *Desire in Language* (New York: Columbia University Press, 1980), 97.

24. Nancy Stark Smith, "Editor Note," *Contact Quarterly* 6, no. 2 (Winter 1981): 2.

25. Kristeva, "Revolution in Poetic Language," 93.

26. Julia Kristeva, "Women's Time," in *Feminist Theory: A Critique of Ideology,* ed. Nannerl O. Keohane, Michelle Z. Rosaldo, and Barbara C. Gelpi (Chicago: University of Chicago Press, 1982), 34.

27. Smith, "Dance in Translation," 46.

28. Jacqueline Rose, *Sexuality in the Field of Vision* (London: Verso, 1986), 146.

13

Auto-Body Stories

Blondell Cummings and Autobiography in Dance

Meaning in Motion: New Cultural Studies of Dance, ed. Jane Desmond (1997).

As I advance in these memoirs, I realize more and more the impossibility of writing one's life—or rather, the lives of all the different people I have been. Incidents which seemed to me to last a lifetime have taken only a few pages: intervals that seemed thousands of years of suffering and pain and through which, in sheer defense, in order to go on living, I emerged an entirely different person, do not appear at all long here. I often ask myself desperately, what reader is going to be able to clothe with flesh the skeleton that I have presented? I am trying to write down the truth, but the truth runs away and hides from me. How find the truth? If I were a writer, and had written of my life twenty novels or so, it would be nearer the truth.

—ISADORA DUNCAN, *MY LIFE*

How does this statement, written near the end of her autobiography, reflect on the lively account of art and love that Isadora Duncan has given her reader? Faced with the daunting task of creating a coherent literary account of her life, Duncan tries to tell her story only to realize (some 300 pages later) the impossibility of such an attempt.[1] She claims, instead, that were she a novelist, the "truth" of her life would be found in her novels, not in her autobiography. In "Writing Fictions: Women's Autobiography in France," Nancy Miller tackles this issue of "truth" in autobiography and proposes a new reading similar to the reading that Duncan alludes to. Although Miller calls for a "double reading—of the autobiography with the fiction," she is quick to note that her dual reading is not suggesting (as others have) that all women's fiction is autobiographical. Rather, what she proposes is "an intratextual practice of interpretation which . . . would privilege neither the autobiography nor the fiction, but take the two writings together in their status as text."[2] Miller concludes the chapter with her usual panache by declaring: "The historical truth of a woman writer's life lies in the reader's grasp of her intratext: the body of her writing and not the writing of her body."[3]

But what if the body of her writing is the writing of her body? What if the female signature that we are trying to decipher is a movement signature? What if its "author" is a dancer? At the risk of distorting Miller's comments by switching their context from writing to dancing—from the literary muse to the moving one—I want to explore some ways in which autobiography is staged in dance, not so much to focus on the nature of identity per se, as to examine the complex ways in which dancing can at once set up and upset the various frames of the self. How does the presence of a live body create a representation of identity that differs from literary autobiography? How closely intertwined with its own physical reality is the "self" of dance?

While feminist critics concerned with the representation of women in film, art, and popular culture have dubbed the 1980s the decade of the body, those working in literary theory tend to see these years as framing various debates over the nature of identity and the social construction of gendered writers and gendered readers.[4] So far, few feminist scholars have tried to connect the two realms in order to address issues of identity by looking at the representation of the performing body within the context of gender and race. In this essay, I use the frame of autobiography in dance as my own intratext—of writing and dancing—in order to explore the complex issues involved in representing a self through the dancing body. Beginning with a rereading of Isadora Duncan's *My Life* in terms of her actual dancing, I will discuss the ways in which feminist approaches to autobiography have shifted their focus from seeking to identify (or constitute) a "self" in the name of "woman," to questioning the very possibility of a unified writing subject. Turning to contemporary dance and focusing on three works choreographed by Blondell Cummings, I ask what it might mean to represent these conflicting positions within a live performance.

The emphasis on fluid and constant motion in many contemporary forms of dance (such as contact improvisation) suggests an intriguing analogy to recent explorations of the autobiographical self. Duncan's autobiography is framed by a rhetorical stance that asks how she is to find the "'truth" of her "self" among all the different people she has been. This ambiguity of identity can be seen as reflecting the radical nature of an art form whose very medium insists on changes in location, on moving through spaces. Nonetheless, the physical presence of a dancer's body refuses any loose assumptions about the playful postmodern multiplicity of dancing by relentlessly insisting on those cultural moorings—the social implications of gendered, racial, and historical ties—that the live body can never escape. The existential questioning with which Duncan—a white, middle-class bohemian artist from the early twentieth century, interrupts her conventional autobiographical voice holds very different meanings in a solo dance by Cummings—a black, middle-class, contemporary choreographer. By looking at issues of identity and representation within a discussion of the body in dance, I hope to keep these differences in mind by focusing on how they are played out on the stage.

Referring to a moment in the beginning of her choreographic career, when her family had just arrived in Paris, Duncan writes:

I spent long days and nights in the studio seeking that dance which might be the divine expression of the human spirit through the medium of the body's movement. For hours I would stand quite still, my two hands folded between my breasts, covering the solar plexus . . . I was seeking and finally discovered the central spring of all movement, the crater of motor power, the unity from which all diversities of movements are born, the mirror of vision for the creation of the dance.[5]

These sentences, which are woven into more explicitly autobiographical facts, such as when Duncan went to school and the economic plight of her family after her mother's divorce, establish the mythopoetic voice that carries the narrative themes of *My Life*. Again and again, Duncan recites a litany of inspired performances in which her body becomes a medium for her soul, registering with Cixousian euphoria the swells of ecstasy— both her own and the audience's—that her performances create. Although Duncan calls her dance performances "representations," she never discusses them critically as a representation of the self and only rarely expresses any ambivalence about who she is in terms of her dancing. While her memoir comments on the changing selves of her life experience, her meditations on dance reveal her most fervent belief in a joyous, unified expression of the self through movement.

Sorting through Duncan's zealous expressions of her selfhood in *My Life*, Patricia Spacks analyzes Duncan's autobiography as a psychological portrait and looks for the psychic attributes of what she calls the "female imagination," "the ways of female feeling, the modes of responding, that persist despite social change."[6] In *The Female Imagination* Spacks interprets Duncan's autobiography as a narcissistic tale of the artist as a visionary, seeing it as emblematic of woman's need to resist societal constrictions by way of her creative imagination. "The woman as artist may help to illuminate the woman as woman."[7] Not attuned to the potency of Duncan's experience as a dancer, Spacks reads *My Life* only for a coherent portrait of the artist as a visionary and the visionary as a woman. "The woman's most potent fear is likely to be of abandonment, her most positive vision, of love . . . She dreams of herself as beautiful, therefore beloved; as powerful because beloved."[8] Spacks insists that Duncan's construction of the monumental self in *My Life* is adolescent, and she searches Duncan's "tawdry prose" for the discrepancies between Duncan's vision of her dancing and the "facts" of her loves and woes in a way which subsumes Duncan's connections with dance in her own analysis of a "female imagination." Spacks continues: "The disproportion between the way she sees and the way she reveals herself creates much of the interest of her autobiography, testimony to a mind that refuses to accept the domination of external circumstance. Her vision more compelling than any conceivable reality, she declares her ultimate power to deny facts, transforming them into myth."[9] In giving us a portrait of Duncan as an obsessive artist, Spacks skims over the cracks in Duncan's writing, reinforcing a vision of the artist as a creative genius working outside of society and never probing the social constructions underneath that facade.

Taking my cue from Miller's intratext, the "double reading—of the autobiography with the fiction," I propose to read *My Life* in conjunction with what we know of Duncan's actual dancing; not in order to validate her mythopoetic voice by citing reviewers' praises of her dancing persona, but rather to point to the possibility of a different kind of attentiveness in reading autobiography. In addition to the obvious translations from a literary context to a performance one, the differences between Spacks's and my readings of Duncan's autobiography illustrate a shifting approach to issues of identity in feminist studies. Published in 1975, Spacks's *Female Imagination* came from a women's studies tradition that sought to analyze women's writing for the uniquely "female" perspective created by the marginalization of women in Western society. Even while she is remarking on the tensions between Duncan's desire and the socially defined possibilities for women at the time, Spacks is interested, finally, in locating a specific female subjectivity. I am less interested in defining the characteristics of a female signature per se, than in exploring the intratextual autographs of writing and dancing—in other words, I want to look at the ways in which the performing body physicalizes the autobiographical voice to produce a representation of subjectivity that is at once whole and fragmented.

Unfortunately, there are no known films that could help dance scholars re-create Duncan's dancing. Most reconstructions of her solos are based on the memories of her six adopted "daughters," especially Irma, Anna, and Theresa.[10] Nevertheless, the wealth of photographs, drawings, paintings, and written descriptions by her contemporaries bear witness to Duncan's extraordinary performing presence and give us possible clues as to what her dancing was like. Take, for instance, a remarkable description of the first time he saw Duncan dancing by Gordon Craig, son of the famed British actress Ellen Terry and one of Duncan's lovers:

> Quite still . . . Then one step back or sideways, and the music began again as she went moving on before or after it. Only just moving—not pirouetting or doing any of those things which we expect to see, and which a Taglioni or a Fanny Elssler would have certainly done. She was speaking in her own language—do you understand? Her own language: have you got it?—Not echoing any ballet master, and so she came to move as no one had ever seen anyone move before.[11]

Craig's written evocation connects with Duncan's own passages in *My Life* to represent the writer as dancer and the dancer as writer. The language of Duncan's dancing, which Craig describes as "her own language," parallels Duncan's description of waiting for the movement to start in her solar plexus—that "crater of motor power." It is also important to note that Craig fuses dancing and writing in order to give Duncan a certain authority over her own text.

Duncan's mythologizing of her experience in *My Life* can be heavy-handed at times: "I was possessed by the dream of Promethean creation that, at my call, might spring from the Earth, descend from the Heavens, such dancing figures as the world had never seen."[12] However, one can learn to read beyond the tone of her writing and into her dancing. Spacks describes Duncan's allusions to Prometheus in the passage quoted earlier as "conventional romantic rhetoric," paradoxically placing Duncan in the historically masculine category of the artist as tragic hero.[13] When read next to a well-known photograph by Edward Steichen of Duncan standing in the Parthenon, however, her reference to "Promethean creation" not only suggests an invocation to Zeus—at once a challenge and an appeal to "see me"—but also makes me aware of the physical implications of that invocation: the lines of movement streaming through Duncan's body; her outreached arms calling energy from the skies, and her legs receiving a grounded support from the earth. Even the passage in which Duncan describes how she stood in the studio waiting for inspiration affords the reader who looks beneath its mythic veneer an insight to the importance of breath and central chest initiation of her movements. It was Duncan's strength of vision that gave her the physical and moral fortitude to actually go out there on stage and dance. Acknowledging the importance of her dancing self enables the reader of *My Life* to look for another story—a movement story—threaded among the pages of her autobiography.

Giving little weight to Duncan's extraordinary achievement in radicalizing the theatrical dancing of her time, Spacks simply condemns Duncan for recording so convincingly her illusions about her art: "As an autobiographer, Isadora Duncan is dreamer rather than observer of her life: not an artist despite all her assertions of artistry."[14] Read within the context of her dancing, however, Duncan's autobiography reveals the very real tensions between her need to justify her work to a society that she feels has misunderstood her art and her desire to share the experience of creative momentum that sponsored her dancing. To efface that dancing body from her writing is to negate a powerful force in the creation and representation of Duncan's life.

Doubly circumscribed by the theatrical frame of her dancing experience and the literary frame of her writing, Duncan's autobiography is riddled with intriguing gaps produced by her shifts in identity. Inspired by the memory of a successful performance, Duncan proclaims the universality of her mission and refers to her work as art and herself as an artist in order to highlight the aesthetic and spiritual aspects of an art form based on the display of bodies, which had strong connotations of entertainment and still carried traces of an earlier association with prostitution and loose morals. The fact that she rarely calls herself a dancer—though she writes of the dance—points to Duncan's acumen with regard to the cultural milieu in which she performed, as well as her attentiveness to the subtle precariousness of a publicly defined identity for women. At times, this strident sense of individualism carries her along for pages, bolstering her confidence in her mission. Other times, however, Duncan disrupts the self-congratulatory tone of her writing by directly confronting her readers with a speech aimed at defending her unorthodox lifestyle in the name of art. Her usual exalted, self-assured pace is broken up by periodic moments of introspection when Duncan is likely to ask, "Where can I find the woman of all these adventures? It seems to me there was not one but hundreds."[15]

Discussing the difficulty of translating the memory of one's life experience into a literary medium and the impossibility of completely escaping the influence of others' perceptions of who you are, Duncan allows her readers to see the gaps in her identity; these black holes of absence in the otherwise smooth narrative of her extraordinary presence. Writing her life story is difficult for Duncan; for it is on the autobiographical stage, more so than on the dancing one, that her various identities—like so many illustrious ghosts—emerge to confront and question one another. The act of writing places a shadow over her dancing: "Words have different meaning. Before the public which has thronged my representations I have had no hesitation. I have given them the most secret impulses of my soul. From the first I have only danced my life."[16]

Duncan feels more in control of her self-representation when she is dancing than when she is writing. Her supreme confidence about the authenticity of her movement expression contrasts dramatically with her ambivalence about writing a life. Duncan's preferred means of self-expression is clearly the language of dance. In *My Life,* Duncan tries to find words that can translate her elated experiences of dancing to her readers. What she finds, however, is that in spite of a dramatic, mythopoetic voice, the project of writing one's life exposes the fragility not only of the writing self, but also of the dancing self. As readers, we can negotiate this rocky languagescape by redirecting our goal of looking for a coherent self in the autobiographical signature into a more open, double reading, which might examine how writing and dancing combine to create different, interwoven signatures.

In his essay "Self-Invention in Autobiography: The Moment of Language," Paul Eakins coins a phrase that is particularly resonant in the present context.[17] Discussing the realization of selfhood through language, Eakins refers to this process as "the performance of the autobiographical act." Eakins's use of a theatrical metaphor in discussing this "art of self-invention" is echoed in much of the recent spate of feminist scholarship on autobiography. In this new body of literary work, autobiography is treated less as a truthful revelation of the singular inner and private self than as a dramatic staging—a representation—of the public self. What this performance paradigm emphasizes is the acutely self-conscious public display inherent in the act of penning one's life, especially for women, who must deal with a double jeopardy: they are both on display and often never really feel in control of the terms of that representation. Even though current theory is less interested in reading autobiography as a mirror of women's experiences, we can still ask: what does it mean for women to write the stories of their lives?

The outpouring of women's autobiographies in the twentieth century has been celebrated by feminist scholars as an awakening—a speaking of life stories that have historically been silenced. Collections of critical essays such as Jelinek's *Women's Autobiography,* Mason and Green's *Journeys: Autobiographical Writings by Women,* Benstock's *The Private Self: Theory and Practice of Women's Autobiographical Writings,* Stanton's *The Female Autograph,* and Smith's *A Poetics of Women's Autobiography* all comment on the growing feeling of emancipation from the scripts (mostly by men) that have traditionally written women's lives. More than a factual document or realistic description of their lives, women's autobiographies often create a selfhood by virtue of that very process (performance?) of writing. The struggle to mediate between private ambitions and public conditions may fragment a woman's sense of her self, but if these layered bits of experience do not add up to the traditional depiction of one grand unified identity, they nonetheless reveal a productive authority—a writing self. In much of the feminist scholarship on autobiography, "voice" is seen as a metaphor for the act of inscribing one's self in the world. "To find her own voice" implies a great deal more than expressing a thought or opinion: it also carries a healthy blend of satisfaction and bravado. The whole world is a stage, the autobiographical self may be a representation, but it is her voice. In the coda at the end of her book, Sidonie Smith speaks of the contemporary woman autobiographer: "Fashioning her own voice within and against the voices of others, she performs a selective appropriation of stories told by and about men and women. Subversively, she rearranges the dominant discourse and the dominant ideology of gender, seizing the language and its powers to turn cultural fictions into her *very own story* [emphasis added]."[18]

It is, of course, important to celebrate women's finding their voices—as much of women's literary criticism so joyfully does. However, with the influence of poststructuralist thought on feminist theory and the internal debates concerning whether "woman" is not, in fact, completely a social construction, feminists have begun to question what it means to call something our "own." While the written signature is conventionally associated with authorship, performances are less clearly signed because they are based on an indeterminate dialogue between performer and audience. Dance performances are an extreme example of fluidity of authorship, since it is virtually impossible for a choreographer to transpose exactly his or her movement onto another body. This past decade has witnessed an increase in autobiography included within the context of dance. The various connections between the writing self and the dancing one—the movement and the text—can range in these performances from a loose juxtaposition of sound and gesture (as in the solo work of Ishmael Houston-Jones and Simone Forti), to a carefully orchestrated tableau that meshes these verbal and physical elements to produce an intricate web of movement and meaning (as in the recent work of Bill T. Jones and Arnie Zane dance company). Translating reader-response theory into the performance context, one could say that not only is each dance "read" and interpreted by audience members, it is constantly "read" and reinterpreted by the person performing those movements. In many ways, then, the presence of the performing body can challenge and stretch even the most recent explorations of the autobiographical self. The act of performing itself (or one's self) foregrounds the fact that the self is also always reinvented by a physical body that cannot be so easily or neatly fragmented. In the very act of performing, the dancing body splits itself to enact its own representation and simultaneously heals its own fissure in that enactment.

Reading *My Life* next to Duncan's dancing provides us with an intra-text—of the body and the writing—which can refocus our thinking about the autobiographical self. By inserting the dancing body into a study of autobiography, I do not mean to reduce women (once again) to being *only* their bodies. I am aware that phrases such as "speaking through the body" which can be envisioned as a means of authorizing the "self" in dance, can also connote social inscriptions which reflect the powerlessness of hysteria and summon up historical moments when women did not have the option to use their voices assertively—when their only option was to "speak through the body." But I think it is important not to shy away from a theoretical engagement with the female body and its representations in dance just because they comprise a network of layered contradictions and cross-referenced significations.

One of the earliest published accounts of Blondell Cummings's choreography appeared in the March 14, 1971, *New York Times*. Anna Kisselgoff, the *Times*' dance critic, was reviewing an afternoon showcase of young choreographers that took place at the New School in New York City.

> Particular promise was shown in "Point of Reference" by Blondell Cummings who composed a touching encounter between herself, a twenty-two year-old black girl born in South Carolina, and Anya Allister, also twenty-two, a Jewish girl born in Russia. Each girl recited her biographical information on tape. The honesty of the movement matched the direct statement about minority background.[19]

While Cummings's publicity statements mark 1978 as the year she began to choreograph regularly, it is telling how many of the elements that Kisselgoff mentions in this early dance are still motivating concerns in Cummings's dance making almost two decades later. The theatrical correspondence between the dancers, their movements, and taped biographical stories, the "honesty" of the emotionally vivid gestural movements, and the juxtaposition of different cultural and racial backgrounds have informed Cummings's work throughout her choreographic career.

Cummings spent most of the 1970s working with Meredith Monk/The House—a performance ensemble that blended music, movement, and text to present imagistic theater rituals. While she was developing one of the company's seminal pieces, *Education of the Girlchild,* Monk asked the various performers to create a stage persona that embodied an important aspect of their own identities. In an interview with Marianne Goldberg, Cummings describes the process of shaping her particular character: "I tried to find a way of representing an archetypal figure that I would understand from a deep, personal, subconscious point of view that at the same time would be strong enough to overlap several Black cultures."[20] Cummings's character in *Education of the Girlchild* is autobiographical in that it was developed directly from Cummings's personal experience of African-American cultures. These memories and sensations were then distilled into repetitious movements (as in her continuous swaying during the traveling section) or large, emotional gestures (such as her silent compulsive scream). They are meant to strike the viewer as archetypal, somehow so basic that they could be a part of everyone's experience. This movement from memory to gesture, from a specific life experience to a formal movement image, underlies much of Monk's work with The House, and is also the central source in Cummings's own work. As Linda Small predicted in a 1980 article on the then-emerging choreographer, Cummings was to "become recognized for her ability to recycle experience into art."[21]

This comment by Small pivots on an assumption about autobiography that is valuable to take up here. When she coins the phrase "recycle experience into art," Small suggests that Cummings is taking the raw material of a life experience and representing it through formal "artistic" means. But as already noted, Eakins's use of the trope of performance to discuss autobiography reflects just how layered with representation the self already is. Even in the "raw" experience of life, the "self" is performed; autobiographical performances are often complex ways of consciously taking responsibility for the terms of that experience. Yet it is critical to realize that within the context of a dance performance these different levels of representation are contained within one physical, racial, and gendered body.

In 1978, Cummings began a collaboration with writer Madeleine Keller that exploded into the multidimensional performance piece called *Cycle.*

She was working as an arts administrator with the now-defunct CETA program, and her organizational abilities were funneled into this mammoth artistic project that included group workshops, taped interviews, visual and literary contributions from a widely diverse cross-section of people, as well as a solo performance by Cummings and a video document. The interconnecting theme was individuals' reactions to women's menstrual cycles. The name *Cycle* refers not only to the menstrual cycle but also to the way in which ideas and images are recycled throughout the piece. Cummings recalls that the genesis of the whole project took place in the back seat of a car while she was on tour with Meredith Monk/The House. Curled up in agony because of her menstrual cramps, she declared that some day she would make a performance piece based on this experience. The momentum of the project peaked in August 1978 when Cummings performed her solo at the Warren Street Performance Loft, New York City.

Cycle proved to be a catalyst in Cummings's choreographic career not only because it lent inspiration and a name to Cycle Arts Foundation—the multifaceted arts organization that supports her choreographic projects and collaborations—but also because it affirmed her artistic process. Taking a subject that she was intimately connected to, Cummings created a variety of forums in which to collect other people's reactions to this same issue. In an interview, Cummings spoke about her desire to appeal to multiple cultures, to transform her personal interest into an experience that many people could relate to. *Cycle* was an appropriate vehicle for this work. For Cummings, a topic such as menstrual cycles could potentially involve women from practically every class and cultural experience. It also affects women in an age range of about forty years, and most women can talk about it with the confidence and authority of being an expert in the matter. Finally—significantly—this piece even allowed her mother to interact with Cummings's artistic projects—a realm of her daughter's life in which she rarely actively participated.

Cummings is interested in finding a way to universalize or, at least, extend her particular concerns in order to allow many people to identify and engage personally with her work. For instance, *Cycle* was not meant to speak just to women. Cummings believes that men, by way of their family or friendly connections to women, are implicated in this topic of menstrual cycles as well. Cummings does not want to essentialize or separate women from men. In this sense, her desire to expand a personal issue into an umbrella that could cover many people's experience suggests that she feels that the personal is not only political, but also can create cross-cultural affinities.

Although her work is not always explicitly autobiographical, Cummings's solo choreography repeatedly presents the audience with links between the character she is portraying and her own self. As one reviewer explains: "[She] conjures up both a personal history and an entire culture."[22] Unlike the genre of art/life performances that seek to blur the distinctions between representation and "real" life, Cummings uses performance as a formal means to explore more general cultural and psychological influences (friendships, relationships, working, money) that shape her life. Yet specific movement material often reappears in subsequent solos. These repetitive gestures combine with an underlying narrative thread (often augmented by bits of personal stories and anecdotes by a woman's voice on the soundtrack) to create a woven fabric of dancing and autobiography. Cummings herself articulates the way these characters evolve from her life experience:

> My characters might seem like they're coming out of the blue, but they take a long time to develop . . . I've done a lot of traveling alone, which has made me a real observer, real interested in detail, and in basic but universal things—food and eating styles, friendship, the menstrual cycle. Sure my pieces come from being a woman, black and American, but they're mostly concerned with the human condition.[23]

Despite that fact that Cummings tries to abstract personal material into portraits that have a wider connection to her audience, she has a vivid and quirky movement style that leaves little doubt that she is performing her own story. Cummings's performing presence is intensified by her quick hand gestures and split-second changes of facial expression that contrast dramatically with her slower, more fluid shifts of weight. While she wants to affect audience members with a broad range of life experiences, Cummings does not dissolve into a non-differentiated character in an attempt to be everything for anybody. Her dancing rarely uses the abstract and formalized positions and movement styles of more traditional dance techniques. Often the audience assumes that her portraits are dramatic extensions of the various facets of her life. This autobiographical association in her work is accentuated by the fact that when she is onstage, she is often dancing alone. Although she has choreographed for her own company and the Alvin Ailey Repertory Ensemble, among others, Cummings rarely appears in these group pieces. When she is dancing, there is often the sense that she inhabits a private space, moving around and through her world with the intuitive frankness of a woman alone in her apartment. Cummings speaks of her solo work with a hint of existential resolve:

> I feel strongly about solo work, because I think that basically we are soloists. And yes, we couple with other people, we socialize with other people; but you're born alone and you go through certain periods of your life that change and the only thing that is consistent is you—yourself. When you die, you die alone. I feel that when one is being solo, it allows the solo sorts of self to be able to identify with that person and hear that inner voice.[24]

Significantly, it is the images, voices, gestures, and memories of other people that filter throughout one of Cummings's most popular solos, *Chicken Soup* (1981–83). Danced independently, or as the first section in the evening-length collection of solos called *Food for Thought, Chicken Soup* presents Cummings as a woman whose life revolves around the community and loneliness of the household kitchen. The first image is the back of a woman dressed in a long white skirt and white shirt, swaying from side to side with her shopping bag in hand, just as if she were walking down a country lane on her way to market. This image dissolves into another picture of a woman seated primly on the edge of a chair. As a nostalgic, wistful melody plays, her face and hands become animated with a variety of gossipy—"Oh, you don't mean it!"—expressions. During this silent, cheerful chatter, Cummings begins to rock in a movement so old-fashioned and yet so hypnotically soothing that it is hard to imagine that she will ever stop. As Cummings banters away with herself, a woman's voice reminisces in a calm, thoughtful manner. Phrases such as "the kitchen was the same" melt into the tableau of the woman rocking in the chair. The constant repetition of rocking makes time seem somehow irrelevant. Soon, however, the pleasant conversation turns to one of grief and pain, and Cummings's body encompasses the change with full central contradictions. The quick, flickering hand gestures, which traced years of passing out cards and cups of tea at a bridge table, get caught for a moment in a posture of pain or anger and then release back into the repetitious flow of rocking and talking. Joining the music on the soundtrack, a woman's voice haltingly describes afternoons spent around the kitchen table talking of "childhood friends, operations, abortion, death, and money." It seems as if the scene we are watching is her memory. Participating in the merged memory of voice and body, Cummings's character is selectively responsive to these words, periodically breaking into a stop-action series of emotional gestures that mime the spoken words and have become a trademark of her work.

"Moving Pictures" is the phrase Cummings uses to describe her uncanny ability to segment movement into a series of fast stop-action bits that give the impression of movements seen under a strobe light or of a filmstrip seen frame by frame. Cummings explains their genesis by telling a story about her childhood fascination with photography and the excitement of getting her first camera. This movement technique is the result of grafting photographic images onto the kinetic energy of dance. By freezing her movement in an evenly rhythmic succession, she gives the effect of being in a strobe light, without the flickering darkness. In this choreographic process, Cummings forces the viewer to take a mental picture, so to speak. The zest and physical intensity of Cummings's living body coupled with the timeless quality of photography—its overwhelmingly memorable specificity of character— creates a fascinating conflict between stillness and movement, death and life. Reviewing an early concert of Cummings's work, Burt Supree, a dance critic for the *Village Voice,* writes of her "silent wildness." "She's most astonishing, though, in a section where she moves as if caught in the flicker of a fast strobe, no sounds coming from her gaping mouth, sliding from worry to fear to screaming terror, blending into laughter which merges again into wailing."[25] Cummings describes her unique movement images as "an accumulation of one's life" and speaks of how they are pregnant with memory for her. Interestingly enough, she also discusses these "moving pictures" as autobiographical, not because they have become a signature style of moving which can be found in almost every solo she has choreographed, but because they are a way of picturing herself with an outside eye. At once the photographer and the image, she creates an unusual mode of self-reflexivity in dance.

While Isadora Duncan actually needed to write her autobiography in order to see herself with an outside eye and only realized in retrospect that "from the first I have only danced my life," Cummings has found a method of including this process of self-reflection into the dancing itself. The exalted and unified dancing self that is so emblematic of the autobiographical voice in *My Life* has been transformed by time, culture, and aesthetics into a fractured combination of image, gesture, and movement in Cummings's dancing. How are we to find a single "self" amid all these split-second portraits of women crying, rocking, laughing, and talking?

Chicken Soup continues. Stepping away from the picture gallery of women that she animates in the rocking chair, Cummings sinks to the floor and picks up a scrub brush. Her body bobs with the rhythm of her work, and the action of the bristles across the floor creates a swish swish accompaniment. The audience sees her in profile; her body stretching and contracting with the strong, even strokes of her arms. The broad sweeps of her movement are more important than the task of cleaning the floor. Although the image could be one of contracted menial labor, there is a caring, authoritative quality in Cummings's motion that suggests that this work is immensely satisfying. Cummings notes: "There is poetry to scrubbing the floor. Scrubbing the floor is scrubbing the floor, but the way you scrub it can reflect your own physicality, your own background, your own culture."[26]

The direct, spare physicality and its affirmation of life in work diffuses when Cummings trades her brush for a long black scarf. As a nostalgic hummed melody floats into the scene, Cummings swirls the scarf in the air and crosses the stage with joyous, exalted skips and leaps. This moment of whirling happiness fades into a sad sweep of the scarf as Cummings walks to the back of the stage and waves good-bye. Loss and mourning crush the previous gaiety. Her heavy, tired body is dwarfed by the shadow of herself projected on the background. The figure, swelled by grief, looms behind Cummings. Then, the emotional tides change once again as a chicken-soup recipe is recited and Cummings picks up a cast-iron frying pan with all the assurance and sassiness of a woman who could cook in her sleep. Like a simmering soup, there is a constant rhythm and bubble in her body. Chopping, mixing, and frying actions are embodied by full motions that spread through her body and down into her feet as well. With cooking coursing through her body, Cummings comments on the images she has made by a series of wonderfully comic facial expressions. Innuendo wafts, like the imagined aroma of her cooking, in and around this figure, and when the recipe directs her to "simmer until tender," Cummings ironically, and with a knowing smile directed to the audience, shimmies her hips.

Chicken Soup is generally referred to as, in the words of one critic, "a fond memory of black rural life."[27] Considering Cummings's very urban experience, one might wonder whose memory this is and where it comes from. It is often difficult to discern what parts are remembered and which ones are invented, particularly when the memory serves as a basis for a work of art. In an article called "The Site of Memory," Toni Morrison discusses how memory influences her writing, merging fiction with autobiography. She describes how she fills an "image" of her relatives with a "memory" of them. "These people are my access to me; they are my entrance into my own interior life. Which is why the images that float around them—the remains, so to speak, at the archeological site—surface first, and they surface so vividly and so compellingly that I acknowledge them as my route to a reconstruction of a world, to an exploration of an interior life that was not written and to the revelation of a kind of truth."[28] I think that memory serves a similar purpose for Cummings in *Chicken Soup* by allowing her to connect to women in her history and to participate in their worlds. Seeing her gossip in a chair or shake a skillet, I feel as if this is the first time, as well as the hundredth time, Cummings has gone back inside these images to merge past and present, dancing bits of stories from all these women's lives.

When Cummings introduced *Chicken Soup* during an informal lecture demonstration at Franklin and Marshall College in the fall of 1987, she spoke of her interest in food and how she could guess someone's characteristics just by looking in their refrigerator. Cummings described *Chicken Soup* as a solo about women—many different women—who use food to nourish and connect to other people. Her intention was to make a dance that spanned a variety of cultures—Jewish, African-American, Italian—and that desire is reflected in her choice of texts, which include pieces by Grace Paley, as well as a recipe from *The Settlement Cookbook*. Despite this multicultural tapestry in the text, the dance is generally received as being specifically about black women. In fact, when Cummings presented the work on television in the *Alive from Off Center* program during the summer of 1988, the cover of the *New York Times'* television section announced her work as a vision of "traditional roles of black women in America."[29] A curiously intrusive interference by the television producer had Cummings performing the dance in a generic Formica kitchen, wearing a housedress and a flowered apron. The effect, especially to someone who had seen the solo in a theater space, with no set and white costuming, is quite bizarre. The tacky television realism stages a very narrow definition of "traditional roles of black women in America," removing the wonderful ambivalence of Cummings's earlier version of this dance. Unlike the stage portrayal of this solo, where it is unclear whose memories she is dancing, the television production reduces this woman to a generic two-dimensional figure who is trapped in the specific context of her own spic-and-span kitchen.

The publicity for this video underlined how many reviewers discussed *Chicken Soup* as exploring a specifically black heritage. This insistence on viewing the dance only within one cultural tradition—the one referenced by her race—disturbs Cummings. In an interview, she spoke of wanting to sound a resonant note in everyone's background—to create a common memory.

> What happens for me is that it [the sense of familiarity] stops when you start saying that you see me as a black person in the chair because then it might stop your ability to have it go back into your own background. Because if you see it as black and you're not black, then it seems to me you will not allow yourself the same liberty to identify with that character and then you start bringing all the references to a black person and why that makes that black.[30]

The issues of identification that Cummings touches on in this statement are rife with complexity. Self versus other, difference versus sameness, individuality versus community—these polarities are deeply rooted in this culture's social, political, and religious epistemologies. The last few decades in America have witnessed celebrations of sameness in the political industry and difference in those strangely allied realms of intellectual theory and fashion. Most feminists have begun to negotiate between the need for recognizing crucial racial, class, and cultural differences among women and the persistent feeling that women share some sort of affinity, if only in their common awareness of the practical risks of being a woman in today's society. Cummings is caught in this sticky web of identifications, for although she claims she wants to create a "universal" image of a woman that anyone could relate to, she has also described with tears in her eyes the moving and self-affirming experience of dancing *Chicken Soup* for a predominantly black audience in the "Black Dance America" series at the Brooklyn Academy of Music. "It was wonderful . . . And I thought to myself, so this is what it is all about!"[31]

Cummings is a woman and she is black, but her dances can frame that identity very differently. *Basic Strategies V* (1986) is the last section of a cycle of dances called *Basic Strategies,* which explores how people deal with work and money. *Basic Strategies I–III* were originally created for college dancers, and *Basic Strategies IV* was commissioned by the Alvin Ailey Repertory Ensemble. Many of the movements in these earlier pieces are repetitive motions loosely based on a work activity. Mixed in with the music soundtrack are voices telling stories of a business success or describing an early memory. *Basic Strategies IV* is prefaced with a still tableau of arranged figures. Although they are all dressed in white, some characters are recognizable as a nun, a nurse, a farmer, a soldier, and a hospital attendant. The dancing begins as a clump of these figures in white shuffle across the stage chanting "For love or for money." Breaking off from the group, several dancers come to the center of the stage to mime a work activity as a voice on the soundtrack describes a memory of that figure. The realism of story and gesture in these early *Basic Strategies* is replaced in *Basic Strategies V* with a formal juxtaposition of the movements and their contexts.

Basic Strategies V begins with a group section and ends with a solo for Cummings. Although I want to concentrate on the complicated images in her solo, I will take some time to sketch in the first part of the dance, for it sets up many of the double readings within the dance. Originally commissioned by Williams College and the Massachusetts Council on the Art and Humanities, *Basic Strategies V* is a collaboration with the writer Jamaica Kincaid and composer Michael Riesman. In what Cummings terms her process of "collage," this work layers sets, costumes, music, taped texts, and movement to create multiple references of self and community. Unlike *Chicken Soup*, however, *Basic Strategies V* uses the texts, sets, and costumes not as background accompaniment for the dancing, but rather as primary elements that create the basic irony and dramatic tension in this piece and make it so compelling to watch. The remarkable text by Kincaid, who was born in St. John's, Antigua, focuses the dancing in the first group section. The fluid and rhythmic carrying, pushing, pulling movements are juxtaposed to a story (spoken by a woman's soft voice) that braids a history of her people with a history of an Anglican colonial cathedral. The slaves built this cathedral for their masters, but now the descendants of both the slaves and their masters worship there. Noting the ambiguity of her history, the narrator's liquid voice on the sound tape loops back on itself repeatedly:

> My history before it was interrupted does not include cathedrals. What my history before it was interrupted includes is no longer absolutely clear to me. The cathedral is now a part of my history. The cathedral is now a part of me. The cathedral is now mine.[32]

It is never entirely clear how the story of the cathedral relates to the dancing on stage. This section, which is subtitled *Blues II,* is cast in a cool, blue light with a large luminous moon in the background. Dressed in nondescript dance clothes, Cummings's dancers seem much more abstracted than in the earlier versions of *Basic Strategies*. Moving back and forth across the stage while they stay low to the ground, squatting or walking, their movements seem to serve as a background texture for Kincaid's words. Toward the end, a recognizable character of an older person crosses the stage, gradually growing more and more hunched over with the passing of each small shuffling step.

During a brief interlude, Kincaid's second text begins. Although it is read by the same smooth voice, this one is much less personal and describes with encyclopedic detail the habitat, production, and reproduction of the silkworm. Coming after the storytelling intimacy of the first section, this new factual tone strikes an odd, almost dissonant chord. Read like an article from *National Geographic,* the information seems tame enough, if somewhat irrelevant. As the interlude finishes and Cummings's solo begins, however, the context changes and the spoken text transforms into a series of metacommentaries on the politics of colonial enterprise, cheap Third World labor, and the production of Western luxuries.

At the beginnings of her solo, *Blues II,* the lights fade up very slowly to reveal a statuesque Cummings, wearing a shimmering black evening gown and cape. Slowly raising and lowering a champagne bottle and fluted glass, she turns in a curiously disembodied and vague manner, as if she were a revolving decoration in the middle of the ballroom floor. Her impassive face and glittering dress are reflected in the large mirrors that fan out to either side of her. Functioning as a kind of *Huis Clos,* these mirrors confine her movements, meeting each change of direction with multiple reflections of her body. Sometimes Cummings moves with proud, grandiose strides, covering the space with a confident territoriality. Other times, she seems possessed, pacing the floor in this prison of mirrors only to meet up with another reflection of the woman she once was—intended to become.

On one level, these mirrors function as reflections of common cultural representations of women. Glamorous in the evening gown that connotes a romantic lifestyle and independent income, Cummings's many mirrored figures are visually more enticing than the body they reflect. In a way, Cummings seduces the viewers through these images in order to disrupt our visual pleasure and, presumably, the economy that supports it. For instance, in the midst of a waltzy section, where she is swirling around the stage, she abruptly drops to her knees and, drawing her skirt over her face, begs for money. This split-second transformation of her body from ease to despair and back again reminds the viewer of the fragility of that seductive world. This early fracture is quickly smoothed over by the romantic music and Cummings's lyrical dancing. But the crack in the illusion widens as slides are projected on a screen above her head. Alternating images of Third World famine refugees with Western signs of wealth and power (i.e., Ralph Lauren advertisements), these slides throw Cummings's whole persona into question. Is she attempting to buy into these white, patriarchal images? Is she happy? Or is this whole scenario a tragic pretense? At this point in the solo, Cummings launches into an energetic stream of repetitive actions that pull her back and forth across the stage. The lively rhythm of her feet and hand gestures soon borders on mania as the tranquility of the earlier dancing gives way to a literal dis-ease with the costume. Eventually, she takes off the black dress and in the closing moments of the dancing she sits on a chair in her underwear, restlessly gesturing and pointing, in an effort to "speak" her tangled emotions.

Seen within the context of Kincaid's texts and the slides, the apparent glamour of Cummings's persona is undercut by the insistent issues of race, class, and gender. The pristine image of self-involvement—the private satisfaction initially projected by the mirrored glittering gown, champagne bottle, and solipsistic dancing—is clouded by the recognition that both idealistic (advertising) and realistic (photojournalism) images pervade the very fabric of our consciousness. Confronted at every turn with the cultural reflections of who she is, the woman in *Blues II* is fragmented into a series of confusing and conflicting images.

Once the gown and all that it represents has been taken off near the end of this solo, the persistent question of *who am I?* seems to remain for the character. Although Cummings intended that this disrobing should suggest a symbolic stripping away of cultural masks to reveal basic human needs and emotions, there is little sense of resolution or closure. Amidst the bombardment of media images, the woman without the dress is still searching for a single identity that fits. Restlessly turning her head or bent over with an extreme expression of pain, she tries on the very same gestures of hugging, talking, and rocking a baby, which seemed so solidly soothing in *Chicken Soup*. Yet in this new context, these movements are not quite so comfortable, and the woman onstage flits through a seemingly endless succession of gestural memories until finally the music stops and the lights fade out.

These two solos—*Chicken Soup* and *Blues II*—enact a struggle also found in many contemporary women's autobiographies. In *Chicken Soup*, the body is represented as the condition of the self, the place from which memories arise. The still photographic images of the first tableau and the vague reminiscences of the voice provide a setting appropriate to an expression of a woman's community. Gestures of rocking a baby, cooking and eating, waving good-bye, and grieving are consciously portrayed with a belief in their universality—in the archetypal engagement of women in community. In this dance, the body is opened up very wide and presented as a well of remembering and knowing. In *Blues II*, however, the dancing figure is less comfortable with her embodiment. Although some of the movements are similar to *Chicken Soup*, there is an increasingly restless quality in their motion that creates a sense that this female character would like to escape her own skin. Surrounded at every turn by reflections of her body (which she is unable to control or escape and which insistently clash with one another), as well as the slides and the soundtrack, this woman seeks to disengage her body from these pervasive images by taking off her gown. Yet, black and female, her body has been "written" over in so many ways by these background images of black women in her culture that it is still difficult to find an "original" signature.

While both solos begin with distilled, almost photographic images of women that are recognizable as cultural icons (woman as nurturer and woman as beautiful object), Cummings's *Chicken Soup* solo presents a person who can effectively connect with her memory to create images of herself, for herself. This character is a movement storyteller; she speaks through her body. Scholars of African-American literature often connect autobiography to a cultural experience of storytelling in the black community. Presented in the context of a dialogue with the community audience, "telling one's own story" is an empowering act which affirms a selfhood in connection with other people. In the section titled "Writing Autobiography" in her recent book, *Talking Back: Thinking Feminist, Thinking Black,* bell hooks also locates her own autobiographical impulse in that tradition. "Within the world of my childhood, we held onto the legacy of a distinct black culture by listening to the elders tell their stories. Autobiography was experienced most actively in the art of telling one's story."[33]

This ability to tell one's own story is missing in *Blues II.* The potency of this dance lies in the very fact that there does not seem to be any possibility of communication—any community to whom to tell this life story. The gowned woman in this dance is at once connected to and disconnected from the many narratives suggested by the visual images and Kincaid's texts. Because her body is a figurative screen for the contradictory meanings of these visual images and the powers who control their representation, it is impossible for her to find a useful identity or a comfortable way of moving. Physically dwarfed by the mirrors and the slides, the woman drifts through this mélange of cultural representations like a ghost through a maze. The mirrors amplify her spatial (and psychological) disorientation, reflecting and fragmenting the visual definition of her self. As a result, her internal physical equilibrium is disrupted and she either floats aimlessly about the stage or rushes frantically from one reflected image to another in a bewildered attempt to find one that looks right. Whether she is physically inert or psychically distraught, the dancing seems to be compelled by a restless searching for a visually and physically satisfying self. Even when she rejects the "lie" of the dress, even when she takes off the costume of "high" culture, there is no reassuring "natural" self underneath it all. The dance ends without closure, continuing its ambivalence about the intertwining issues of race, culture, gender, and identity.

Although critics often interpret *Chicken Soup* as a nostalgic portrait of the lost companionship of a women's community, and *Blues II* as a vision of the pressures and conflicts embedded in the identities of middle-class African-American women, it would be reductive to imply that these characters are simply derived from Cummings's immediate experience. Like all autobiographical material, they are representations. As hooks points out, autobiography "is a very personal storytelling—a unique recounting of events not so much as they have happened, but as we remember and invent them. [My autobiography] seemed to fall in the category of writing that Audre Lorde in her autobiographically based work *Zami,* calls bio-mythography. As I wrote, I felt that I was not as concerned with accuracy of detail as I was with evoking in writing the state of mind, the spirit of a particular moment."[34]

If we cycle back to the beginning discussion of Isadora Duncan's autobiographical "intratext" (of the dancing and the writing), Lorde's term *biomythography* stands out as particularly intriguing. I like how it emphasizes the activity of writing one's body and the mythic dimensions inherent in performing this representation. As she stood still in front of her famous blue curtains, Duncan must have appeared as a grand figure onstage; a being not unlike the mythic dancing self whom she describes in *My Life.* Yet her writing reveals the conflicts between her self-representation as an artist and her personal sense of herself as a woman, and the prevalent cultural images and ideologies about women that circulated during her lifetime. Read together, these two autobiographical texts suggest the inevitable contradictions within a representation of any self, biomythological or not.

Seven decades and several cultural revolutions later, Blondell Cummings expresses this very tension as a central theme in her solo dance performances. The resulting portraits of women represent a struggling identity that can only be pieced together through the negotiation between the inner voices of memory, bodily experience, and public representation. Wresting the power of seduction and colonialization from the media images projected above her head, Cummings shows not only the cracks and flaws in these cellophane narratives but also the possibility of other stories emerging from their gaps. Her disrobed figure at the end of *Blues II* has refused the closure implicit in the commodified image of a glamorous woman complete with champagne bottle. She may not have yet found another ending; but, at the very least, she is looking forward to writing many more stories.

The strategy of reappropriation in order to fit a cultural experience or personal need is echoed in an excerpt from Ralph Ellison's "The Little Man at the Chehaw Station," which Houston A. Baker cites as an epigraph to his book *Blues, Ideology, and Afro-American Literature: A Vernacular Theory:*

"So perhaps we shy from confronting our *cultural* wholeness because it offers no easily recognizable points of rest, no facile certainties as to who, what or where (culturally or historically) we are. Instead, the whole is always in cacophonic motion."[35] In the introduction, Baker uses the image of blues music as a kind of "cacophonic motion," which illustrates at once the historic specificity of an African-American heritage and the multiplicity of its subjects. "To suggest a trope for the blues as a forceful matrix in cultural understanding is to summon an image of the black blues singer at the railway junction lustily transforming experiences of a durative (unceasingly oppressive) landscape into the energies of rhythmic song. The railway juncture is marked by transience . . . and is simply a single instance in a boundless network that redoubles and circles, makes sidings and ladders, forms Y's and branches over the vastness of hundreds of thousands of American miles."[36]

Taking my cue from Baker's metaphorical understanding of African-American identity in terms of the blues and the blues in terms of incessant motion, I want to suggest another way to look at the woman in Cummings's *Blues II*. Some feminist scholars object to a representation of autobiography that situates identity as inherently fractured and multiple, insisting that this decentered subject loses any viable connection to a political community. Seeing instability only in terms of its rather frightening psychic consequences, these scholars are nonetheless hard-pressed to find a representation of the unified self that does not seem romantically nostalgic. But what if we switch tracks and look at instability as motion—as the beginning of a dance. While at the same time that the woman character in *Blues II* can be seen as drowning in the existential refractions of too many self images, there is a certain fluidity and ease of movement from one mirror to the next, an internal shifting of weight and context. If we think of *Blues II* in terms of Baker's use of the blues (another intratext), we can position Cummings's dance at the intersection of several cultures while still figuring its connection with an African-American community. If the blues give us a rich image of incessant motion within a culturally specific identity, *Blues II* suggests its logical sequel—in dance.

NOTES

1. There is some speculation as to whether Isadora Duncan actually wrote her own autobiography or whether it was mostly written and edited by Duncan's close companion Mary Desti. For the purposes of this essay, the authenticity of this work is not of primary concern. Mostly, I am interested in the changes in tone from the self-assured mythopoetic voice to the questioning one. Even if Duncan did not actually write *My Life*, it has certainly become part of her history.

2. Nancy Miller, "Writing Fictions: Women's Autobiography in France," in *Sub-*

ject to Change: Reading Feminist Writing (New York: Columbia University Press, 1988), 60.

3. Ibid., 61.

4. See, for example, a special issue of *The Drama Review* on movement analysis, particularly Elizabeth Kagan and Margaret Morse on "The Body Electronic," *Drama Review* 32, no. 4 (Winter 1988): 164–80.

5. Duncan, *My Life,* 75.

6. Patricia Meyer Spacks, *The Female Imagination* (New York: Alfred A. Knopf, 1975), 3.

7. Ibid., 160.

8. Ibid.

9. Ibid., 163.

10. For more information about the historical sources on Duncan see Deborah Jowitt, *Time and the Dancing Image* (New York: William Morrow, 1988), 69–102.

11. Quoted in Francis Steegmuller, *Your Isadora* (New York: Random House and the New York Public Library, 1974), 23.

12. Duncan, *My Life,* 213.

13. Spacks, *The Female Imagination,* 161.

14. Ibid., 163.

15. Duncan, *My Life,* 2.

16. Ibid., 3.

17. Paul Eakins, *Fictions in Autobiography: Studies in the Art of Self-Invention* (Princeton, NJ: Princeton University Press, 1985).

18. Sidonie Smith, *A Poetics of Women's Autobiography* (Bloomington: Indiana University Press, 1987), 175.

19. Anna Kisselgoff, "Music's Absence Marks Five Dances," *New York Times,* March 14, 1971.

20. Marianne Goldberg, "Transformative Aspects of Meredith Monk's 'Education of the Girlchild,'" *Women and Performance* 1, no. 1 (1983): 21.

21. Linda Small, "Best Friend Forward," *Village Voice,* March 10, 1980.

22. Paula Sommers, "Blondell Cummings: Life Dances," *Washington Post,* November 30, 1984.

23. Ibid.

24. Interview with the author in New York City, February 7, 1989.

25. Burt Supree, "Worlds Apart," *Village Voice,* December 17–23, 1980.

26. Quoted in Debra Cash, "Blondell Cummings: Melds Two Worlds of Dance," *Boston Globe,* January 1986.

27. Nancy Goldner, "Electric Cooking," *Saturday Review,* May/June 1983, 37–38.

28. Toni Morrison, "The Site of Memory," in *Inventing the Truth,* ed. William Zinsser (Boston: Houghton Mifflin, 1987), 115.

29. *New York Times,* August 7, 1988.

30. Interview with the author, February 7, 1989.

31. Interview in Michael Blackwood's film *Retracing Steps,* 1988.

32. Jamaica Kincaid, 1987. This text was commissioned especially for Cummings's dance.

33. bell hooks, *Talking Back: Thinking Feminist, Thinking Black* (Boston: South End Press, 1989), 158.

34. Ibid., 157–58.

35. Houston A. Baker Jr., *Blues, Ideology, and Afro-American Literature: A Vernacular Theory* (Chicago: University of Chicago Press, 1984), 1.

36. Ibid., 7.

14

Femininity with a Vengeance

Strategies of Veiling and Unveiling in Loïe Fuller's Performances of Salomé

Traces of Light: Absence and Presence in the Work of Loïe Fuller (2007).

> To put on femininity with a vengeance suggests the power of taking it off.
> —MARY RUSSO, "FEMALE GROTESQUES: CARNIVAL AND THEORY"

In a move that seems to be universally interpreted as a big mistake, Loïe Fuller produced her own version of the Salome myth in 1895 and cast herself in the title role. This *création nouvelle* was billed as a "pantomine lyrique en deux actes," and ran for less than two months at the Comédie-Parisienne. Most critics panned the play. Jean Lorrain, who had previously been a real fan of Fuller's work (describing her as "the beautiful girl who, in her floating draperies, swirls endlessly around in an ecstasy induced by divine revelations"), penned vituperative remarks that were personally insulting and just plain mean.[1] Various other reviewers (with the notable exception of Roger Marx) registered their disappointment in this new creation by La Loïe. Even late twentieth-century scholars, writing from a perspective of at least historical, if not critical, distance tend to dismiss this fin-de-siècle work as a limp, nostalgic gesture toward the expressive (melo)dramas with which Fuller began her career. Despite the troubled results of her first foray, twelve years later Fuller took on this decadent icon once again—this time when she was forty-five. *La Tragédie de Salomé* premiered on November 9, 1907, at the Théâtre des Arts. Although the press reviews for this production were not as personally or professionally damning, the production was a commercial failure and closed after a short run.

Most Fuller scholars chalk these two failed attempts to play Salome up to a bizarre lapse in Fuller's usually astute professional judgment. If they talk about these *Salomé* productions at all, it is usually to discuss Fuller's innovative use of underlighting in the 1895 version, documenting how Fuller developed the spectacular *Fire Dance* from the production's *Sun Dance* and toured it and other shorter dances independently of the original pantomime. I, however, find myself intrigued by Fuller's desire to repeatedly reinvent this biblical temptress, precisely because the whole enterprise does not quite make sense. I mean really—why, after having studiously avoided the dancer-as-seductress stereotype so rampant at the end of the nineteenth century, did Fuller decide to enact one of the century's most notorious femme fatales? What was she trying to accomplish? Why was she compelled to take on Salome not once, but twice? What strategic uses of the veil are implicated in these stagings? And what, indeed, was she interested in uncovering, or rather discovering, in herself and in her work by "becoming" Salomé?

These are some of the questions that animate this essay. I believe that an in-depth comparison of her 1895 and 1907 stagings of *Salomé* can illuminate an important shift in Fuller's oeuvre. Not only does each production reveal a singular approach to the subject matter, but each one also reflects a different feminist strategy for confronting and intervening in misogynist representations of sexualized women. Put very simply for the purposes of comparison in this introduction, Fuller's first *Salomé* revised the traditional narrative to create a mystical, "chaste," younger Salome, who dances in order to save John the Baptist. Here she replaced the deadly seductress with a more positive role model. Interestingly, in her second attempt, Fuller returned to a more traditional portrayal of Salome as a desperate, desiring woman. For this 1907 staging of *La Tragedie of Salomé*, Fuller played with the many known cultural representations of this iconic woman, miming a different approach to the legendary figure within the production's two acts. This production incorporated both the emotional and the campy in an ironic juxtaposition of citation and expression.

By 1895, Fuller's extraordinary success was predicated on her fluid imaging of cloth and color. Veiling her body, her expansive silks created visions that remained in a comfortably abstract, albeit dynamic, realm. As Mallarmé's "no-woman," Fuller effectively separated herself from the frames of female characterization and traditional narrative (where the public, performing woman usually ended up desperate—or dead). When she enacted Salome, however, Fuller was forced to confront not only her public's assumptions about who she was, but also the myriad literary and visual representations of this legendary figure swarming—like so many insects—across late nineteenth-century stages, as well as in private salons. For the first time since establishing her signature as the original "Serpentine Dancer," Fuller had to revise her performative identity. That she chose to play out her femininity with a vengeance tells us quite a bit about the woman behind the veil.

Rhonda Garelick's chapter on Loïe Fuller in her book, *Rising Star: Dandyism, Gender and Performance in the Fin de Siècle*, is entitled "Electric Salomé: The Mechanical Dances of Loïe Fuller." Although this chapter, which focuses on Fuller's presence at the 1900 Paris Exposition, playfully references the cultural trope of Salome as a dancer who "unveils," Garelick never discusses Fuller's performances of this female legend in any depth. Instead, she holds to the common perspective, which juxtaposes Fuller with the "other" more provocative women performers, such as the Orientalized belly dancers parading through the Parc du Trocadéro:

> Fuller, it should be recalled, never took her clothes off, never gyrated, and never shocked respectable people . . . True, she was foreign in France, but hailed only from unsensual America, a country that had (and still has) a reputation for sexlessness and a kind of sanitized heartiness very removed from either Oriental or European passion. Hers was the dazzle not of the body but of machinery, technology, and Yankee ingenuity. In the French imagination, Fuller's appeal was always closer to Thomas Edison than to Josephine Baker's.[2]

Certainly it was true that Fuller was very much associated with what Garelick calls "Yankee ingenuity," especially in the context of the 1900 exposition. It is also true that she had a reputation for "cleaning-up" the Folies Bergère, enabling the management to create matinees innocent enough for women and children to attend. But, as Current and Current point out in their book *Loïe Fuller: Goddess of Light,* by her second season at this nightclub, the director had reincorporated a number of "girlie" acts around Fuller's expanded repertoire. These included women such as "La Belle Otero," a well-known courtesan whose private life and public postures onstage referenced one another. Despite the highly sexualized frame of the other acts in the Folies Bergère, from the beginning of her celebrity status in Paris, Fuller was consistently cast as frank and without pretense or feminine wiles. Indeed, reviewers would frequently point out her charming naiveté. For instance, a reporter from London's *Strand Magazine* portrays Fuller as a simple "bonnie, blue-eyed little woman, plain in her dress, and with a sweet frankness of manner and speech."[3]

Of course, Fuller consciously played into this characterization of her offstage persona. In a famous passage from her autobiography, Fuller writes of her effect on little children who are frequently delighted with her fairy-like performances and whose imaginations, she asserts, are "easily kindled by suggestions of the supernatural."[4] So believable is her fairy-like incarnation, that these children have a difficult time understanding Fuller's transformation back into an ordinary woman. Citing the example of one little girl who recoiled with horror (Fuller's words) when she was introduced to the dancer backstage, Fuller reports that she tried to keep up the illusion by telling the girl that she was merely the fairy's emissary.

> The mother and child found their way to my dressing room . . .
> The child's eyes opened wider and wider. The nearer I came the further she shrank away.

Quite astonished her mother said: "What is the matter dear? This is Miss Fuller, who danced for you so prettily a few minutes ago. You know you begged me so hard to bring you to see her."

As if touched by a magic wand the child's expression changed.

"No, no. That isn't her. I don't want to see her. This one here is a fat lady, and it was a fairy I saw dancing."

If there is one thing in the world of which I am incapable, it is consciously to cause anyone pain, and, with my love of children, I should never have been happy again if I had caused my little visitor to be disillusioned. I endeavoured therefore to be equal to the situation, and I said to the child:

"Yes, my dear, you are right. I am not Loïe Fuller. The fairy has sent me to tell you how much she loved you and how sorry she is not to be able to take you to her kingdom. She cannot come. She really cannot. She told me just to take you in my arms and give you a kiss, a good kiss for her."

At these words the little one threw herself into my arms.

"Oh," she said, "kiss the pretty fairy for me and ask her if I can come again to see her dance."

There were tears in my eyes as I replied:

"Come as often as you like, my dear little girl. I hear the fairy whispering in my ear that she would like to dance for you all the time, all the time."[5]

Similar references to Fuller's sweet, magical incarnations crop up in almost every historical source on La Loïe, many of which, like Margaret Haile Harris's exhibition catalogue, refer to her as a "magician of light."[6] Embedded in these various reports is an interesting contradiction in terms. Fuller is at once portrayed as a "naturally" unpretentious woman offstage, and as someone who can radically transform herself into a fairy or a flower onstage by means of the artifice of cloth and light. Ironically, although many cite Fuller's ability to transform herself by taking on a veil, few will acknowledge the possibility of Fuller's using her extensive theatrical capacities to take off that veil. It seems to me that there must have been something about her offstage persona that limited the public's ability to envision Fuller's performances in any other light.

Indeed, the obsessive iterations of Fuller's dancing persona as chaste, correct, and *sans coquetterie érotique,* belies a certain anxiety concerning other possibilities. Referring to her presence in the 1900 Paris Exposition, Garelick asserts that "Fuller was a veil dancer who never really *un*veiled."[7] Here Garelick, like many cultural historians intrigued by Mallarmé's references to Fuller, generalizes Fuller's dancing as a series of increasingly sophisticated and technologized Serpentine dances, conveniently airbrushing out Fuller's 1895 performances in which she did, in fact, unveil herself—as Salome: "Fuller's performances provided a white-washed, apparently de-eroticized version of some of the more lubricious veil dances being performed across the exhibition park at the Trocadéro."[8]

Interestingly enough, there is also very little material on her first performances of Salome in Fuller's autobiography, *Fifteen Years of a Dancer's Life*. On these pages, her own narrative moves very quickly from her early successes at the Folies Bergère to a recitation of all the famous people she has met. Much of this is organized as a series of vignettes about her encounters with artists, philosophers, kings, and queens, and seldom tells us much about her performing career. Even so, occasionally a certain story can be illuminating in surprising ways. For instance, in the middle of chapter 15, "Several Sovereigns," Fuller recounts an extraordinary incident. Subtitled "Massaged by Royal Command," this anecdote describes Fuller's first encounter with the Archduchesses of Austria. This recollection is worth quoting in full, as it reveals Fuller's awareness of, and responses to, a markedly voyeuristic gaze:

> I was once at the Swedish gymnasium at Carlsbad, where machines with electrical vibrations shock you from head to foot. I was just about to dress myself when one of the women of the place came to me, and said:
>
> "Won't you please return to the hall, and pretend to take the electric treatment again in order that the archduchesses, who are there with a whole crowd of court ladies, may see you?"
>
> I replied: "Tell the archduchesses that they can see me this evening at the theatre."
>
> The poor woman then declared to me that she had been forbidden to mention their Royal Highnesses, and that they had bidden her get me back into the hall on some pretext or other.
>
> She was so grieved at not having succeeded that I returned to the machines, and had my back massaged, in order that the noble company might look at me at their ease, as they would survey an interesting animal.
>
> They looked at me, all of them smiling, and while they viewed me I never turned my eyes away from them.
>
> The odd thing was that they did not know that I knew them. I was, therefore, as much amused by them, and without their perceiving it, as they were amused by me.[9]

Clearly Loïe Fuller did not mind being naked in front of a group of titled ladies. Splayed out in all her fleshy glory, she watches the duchesses watching her. In fact, she seems to derive a certain amount of satisfaction from the whole scenario. While I will try to refrain from projecting too much into the situation, I think that it is fair to say that, at the very least, this narrative demonstrates Fuller's acute awareness of her audience, and her interest in not only positioning herself as the object of (in this case) the female gaze, but also intervening in that power dynamic by looking back. Compared to the super-sexualized displays at the Folies Bergère, Fuller's dancing may have seemed relentlessly "chaste," as many reviewers have attested. But that posture of asexuality obviously wasn't the only one stoking the fires of her artistic imagination.

Before turning to an analysis of Fuller's 1985 *Salomé*, I would like to introduce a theoretical discussion that provides a useful framework for thinking about these two apparent anomalies in Fuller's oeuvre. In the mid-1980s, as feminist theory was grappling with questions of theatricality and performance, Mary Russo wrote a short essay that was published in Teresa de Lauretis's seminal collection, *Feminist Studies/Critical Studies,* and from which I take the epigraph to this chapter. This piece remains, for me, one of the most savvy, succinct analyses of the libratory possibilities of "making a spectacle" of oneself for women inclined toward theatrical gestures. Russo's essay begins with a proscription that resonates with many women who came of age in the twentieth century.

> There is a phrase that still resonates from childhood. Who says it? The mother's voice—not my own mother's perhaps, but the voice of an aunt, an older sister, or the mother of a friend. It is a harsh, matronizing phrase, and it is directed toward the behavior of other women:
> "She" [the other woman] is making a spectacle out of herself.
> Making a spectacle out of oneself seemed a specifically feminine danger. The danger was of an exposure . . . For a woman, making a spectacle out of herself had more to do with a kind of inadvertency and loss of boundaries: the possessors of large, aging, and dimpled thighs displayed at the public beach, of overly rouged cheeks, of a voice shrill in laughter, or of a sliding bra strap—a loose, dingy bra strap especially—were at once caught out by fate and blameworthy. It was my impression that these women had done something wrong, had stepped, as it were, into the limelight out of turn—too young or too old, too early or too late—and yet anyone, any woman, could make a spectacle out of herself if she was not careful.[10]

Working through theories of the carnivalesque by way of the work of Mikhail Bakhtin, Russo delineates both the cultural stakes (what she describes as a double jeopardy) and the political possibilities of claiming the limelight. "The figure of the female transgressor as public spectacle is still powerfully resonant, and the possibilities of redeploying this representation as a demystifying or utopian model have not been exhausted."[11] The intersection of carnival theory with feminist theory produces a cultural analysis of the female body as a "grotesque" body. This body is open and permeable, the body of process and change (the "becoming" body). This inherently female body is opposed to the classical (male) body that is contained, hard and timeless—just like a smooth, white marble sculpture. Rather than try-ing to (hopelessly and often dangerously) pursue a "perfect" classical body, women, Russo suggests, might do well to explore a strategic deployment of this grotesque and excessive body as a sort of feminine masquerade. Playing with the symbolic and cultural representations of women while also attend-ing to the experience of living in a woman's body might well produce some interesting and potentially subversive spectacles. Here Russo quotes Luce Irigaray's famous passage on mimesis:

> To play with mimesis is thus, for a woman, to try and recover the place of her exploitation by discourse, without allowing herself simply to be reduced to it. It means to resubmit herself—inasmuch as she is on the side of "perceptible," of "matter"—to "ideas," in particular to ideas about herself, that are elaborated in/ by masculine logic, but so as to make "visible," by an effect of playful repetition, what was supposed to remain invisible: the cover-up of a possible operation of the feminine in language. It also means to "unveil" the fact that, if women are such good mimics, it is because they are not simply reabsorbed into this function.[12]

What Russo is getting at here developed over the next decade into fem-inist discussions of gender as performative. Theorists such as Teresa de Lauretis, Judith Butler, Iris Marion Young, and Elizabeth Grosz (as well as many other scholars from a variety of fields), began to articulate the ways in which gender and sexuality are implicated in and as embodied performance. To speak of gender or sexuality as performance is not to imply, however, that these experiences are merely theatrical tics—something that is as easy as putting on or taking off a hat or a scarf for effect. As anyone who has any experience in the performing arts understands—acting, dancing, playing music, singing—all these disciplines require elaborate psychic and physical preparation. What this enactment paradigm does suggest, however, is the possibility of playing it other ways.

Fuller's French reputation was very much cemented to a portrayal of Fuller as a frumpy American matron. At the cusp of the twentieth century, her particular mix of talents—the combination of typically masculine in-terest in electricity, lighting design, and scientific experimentation, and the typically feminized vocation of performing on public stages (especially as a dancer)—seemed in some odd way to render her androgynous. It is almost as if these masculine and feminine aspects of her persona cancelled one an-other out to render her neuter—or lesbian. For underneath many of these discussions concerning her appearance runs an old-fashioned subterranean current of misogyny and homophobia that seems to assume the reason Fuller did not flaunt her stuff on the stage of the Folies Bergère is connected to her physique (her not having the girlie body that would presumably at-

tract men), which, in turn, is connected to her preference for female intimacies. The logic here is twisted, and reflects the critics' limited mindset more
that the historical record.

Strangely myopic, these critics tend to pass over the photographic and
published evidence of her early career to homogenize Fuller's appearance as
plain (or pointedly "not beautiful"), and her body as stocky (or downright
"fat"). Actually, for her time, Fuller was considered cute and fetching in her
twenties, pretty in her thirties, and still attractive and plump, perhaps, but
certainly not obese, well into her forties. As just noted in the episode "Massaged by Royal Command," and as we shall see in our discussions of Fuller's enactments of the Salome legend, being a lesbian does not necessitate
a renunciation of a highly feminized, performative sexuality. Au contraire.

The Dance Research Collection at Lincoln Center Library houses a series
of souvenir cards of Fuller's early theatrical career. I would like to compare
two in particular. One is a well-known image of Fuller in a breeches role,
such as the one she played in the 1886 New York performances of *Little
Jack Sheppard*. The other is a lesser-known photograph of Fuller posing
coyly behind a large open Japanese fan. This soubrette shot shows a young
Fuller bare shouldered, with only a pearl chocker and jeweled headband
on. The assumption, of course, is that she is naked behind the fan; her smile
serving as the invitation for the (presumably, but not always, male) viewer
to investigate further. This image, which is basically a classic nineteenth-
century pinup postcard, contrasts nicely with the one of Fuller dressed as a
boy. Here too, she smiles seductively, but in that knowing, slightly tongue-
in-cheek manner that makes male drag so powerful.

The masquerade of the various well-known breeches roles in the second
half of the nineteenth century created an interesting liminal place for the
imaginative performer. True, these "tights" roles were often guises to flaunt
and further sexualize the female performer by revealing her "handsome"
thighs.[13] But they could also serve to extend the possibilities of roles for an
actress. In this photo, Fuller is standing in a firm, wide stance, her weight
leaning back into her right leg in a rather self-satisfied way. Who knows,
maybe she had just read her reviews in the *Times,* which complimented her
on her believable acting: "Miss Loïe Fuller, as the hero of the piece, does
this little bit very neatly, and indeed Miss Fuller's impersonation is very
commendable throughout the play. She looks like a boy, as few women do in
breeches, and she acts like one, which is still less frequently accomplished."[14]

One of the few pieces of Fuller scholarship to address La Loïe's ability to
play convincingly across soubrette and breeches roles is a short paper given
at the 2000 Society of Dance History Scholars conference and subsequently
published in the proceedings. Written by Tirza True Latimer, it is entitled
"Butch-Femme Fatale." In this piece, Latimer focuses on Fuller's dual mas-
querades as evidence of Fuller's lesbian identity.[15] The reductive reading of

the performance/life equation, where critics interpret performances or texts as direct signs pointing to the author's "true" identity, is less interesting to me in this context. Instead, I would like to focus on the multiple refractions of images formed by the three-way mirror of Fuller's ironic participation in the traditional frames of theatrical representation. I draw attention to Fuller's masquerade, as well as her Sapphic proclivities, not in order to confirm her status as a lesbian (which was never really in question anyway), but rather to foreground her early theatrical experiences in "playing with mimesis." These, I believe, served as a theatrical foundation for her later attempts to perform across the hyper "feminine" positions of desire in Salomé.

It is generally acknowledged that, when Loïe Fuller presented her Serpentine dance at the Folies Bergère, she had created a radical new approach to dancing entertainment. Sure, there had been elaborate lighting effects staged before. And too, serpentine dancers had appeared in Paris even before Fuller's arrival. Fuller's use of torque and momentum, combined with her active engagement with the lighting, put her performances in a category all their own. When Fuller decided to interpret Salome, however, she was working with a cultural stereotype based loosely on a biblical narrative that had been inscribed and reinscribed (written, painted, enacted) repeatedly over the course of the latter half of the nineteenth century. As Elaine Showalter notes in her chapter on "The Veiled Woman" in her book, *Sexual Anarchy*:

> The most popular veiled woman of the fin de siècle is Salome, the dancing daughter of Herodias. In France, Salome became an obsessive icon of female sexuality for Flaubert, for the artist Gustave Moreau, who did over seventy drawings of her, and for the novelist Joris-Karl Huysmans, who wrote about Moreau's 1876 painting of Salome in *À Rebours* (Against Nature [1884]) as the "weird and superhuman" object of his hero's fantasies of feminine evil.[16]

If Moreau's paintings laid an iconographic foundation for future Salome images, Oscar Wilde's infamous play, published in 1895 with illustrations by Aubrey Beardsley (but staged only in 1896), represents one of the most famous literary interpretations.

The "original" story of Salome dancing before Herod and his court appears in the New Testament, in Matthew 14. Presented as a retelling of a past event, the narrative gives only the barest details of the event. Indeed, two brief sentences capture the nexus of her role: "But with his birthday celebrations the daughter of Herodias danced before the guests, and Herod was so delighted that he took an oath to give her anything she cared to ask. Prompted by her mother, she said, "Give me here on a dish the head of John the Baptist."[17] The specific details then about Salome's motive or even about her dancing display, were left up to the fin-de-siècle artists and writers to supply. And supply they did.

One of Gustave Moreau's Salomé paintings, a watercolor entitled *The*

Apparition, was the major sensation of the 1876 Paris Salon. In his novel *À Rebours,* Huysmans's protagonist contemplates Moreau's painting to the point of obsession. His description of the work of art is embellished by grotesque as well as erotic details:

> She is almost naked; in the heat of the dance her veils have fallen away and her brocade robes slipped to the floor, so that now she is clad only in wrought metals and translucent gems. A gorgerin grips her waist like a corselet, and like an outsized clasp a wondrous jewel sparkles and flashes in the cleft between her breasts; lower down, a girdle encircles her hips, hiding the upper part of her thighs, against which dangles a gigantic pendant glistening with rubies and emeralds; finally, where the body shows bare between gorgerin and girdle, the belly bulges, dimpled by a navel which resembles a graven seal of onyx with its milky hues and its rosy finger-nail tints.[18]

Here is a classic Salome scenario—one in which the dancing girl arouses the viewer's sexual desire; the potency of her sensuous display intensifying as she sheds one veil after another.

In contrast to this Salome figure as the object of another's desire, Wilde's Salome is caught up with her own desire for Saint John the Baptist. In Wilde's text (from which the libretto of the Richard Strauss opera of the same name is derived), Salome proclaims her own desire: "I am amorous of thy body, Iokanaan!"[19] Through her archaic-sounding language, Salome ritually evokes the beauties of Iokanaan's body ("Thy body is white, like the lilies of a field . . ."), only to desecrate it as her requests for contact are repudiated by Iokanaan's superior attitude: "Back, daughter of Sodom! Touch me not. Profane not the temple of the Lord God."[20] Practically hysterical with her frustrated desires, the adolescent Salome dances for Herod, in exchange for John the Baptist's head, severed from his sanctimonious denial, which she finally claims by kissing on the mouth. Ironically (and intentionally, of course), Salome's infamous dance of the seven veils is never described by Wilde. It is only indicated in the play text by the following sparse stage directions: "Salome dances the dance of the seven veils."[21] In her book on Wilde, Katherine Worth suggests that Wilde may have been impressed by Fuller's "swirling greens and blues" when he envisioned Salome, whom he described as being costumed in "green, like a curious, poisonous lizard."[22]

Many fin-de-siècle artists interpreted the Salome legend, and I will not attempt to present an exhaustive survey of these representations. So too, the work of Moreau and Wilde can be (and has been brilliantly) discussed in much greater depth than space permits me to do here. I point to these two examples mostly in order to introduce a continuum of the possibilities available to Loïe Fuller when she conceived of her own version. These precedents stretch from Salome's dance as an evocation of someone else's desire, to its being an expression of her own. Respectively, these two poles represent either end of the psychic continuum of object and subject across which Fuller staged her own vision of sexuality and desire.

According to "Miss Fuller's New Dance," a *New York Times* article published in January 1896 to publicize Fuller's American tour, it was Armand Sylvestre, a writer and one of the main librettists at the Folies Bergère, who suggested the role of Salome for Fuller. The article quotes Fuller as saying, upon hearing this remark: "And why can't I be Salome, or whatever her name is, dancing before Herod?"[23] The article continues in its dual description/promotion of the work:

> The outcome was the dignified and dramatic pantomime in which Miss Fuller is the main figure and which she has been presenting at the Palace Theatre, London, and the Comédie Parisienne to crowded houses. It consists of four tableaus, descriptive of the Biblical scene between Herod and John the Baptist. The first represents the prophet visiting Herod, commanding him to put away Herodias, his unlawful wife. Herod refuses at first, but finally accedes partially, and is angry with Herodias. She studies how she may win him back, and decided that the best way will be to have her daughter Salome dance for him. This is done, and upon seeing the dance Herod accedes to the demands of Herodias . . . The pantomine is concluded with Herod's dispatching a servant to behead John the Baptist, Salome entering to protest just after the command has been executed.[24]

In preparing her first *Salomé,* Fuller collaborated with Georges Rochegrosse, a popular salon painter, who did the costumes and helped with the sets; with Gabriel Pierné, who composed the musical score; and with C. H. Meltzer on the libretto. In their book, Current and Current describe Fuller's version as depicting a Salome who is "quite spiritual and essentially chaste," and is a follower of John the Baptist.[25] She dances in order to save his life, rather than out of lust for him. For this lyrical pantomime, Fuller departed from her usual scenic sparseness to incorporate an elaborate palace, complete with a perspectival view of Jerusalem on a backdrop. The visual iconography lent an air of Orientalist decadence reminiscent of Moreau or Flaubert. Nonetheless, one of the key dramatic effects was still the spectacular lighting, particularly Fuller's use of underlighting. "In the floor of the stage are cut six holes, arranged like a triangle. In these openings, which are nearly a yard square, are inserted squares of heavy plate glass upon which Miss Fuller dances. It is impossible to describe the effect which is produced as she circles from one stream of light to another, and her whole performance is said to be a marvel of beauty and grace."[26]

Promoted as the show that would reveal to the world just how great an expressive artist Fuller was, *Salomé* received warm previews. (One wonders if visions of becoming like Sarah Bernhardt, whom Fuller greatly admired and who was, at one point, scheduled to play Wilde's Salome, danced in her head.) Indeed, the *New York Times* quoted at length a feature praising the show in the London *Figaro* on March 17, 1895, two weeks after *Salomé* opened at the Comédie Parisienne:

> As I saw her on the stage of this little theatre—just sufficiently lighted to see the expression of her face—Pierné at the piano, Armand Silvestre and Pierre Berton following the working of the drama in her wonderful dance—it seemed scarcely believable that this small figure, in her ordinary dark walking dress, without the aide of lights or stage accessories, with no word spoken, could move us to the extent she did. Her dance to the sun, her religious dance, her dance of desperation, were all remarkable expressions of the mind, and had such an effect upon us that when she fell at the sight of John the Baptist's head, we all rushed towards her and kissed her . . . The question now is: What will the public think of it? And will the colored lights mar, or will they enhance, the artistic effect? Of course it cannot be expected that Loïe Fuller will dance every night as she danced at that rehearsal. It is with her more a matter of inspiration than step but there are many points in favor of her repeating the greater part in much the same manner.[27]

Apparently, the night that Jean Lorrain went to the Comédie Parisienne, Fuller's performance was less inspired. Nevertheless, the savageness with which he skewered Fuller suggests that much of the problem had to do with Lorrain's own expectations about what Fuller should be doing onstage. In the March 9 entry in his journal, published in *Poussières de Paris,* Lorrain begins his review with the effusive, descriptive language reminiscent of his earlier evocations of La Loïe: "Mystery! The colors and nuances of light illuminate and dim in turn, developing into spirals and then suddenly billowing like wings, opening and closing, and then in the middle of this flood of motion and fabric emerges the figure of a woman, her shoulders and arms deliciously pale, appearing all of a sudden between the enormous petals of a giant violet, or the wings of an incredible butterfly."[28] But soon, Fuller emerged from the mist of her mysterious effect to take on a more dramatic role in this pantomime. "And it was a disappointment." Disillusioned by Fuller's refusal to remain shrouded by the lighting, Lorrain succumbs to his own frustrations. "One perceives too late that the unhappy acrobat is neither mime nor dancer; heavy, ungraceful, sweating and with make-up running at the end of ten minutes of little exercises, she maneuvers her veils and her mass of materials like a laundress misusing her paddle."[29]

Unfortunately, there is little else in the review that actually describes the show. Who else was onstage? What color were the lights? How did the drama unfold? One gets the impression that Lorrain simply stopped watching the show; fixating on his patronizing conviction that Fuller could only appropriately do one thing—sequester herself behind her voluminous silks and mysterious lighting effects. Lorrain concludes his review with a final diatribe: "Luminous without grace, with the gestures of an English boxer and the physique of Mr. Oscar Wilde, this is a Salomé for Yankee drunkards."[30]

For Current and Current, Lorrain's outburst was "understandable." They write: "Short and fat as she was, Loïe hardly had the figure for Salomé, who traditionally was pictured as statuesque. And Loïe could be seen all too well in the Comédie Parisienne, an intimate theater with a small stage, where she was close to her audience in a way that she had never been at the Foiles Bergère . . . Hence she lost that aura of unreality, ineffability, and mystery that had made her seem a creature of poetic charm."[31] One sees too much—too much body, too much flesh, too much expression, too much woman. No longer hidden by the whirling silk of her earlier costumes, Fuller is criticized for her excess, for exceeding the limits of appropriate display; indeed, for making a "spectacle of herself."

Giovanni Lista, in his massive tome on Fuller, also sees this first *Salomé* as a personal and professional failure for Fuller. Combining his critical evaluation of Fuller's work with a bizarre psychoanalytic approach to her biography, Lista puts forward an emotional paradigm to explain the dilemma of her presence in this new piece. In his chapter discussing Fuller's first *Salomé*, Lista describes the "existential drama" of Fuller's life at that time, and the "impossibility of giving free rein to her creative capacities and her vital energy other than by the veiled gestures that serve both to create her effects, but also to negate her female body."[32] The whole question of what is revealed and what is concealed in Fuller's *Salomé* becomes even more complex as Lista draws out of this theatrical experience the emotional subtext of Fuller's life:

> For the first time, she unveiled her capacity for emotion, her femininity, the
> richness of her soul. Against the archetype of the lustful woman, she identified
> herself with the most fragile and feminine woman she could be. The failure of
> *Salomé* was therefore more complete. In terms of her artistic career, she found
> herself condemned to take on again the veil in both the literal sense and the
> metaphoric sense of the word, forever to place her nude body behind a screen
> for others to project their desires or their fantasies. And this is equally true
> of her existential trajectory, because this ultimate negation of her femininity
> will lead her to assume in a definitive manner the homosexual aspect of her
> sensibility.[33]

I want to tread carefully here, for it would be easy to have fun deconstructing these last few sentences. If I read him correctly, Lista is interpreting Fuller's dropping of her Serpentine costume as a metaphor for the unveiling of her closeted femininity (her true self). He also seems to suggest that the "failure of *Salomé*" and a stream of nasty words from one critic (albeit a powerful one), would force Fuller to renounce any pretensions of playing a sexualized character again, thus leading her to confirm once and for all, her homosexual "sensibility." Besides reflecting a series of old-fashioned projections about the nature of female desirability, Lista's take on Fuller is way over the top. He seems to have been inspired by Lorrain to regard her as a Medusa-like, monstrous figure, skewing the historical record considerably in the process.

First of all, Fuller's 1895 *Salomé* was by no means a complete failure. Even the Currents admit (one paragraph after they call Lorrain's disillusionment "understandable") that "she attracted good crowds and gained their hearty applause."[34] Some critics described her expressive movement as "ardent and passionate,"[35] and others found her "natural grace, her clever management of color and her robe manipulation [created] a new and most artistic conception."[36] In addition, the portrayal of Fuller suggested by Lorrain and Lista just does not jibe with contemporary images of her.

Let us look then, at two studio shots from Fuller's 1895 production. One portrays Fuller as an innocent adolescent girl coyly looking out from under a hood. Head cocked, she is smiling and holds out the extra fabric of her multilayered dress, as she steps daintily onto a glass panel that is illuminated from below. Although the black-and-white photograph does not give any sense of Fuller's color palette, the play of shadow and light visible can help us imagine the dramatic possibilities of underlighting. (The closest common analogy to this is the effect that kids get when they project a flashlight under their chins in the dark to create a spooky character.) This photograph is similar to the many variations of Fuller in her Flower Dance costume from *Salomé*. These very popular images show La Loïe dressed in a frock, with masses of flowers in her hair, around her shoulders, and across her dress. These images are part of Fuller's "chaste" Salome legacy.

There is another image, however, which opens itself up to a rather different reading of Fuller's persona. This photograph is one from a series that were made as souvenir cards, printed with "Miss Loïe FULLER" on the bottom. In this shot, Fuller is seated formally on a dais, giving a slightly Eastern flair to the scene. Her arms are resting on the arms of this rough, throne-like structure (both royal and barbaric), and the rigid symmetricality of her body reads as powerful. Here is the picture of a woman who can give orders. Her jaw is set and she drops her chin ever so slightly to look out at the viewer in a challenging manner. There is also a bound quality to her posture; suggesting a contained energy that could very well be destructive were it to be unleashed. This portrait recalls the emotional energy of Wilde's Salome, suggesting the terrifying volatility of adolescence. In any case, these are not images of an actress who would, in the near future, "renounce" her femininity in whatever guise—chaste or ferocious—it takes on.

One of the critics who found Fuller's *Salomé* particularly successful was Roger Marx, an art critic who also worked for the French government, first as Secrétaire des Beaux-Arts and then as Inspector des Musées de Province. In 1889, he organized much of the Paris Exposition, and for the 1900 exposition, he was the curator in charge of selecting paintings. His review of *Salomé* appeared in the April 1 issue of *La Revue Dramatique*. The text was then reprinted in a collection of his writings published in a limited edition art book dedicated to Loïe Fuller, with gypsograph prints (formed by pressing damp paper into a reverse mould of plaster containing colored inks) by Pierre Roche. Marx begins his review by invoking the Salomes of Flaubert, Moreau, and Huysmans. Although other characters—Herod, Hérodiade, and John the Baptist—are similarly portrayed in Fuller's production, her interpretation of Salome is different, Marx informs his readers, "because a miracle of faith replaced the legendary Salome, drunk with blood and voluptuousness, with a mystical Salome—one that is *almost chaste;* it is for John the Baptist that she dances" (emphasis mine).[37] Marx applauds Fuller's dramatic gestures and her ability to play across a whole host of emotions: "on her face, passes in turn joy, pity, anger, fear, anguish, each emotion played out with a compelling energy."[38]

Marx next turns his considerable descriptive powers to the final scene—Salome's dance for Herod. He tells us that Fuller is dressed in a sheer orange silk, with a veil of the same material concealing her face and her chest. She plays with her veil, making figures with the light silk, alternately revealing and concealing her face, depending on her position on the illuminated glass squares. At one point, she slips away. Marx describes her at this point as being "framed in this fine tissue like an idol."[39] The next moment, she reappears in a black lamé dress and plays the *séductrice* (Marx's words), stirring up Herod's passion. "With a devilish coquetterie, she waves her scintillating scarves which reflect the terrifying flare of the underworld . . ."[40]

This is the moment that sponsored Marx's qualifier of Fuller's *Salomé* as "almost" chaste. In fact, she performs this classic seduction dance, not only once, but twice. For when she finds out that John the Baptist has been condemned to death, she repeats the dance—with a difference. Her movements are no longer fluid and graceful, but "jerky and menacing" (*saccadée, menacants*). Bit by bit, her energy fades and she ends the dance with a poignant, final appeal, "weakened by her agony."

By turns sexy and scary, menacing and pleading, Fuller enacts the gambit of classic feminine gestures. Yet I argue that she foregrounds the performativity of this masquerade as well. Not as parody or drag, but rather by making clear to her audience that she is taking on a dramatic role. Fuller's obvious use of underlighting, her willingness to suspend the narrative denouement in favor of dancing spectacle, and her strategic use of repetition all suggest to me that Fuller was intentionally making visible the triangular relationship of character to body. That is to say, she was making visible her movements between being La Loïe (as in her entrance, the only scene Jean

Lorrain liked), quoting classic portrayals of Salome as a femme fatale (did someone say black lamé?), as well as purposefully reinterpreting that role as Loïe Fuller.

Fuller's multidimensional perspectives on Salome are interestingly reflected in a series of images painted for her by students of the École des Beaux-Arts. To celebrate both her 550th performance in Paris and the free performance she gave for them, these art students threw her a party, pulling her carriage through the streets and presenting her with a hand-bound silk folder with commemorative watercolors of Fulleresque images inside. These often exquisite images are housed in the Lincoln Center Library; significantly, three of the images are of Fuller as Salome.

One of the most interesting of these is by a certain Lloyd Warren, who signs himself as an ardent admirer. It is entitled "HAIL! SALOMÉ" and depicts a strong, confident, half-naked woman holding a severed head. We can still see the traces of her most recent movement in the swirl of fabric and jewels spiraling around her waist. Her body is strong and beautiful, and there is an expressive aliveness in this picture that commands attention. This Salome is facing her audience straight on, insisting that we recognize her power and sexual agency. Now, whether this particular rendition was a direct representation of Fuller's show or not is debatable, as apparently Fuller fainted at the sight of John the Baptist's head. Nonetheless, I think the image captures a certain spirit of Fuller's work; at the very least, it portrays a sexy woman with big thighs, suggesting that not everyone who saw Fuller up close thought of her in Lorrain's terms as a "laundress." The other two images of Salome reproduce the Byzantine quality of the scenic elements. One portrays Fuller as a young princess, echoing Victorian renderings of Sappho as both Greek and Eastern. The other is a ludic elaboration of the L in Loïe's name as an Orientalist fantasy in illuminated manuscript.

This last image reflects not only the wake of fin-de-siècle Salomania, but also the ripple effects of its popular relative—the *danse du ventre*. For, along with the ethnographic exhibits in the colonial sections of the Expositions Universelles, came the increasingly theatricalized displays of female flesh loosely labeled belly dancing. In their insightful essay published in *Assemblage* 13, Zeynap Celik and Leila Kinney document how belly dancing moved from its appearance in the "authentic" Muslim villages through being a staple of theatrical events in those exhibitions, to becoming the latest novelty act on the stages of famous Parisians nightclubs:

> For example, while the Islamic quarters in the 1867 exposition were presented with minimal human animation of their architecture, in 1878, theaters were introduced; thereafter, they became indispensable to every Muslim display. In these theaters, music accompanied tableaux vivants from local daily life, in which weddings or shopping at a bazaar, for exampled, were enacted. In spite of

the variety of activities presented, belly dancers formed the core attraction from the beginning, to judge by the coverage they received in official and unofficial accounts of the exhibits and their increasingly elaborate choreography in successive fairs. In 1889 the number of spectators who came to watch the Egyptian belly dancers averaged two thousand per day.[41]

What intrigues me about Celik's and Kinney's postcolonial analysis is the theoretical connection they pursue between the Orientalist framing of belly dancing and the overall mechanism of display already embedded in fin-de-siècle popular entertainment in general. The reasons that belly dancing so flourished in Paris, they argue, is because it "depended for effect upon a deliberate redundancy of representation."[42] That is to say, in this particular confluence of art and life, the dancers became at once symbols of the "authenticity" of Western Orientalist portrayals of an artistic and literary nature, and yet were, in turn, inflected by them: "If anything, they heightened the 'reality effect' of a body of Orientalist imagery already legitimized by travelogues and paintings."[43]

Enter "La Belle Fatma"—a certain Rachel Bent-Eny, of Algerian Jewish origin, who came to Paris from Tunisia with her father, a musician in that colony's 1878 folkloric exhibition in the French capital. Dancing as a child in the invented "native" display, she grew up on the streets of Paris and soon became a star attraction, appearing in the 1889 Exposition Universelle in both the Grand Théâtre and in the "Rue du Caire."[44] By the time Fuller was engaged at the Folies Bergère in the early 1890s, La Belle Fatma was a regular feature at the nightclub, appearing in the ersatz lobby garden. A December 1892 Folies Bergère program featuring "La Loïe Fuller" lists "La Belle Fatma" in the entr'acte as "visible au jardin sans supplement," (complimentary entertainment in the garden) between the shows.

Another interesting, albeit inverted, example of the nineteenth-century funhouse of Orientalist reflection and their mediated refractions, is that of La Goulue—a famous celebrity dancer whose name and image (thanks to Toulouse-Lautrec) were synonymous with such famous belle époque institutions as the Moulin Rouge. In 1895, several months after Fuller's Salomé closed, La Goulue opened her own booth at the Foire du Trone in Paris. Situated between the theater district and the other popular fair attractions— including animals, games, food, and magic lantern travelogues featuring the Middle East—La Goulue's booth featured two large panels painted by Toulouse-Lautrec. Now housed in the Musée d'Orsay, these panels originally banked either side of the entranceway to her show. On the left side is a typical rendering of La Goulue.[45] She is dancing a chahut with her partner, Valentin. On the right side is another portrait of La Goulue performing entitled La Danse Mauresque ou "Les Almées." Here, La Goulue is dressed in a pseudo-Middle Eastern garb, with a black male drummer (complete with turban) and a Middle Eastern-looking woman dressed as a *fathma*, playing the tambourine. Despite the Islamic patina to the setting, La Goulue is doing her usual kick step, cancan routine, and the audience is the typical Montmartre crowd.

This startling confluence of cancan and belly dancing is, of course, precisely the point Celik and Kinney are making in their essay on fin-de-siècle ethnography and exhibitionism. In this example of the staged "density of cultural interchange," what matters is less the cultural differences between East and West (although they are very real, of course), than the ways in which women entertainers (their female bodies) repeatedly become the site of the intersection of colony and commodity. Caught up in this landscape of voyeurism, these women enter a phantasmagoria of stereotype and display. As Celik and Kinney note: "La Belle Fatma [and] La Goulue temporarily vacate one form of identity only to be caught failing to achieve another."[46]

This last line seems to sum up the conflicted position Fuller found herself in when she took on the role of Salome in 1895. While Fuller was attempting to reshape her identity as an abstract dancer into someone known as an equally gifted expressive mime, her audience wanted to see her in the role that made her famous. This is the dilemma of many performing artists. Although a new role for her, Fuller-as-Salome also had to contend with the plethora of Orientalist visions of dancing women being staged throughout Paris at the time. That she made irreverent reference to these various copies of copies is made clear in another publicity postcard from 1895. Here, Fuller is looking as Middle Eastern as we will ever see her. She is dressed in a series of gauzy fabrics draped and tied around her hips and shoulders, and is positioned in a classic "girlie" or serpentine pose, with her feet in profile and her upper body turned to face the viewer. Her hair is covered by a cloth, and she is holding a piece of material across her face, leaving only her famous sparkling blue eyes to tell the viewer that she is laughing heartily at her own masquerade.[47]

Given the complicated geology of Fuller's first *Salomé*—the many cultural layers of innovation, interpretation, reinvention, and reception that have built up, like sediment, over the years—it is difficult not to read George de Feure's poster advertising the 1895 production of *Salomé* as a parable for the "double jeopardy" that Russo points to in her essay "Female Grotesques." Trying to place her signature on a cultural icon with as much baggage as Salome, Fuller finds herself pointing forward, but looking back. The movements of her fabrics and the motion of the active lettering on the poster, all conjure a certain turbulence; an uneasy disjunction that points to the gap between performative gesture and visual iconography that represents the pleasures and dangers of playing with mimesis.

In November 1907, Loïe Fuller produced her second pantomimed version of *Salomé*. Entitled *La Tragédie de Salomé,* it was staged at the newly renovated Théâtre des Arts. Although the technical preparations took much longer than anticipated, the show ran for only a short while. The libretto was written by Robert d'Humière, and, like the more traditional, fin-de-siècle interpretations of Salome, portrayed this legendary woman as seductive and powerful. The music was created by Florent Schmitt, an Alsatian composer, whose musical tastes ran the gamut from Wagner to Debussy, and whose score for Fuller prefigured the raw turbulence of *Le Sacre du Printemps* (1913) by Stravinsky, who was a friend of Schmitt's and to whom the score is dedicated. As in Fuller's early version of *Salomé*, the overall narrative trajectory of the play was segmented into seven distinct tableaux, each of whose raison d'être was less about the dramatic action of the play and more an opportunity to stage fantastic, expressive dances.

The cover of the November 9 program is a weird, but not atypical, blend of Greek and Eastern motifs. There is a decorative series of ancient Greek-looking women bacchants drawn over Doric columns, framing another series of studio headshots of Loïe Fuller costumed in various Egyptian-looking wigs. The seven scenes of the pantomime are detailed in the program notes. In the first tableau, John the Baptist sets the play in motion when he enters Herod's palace and delivers a diatribe condemning Herod's and Herodias's marriage, and the icons, luxury, and (interestingly enough) the "scent" of the harem. As Herod consults with John the Baptist, Herodias schemes. The second tableau is based on *La danse des perles*, a duet between Salome and her mother. Here, yards of pearls are wrapped and draped around Salome, signifying the luxurious and erotic chains of Herod's palace. In the third tableau, Salome performs *La danse du paon* before Herod and Herodias in an extravagant peacock costume. In the climactic moment of the dance, Fuller turns to reveal an iridescent tail of large feathers, which she can open into a fan. This outfit was made with 4,500 peacock feathers—a detail available in the press releases, along with other equally impressive statistics such as her use of 650 lamps and 15 projectors to create 10,240 watts of candlepower.[48]

The next four tableaux are much less frivolous. Indeed, they become increasingly ominous and violent. In the fourth tableau, Salome takes on two serpents that are threatening Herod and Herodias, executing *La danse des serpents* in a manner described as "moitié lutte, moitié incantation," (half-fight, half-incantation). This ritualized battle ends in a frenzied tarentella. The fifth tableau contains the *Dance of Steel*. In this section, the music is described as a "fantasmagorie démoniaque" (fiendish phantasmagoria), and when Salome reappears, it is in a blinding and metallic light. The next, climactic, scene is punctuated by *La danse d'argent*. Here, Salome is dressed in an elaborate, gold and silver sequined robe. She performs a "lascivious" dance for Herod, who grabs her veils, stripping her naked. John the Baptist quickly covers her up—an insubordination that will cost him his head. Suddenly, blood appears to flow over the stage as Salome reappears for a final,

La danse de la peur (the Dance of Fear). In the midst of a furious storm, the head of John the Baptist appears in the sky, driving a tormented Salomé into a *délire infernal.*

This final effect, easy enough to achieve with magic lantern projections, must have referenced, for an early twentieth-century audience, Gustave Moreau's famous painting, *L'Apparition* (1876). In this painting, which was all the rage at the Paris salon that year, a practically nude Salome points an accusing finger at the head of John the Baptist. Although his eyes are fierce, and the bloody entrails flowing from his neck are viscerally frightening, Salome does not flinch or cower. In fact, the energy running from her chest through her left arm and out her finger is like an electrical charge, and it seems that this energy holds the head captive. I evoke this double reading of Moreau's painting in order to foreground the power of Fuller's performance in this final section. Although it is called *The Dance of Fear,* in this climactic moment, Fuller revealed the strength of her mature dramatic persona, interpreting Salome with an impressive dynamism that bordered, at times, on the violent:

> And then we have the *Dance of Fear,* in which she reveals her tragic power, transmitting to her audience actual shudders of terror. All this is breathtaking, strangely captivating, and astonishingly new for those, like us, who have followed the joyous and knowing transformations of this genial creature of light.[49]

Considered by some to be "the triumph of her long career,"[50] Fuller's 1907 *Salomé* was seen by both the journal *Fémina* and the newspaper *Le Temps* as a feminist statement. In his November 5, 1907, article for *Le Temps,* Jules Clarétie writes: "The other evening, I had, as it were, a vision of a theatre of the future, something of the nature of feministic theatre."[51] An acquaintance of Fuller's, Clarétie had been invited to witness a dress rehearsal of the performance, and it was Fuller's ability to shape at once the production from the outside, as a director and lighting designer, as well as from the inside, as a dramatic character, that sponsored his reflections:

> Women are more and more taking men's places. They are steadily supplanting the so-called stronger sex. The court-house swarms with women lawyers. The literature of imagination and observation will soon belong to women of letters. In spite of man's declaration that there shall be no woman doctor for him the female physician continues to pass her examinations and brilliantly. Just watch and you will see woman growing in influence and power; and if, as in Gladstone's phrase, the nineteenth century was the working-man's century, the twentieth will be the women's century.[52]

The marked contrast between Jean Lorrain's remarks about Fuller's 1895 *Salomé,* and those of Jules Clarétie describing her 1907 production are striking. It would be easy, of course, to dismiss my rhetorical balancing act as a futile attempt to compare apples and oranges. For one thing, the shows—produced twelve years apart—were completely different. Schmitt's composition for the 1907 production was infinitely more successful than Pierné's music in 1895. Then too, Fuller took more time to prepare this later show, leaving very little, including her own dramatic gestures, to chance. Whereas those who saw her rehearse in 1895 commented on the improvisational nature of her pantomime, Clarétie described the attention to detail in rehearsals for the 1907 production:

> Then I had the immense pleasure of seeing this Salome in everyday clothes dance her steps without the illusion created by theatrical costume, with a simple strip of stuff, sometimes red and sometimes green, for the purpose of studying the reflections on the moving folds under the electric light. It was Salome dancing, but a Salome in a short skirt, a Salome with a jacket over her shoulders, a Salome in a tailor-made dress, whose hands—mobile, expressive, tender or threatening hands, white hands, hands like the tips of bird's wings—emerged from the clothes, imparted to them all the poetry of the dance, of the seductive dance or the dance of fright, the infernal dance or the dance of delight. The gleam from the foot lights reflected itself on the dancer's glasses and blazed there like a flame, like fugitive flashes, and nothing could be at once more fantastic and more charming than these twists of the body, these caressing motions, these hands, again, these dream hands waving there before Herod, superb in his theatrical mantle, and observing the sight of the dance idealized in the everyday costume. [53]

In addition to all these differences of style and preparation, I would also argue that (ironically) while the narrative of the 1895 version tried to re-envision a decadent femme fatale, one who is a "chaste" and spiritual figure, it was the 1907 return to the stereotype—the seductive and powerful Salome of Moreau—that was proclaimed as "feministic theatre." I find this irony to be both historically and theoretically intriguing. It is particularly extraordinary in light of the fact that the visual traces—the head shots of Fuller in costume—can only be described as patently ridiculous. Crowned in a series of bad wigs, with heavy mascara and pouty lipstick, Fuller looks like a cheap drag queen.

Yet it is precisely the memories of a performance of a drag queen as a legendary female character that provoke me to reconsider these images as traces of embodiment. Ethyl Eichelberger (1945–1990) performed her version of *Clytemnestra* at PS 122, a downtown New York City performance venue, in the late 1980s. Put together on a shoestring budget, with some of the intentionally worst costuming ever seen (layers of cheap acrylic curtains from Goodwill together with fake boobs made from stuffed nylon stockings strung across Eichelberger's tall, bony frame), this was ancient Greek (melo)-drama splayed out in all its twentieth-century vaudevillian glory. Nonetheless, the power of Eichelberger's dramatic pathos resounded, even in the midst of a campy, S&M-inflected pastiche of late 1980s performance art. A tour de force of solo acting, it was like seeing Aristotle duke it out with Warhol. The show was a thrilling experience for those of us in the audience; at times comic and at times intensely moving. I remember vividly recognizing, in the midst of all the flowing gauze and exaggerated gestures, how Eichelberger used characterization (the stereotype) to more fully realize her "self." In that theatrical space that extends from acting to being and back again, lies a transformative power that explains, I believe, an important difference between Fuller's first and second enactments of Salome. Like Eichelberger almost a century later, Fuller played her 1907 *Salomé* with a vengeance, stirring up, in the process, all kinds of viewing pleasures.

NOTES

1. Jean Lorrain, quoted in Richard Nelson Current and Marcia Ewing Current, *Loïe Fuller Goddess of Light* (Boston: Northeastern University Press, 1997), 72.

2. Rhonda Garelick, *Rising Star: Dandyism, Gender, and Performance in the Fin de Siècle* (Princeton, NJ: Princeton University Press, 1998), 116.

3. Quoted in Current and Current, 75.

4. Loïe Fuller, *Fifteen Years of a Dancer's Life* (Boston: Small, Maynard & Company Publishers, 1913), 137.

5. Ibid., 141–42.

6. Margaret Haile Harris, *Loïe Fuller, Magician of Light* (Richmond: Virginia Museum Exhibition Catalogue, 1979).

7. Garelick, 117.

8. Ibid.

9. Fuller, 169–70.

10. Mary Russo, "Female Grotesques: Carnival and Theory," in *Feminist Studies/ Critical Studies,* ed. Teresa de Lauretis (Bloomington: Indiana University Press, 1986), 213.

11. Ibid., 217.

12. Ibid., 223.

13. See Lynn Garafola, "The Travesty Dancer in Nineteenth-Century Ballet," in *Legacies of Twentieth-Century Dance* (Middletown, CT: Wesleyan University Press, 2005).

14. Quoted in Current and Current, 19.

15. Tirza True Latimer, "Butch-Femme Fatale," in *Proceedings for the Society of Dance History Scholars Conference,* 2000, 83–87.

16. Elaine Showalter, *Sexual Anarchy: Gender and Culture at the Fin de Siècle* (New York: Penguin Books, 1990), 149.

17. Quoted in Francine Meltzer, *Salome and the Dance of Writing* (Chicago: University of Chicago Press, 1987), 25.

18. Ibid.

19. Oscar Wilde, *Salome: A Tragedy in One Act: Translated from the French of Oscar Wilde by Lord Alfred Douglas: Pictured by Aubrey Beardsley* (New York: Dover Publications, Inc., 1967), 21.

20. Ibid., 23.

21. Ibid., 54.

22. Katherine Worth, *Oscar Wilde* (London: Macmillian Press, 1983), 64–65.

23. "Miss Fuller's New Dance," *New York Times,* January 24, 1896.

24. Ibid.

25. Current and Current, 80.

26. *New York Times,* March 17, 1895.

27. Ibid..

28. Jean Lorrain, *Poussières de Paris* (Paris: Ollendorf, 1902), 143.

29. English translation from Margaret Haile Harris, 20.

30. Lorrain, 144.

31. Current and Current, 83.

32. Giovanni Lista, *Loïe Fuller: Danseuse de la Belle Époque* (Paris: Éditions Stock, 1994), 218.

33. Ibid., 231–32.

34. Current and Current, 83.

35. Lista, 229.

36. *New York Times,* March 24, 1895.

37. Roger Marx, "Loïe Fuller," *Les Arts et La Vie,* May/June 1905, 272.

38. Ibid.

39. Ibid.

40. Ibid, 273.

41. Zeynap Celik and Leila Kinney, "Ethnography and Exhibitionism at the Expositions Universelles," *Assemblage* 13 (1990): 39.

42. Ibid., 41.

43. Ibid.

44. Ibid., 43.

45. Ibid., 55.

46. Ibid.

47. For an interesting theorization of the serpentine line, see Emily Apter, "Figura Serpentinata: Visual Seduction and the Colonial Gaze," in *Spectacles of Realism: Body, Gender, Genre,* ed. Margaret Cohen and Christopher Prendergast (Minneapolis: University of Minnesota Press, 1995), 163–78.

48. Margaret Haile Harris, 22. Also included in Harris's book is a caricature of Fuller dressed in a silly peacock headdress and tail dressing from *La Vie Parisienne,* November 16, 1907.

49. *Théâtre des Arts,* vol. I, 1837–1920, 469–70. Housed in the Arsenal Archive. Rt 3701.

50. Current and Current, 182.

51. Quoted in Fuller, 282.

52. Ibid.

53. Ibid., 287–88.

DANCING HISTORIES

My first brush with dance history was learning that my mother took Duncan dancing classes at Bryn Mawr College—an all-women's college with a long history of modern dance—where both she and I went to school. Although I did not want to dance like Isadora Duncan, reading her autobiography *My Life* and seeing old college photos of young Bryn Mawr women in Grecian tunics dancing on the lawn below my dormitory was an inspiring legacy as I myself began dancing in college. But because I was so focused on dancing and writing about the contemporary choreography that I was seeing, it took me a while to register that I had, in fact, been gathering important historical perspectives in the midst of my dance training. Throughout the 1980s I had the exquisite pleasure of studying with modern dance teachers such as Betty Jones, Lucas Hoving, Helmut Fricke-Gottschild, Francoise de la Morandière, and Daniel Nagrin at a time when their historical significance and amazing old-school presence seemed to ooze out of their pores. When I began teaching dance history in the early 1990s, the anecdotes from those classes quickly became a way for me to make history come alive for the students. My desire to include a studio component and the integration of embodied knowledge into my history courses opened up a critically creative space where historical fact meshed with intellectual exploration. The four writings included in this section document my personal journey from primarily using historical references to illuminate aspects of contemporary choreography, to venturing directly into late nineteenth-century and early twentieth-century dance. Much to my surprise, I found myself perfectly content to sit in a library or archive and just allow myself to absorb all those traces of the past.

The first piece in this section, "The Long Afternoon of a Faun: Reconstruction and Discourses of Desire," was a talk I presented at the Society of Dance History Scholars 1992 conference on Dance *Re*constructed. This short piece uses contemporary revisions of Nijinsky's *L'après-midi d'un faune* to parse through the issues surrounding movement invention, audience reception, and questions of "authenticity" in dance reconstructions. I compare Marie Chouinard's iconoclastic solo where she is cross-dressed as Nijinsky's faune and Hellmut Fricke-Gottschild's tongue-in-cheek *The Late, Late Afternoon of a Faun* to a more traditional reconstruction of this famous dance by the Joffrey Ballet. Although it was written early on in my academic career, I include this talk here because it serves as an interesting bridge between my discussions of moving bodies and cultural identities in the Feminist Theories section and my later historical investigation of Loïe Fuller's oeuvre.

Both this initial adventure into dance history and the next essay, "Embodying History," use contemporary choreography as a springboard to reflect on how and for whom the past is preserved. Through an in-depth analysis of the historical layers in Bill T. Jones' *Last Supper at Uncle Tom's Cabin/The Promised Land* and Urban Bush Women's *Bones and Ash,* I argue that rewriting the past is particularly important for minority communities, whose contributions are often left out of conventional histories. "Embodying History" traces how two African-American choreographers re-present American history as the stories of their people's struggle and survival in order to frame colonial legacies through contemporary parables. I use Audre Lorde's notion of a "biomythography" to suggest that these epic choreographies create a "collective biomythography," demonstrating the power of dance to embody a cultural heritage.

The next two essays are connected to my biggest history project to date—a book on the work of Loïe Fuller. "Matters of Tact" was an essay I wrote for *Dance Research Journal* based on a series of performative lectures that I had been giving in dance departments around the country. In these dancing/talking events, I juxtaposed an academic discussion of Fuller's oeuvre with my own choreographic interpretations of her work. While reproducing some of Fuller's movement vocabulary such as spinning and spiraling, this performance interrupted any direct sense of reconstruction by projecting shadows of my dancing over the historical images of Fuller's dancing, thereby making visible the layers of interconnection, reflection, and commentary that were threaded throughout this historical project. In the original essay, the layout echoed the performative blend of text and image, but unfortunately I was unable to reproduce that same design here.[1]

"The Tanagra Effect: Wrapping the Modern Body in the Folds of Ancient Greece" was commissioned for a collection entitled *The Ancient Dancer in the Modern World.*[2] This essay is a comparison of the performance careers and writings of four women who were acting and dancing in Paris at the beginning of the twentieth century: Loïe Fuller, Isadora Duncan, Eva Palmer, and Colette. Although stylistically and ideologically their work and artistic legacies are quite different from one another, all four of these women adapted the trope of the ancient Greek dancer to stage their own versions of "natural" or "modern" dancing. Through their words and staged actions, these women created strident feminist manifestos that demonstrated the importance of connecting bodily practices with social positions.

NOTES

1. See the Wesleyan University Press *Traces of Light: Absence and Presence in the Work of Loïe Fuller* website for an interesting reinterpretation of this essay and my performances in the Acts of Passion section.

2. See Fiona Macintosh, ed., *The Ancient Dancer in the Modern World* (Oxford: Oxford University Press, 2010).

[15]

The Long Afternoon of a Faun

Reconstruction and the Discourses of Desire

Talk given at Dance *Re*constructed, the Society of Dance History Scholars conference, October 1992.

Given the panels and discussions during this conference entitled Dance *Re*-constructed, it is perhaps absurdly redundant to begin this paper with the claim that dance is a historical phenomenon. Yet it is precisely in this conference that the self-evident logic of this statement has raised important and sometimes even disturbing questions. What constitutes the dances we are so valiantly trying to reconstruct? Is it the movement? The dancers embodying the movement? The narrative plot? The entire theatrical collaboration including set, costume, libretto, music, dancers, choreography, artistic advisors, and company managers? The social and historical context in which the dance was originally created? All of the above? While my final suggestion may, at first, seem the most satisfactory, it is also clearly idealistic, impractical, and furthermore it reveals the scholarly arrogance that tempts us to contradict the inevitable logic of my first claim—that dance is a historical phenomenon. No matter how hard we try, we can never get back to the "original" dance. We can, of course, attempt to most closely approximate the original conditions of the dance; but, as in the infamous case in which a costume designer meticulously re-created the original weight, texture, and color of a Loïe Fuller costume only to find that no contemporary dancer was strong enough to lift that fabric into the air; that search for authenticity is so often self-defeating.

Despite my interest in problematizing notions of authenticity and originality, I do believe that reconstructions can give us valuable insights into the dancing past. For me, the importance of reconstruction is twofold: one, that it refer to a previous work in a way that foregrounds the historical legacy of a dance tradition, and two, that it open up the possibility of a revision or a reinterpretation of the original work. I suspect that this final statement may seem blasphemous to some scholars in the audience, but before I am condemned as a poststructuralist neophyte, I hope to work out some of the more subtle implications of this pronouncement through a discussion of three contemporary reconstructions of Nijinsky's *L'après-midi d'un faune*. The Joffrey Ballet's production of this Diaghilev classic, Marie Chouinard's

1987 solo called *L'après-midi d'un faune,* and Hellmut Fricke-Gottschild's 1992 dance entitled *The Late, Late Afternoon of a Faun.*

L'après-midi d'un faune was the first ballet that Nijinsky choreographed for Diaghilev's Ballets Russes, and it is remembered for Nijinsky's innovative use of a severely stylized movement vocabulary based on two-dimensional frieze-like positions, angular lines, and a strangely unballetic parallel profile stance. In an intriguingly circular legacy of influence, Nijinsky's theme comes from Debussy's music that accompanied the dance and was, in turn, inspired by Mallarmé's poem of the same name. As the furor over the ballet's premiere makes obvious, however, the reverie of the poetic text and its musical interpretation produces a very different dynamic when it is physicalized onstage. As Lyn Garafola suggests in her extensively researched book on Diaghilev's Ballets Russes, "Where the poem blurs the line between dream and reality, the ballet presents the erotic theme as lived experience: the reality of the Nymphs, like the scarf that sates the Faun's desire, is never in question."[1] Indeed, at first glance the storyline of the dance seems to be a classic narrative of male desire: a faun sees a group of beautiful nymphs and pursues them. The nymphs flee, but one drops a scarf that the faun retrieves and fetishizes, later "making love" to it in the infamous orgasmic ending of the dance. To an audience brought up on such Orientalist fantasies as *Schéhérazade,* the plot in itself certainly would not have produced more than a murmur. The explosive scandal which marked the 1912 Parisian reception of the dance was provoked instead by the way Nijinsky refused the conventional representations of erotic desire, embodying instead a raw sexuality in his dancing presence.

Propelled by the intensity of his own desire, the faun in Nijinsky's dance moves back and forth across the stage with close, careful steps, pivoting into a provocative gesture with each turn. His stark profile alignment foregrounds his torso that is intermittently punctuated by sudden pelvic contractions and oddly fierce extensions of the arms. Suspended in a pose, the faun seems alternately stoic and dangerous, particularly when the violence of his bound desire threatens periodically to erupt. Curiously, his interactions with the nymphs and even his final possession of the scarf do not really interrupt the concentrated autoeroticism of his movement.

The Joffrey Ballet's production of *Faune* is the most traditional reconstruction that I will discuss here. As a company that is committed to preserving in their repertory a number of the Ballets Russes avant-garde masterpieces, the Joffrey Ballet uses their institutional resources to research and replicate the original backdrop, costumes, music, and choreography. In the version produced for *Dance in America,* Rudolf Nureyev, a Russian emigré dancer who was trained at the same theater school as Nijinsky, took on the role of the faun.

In many ways it is amazing to witness the Joffrey's production of *Faune* in order to see the historical traces of Nijinsky's first choreography come to life onstage. The dance begins with Nureyev reclining on the bucolic hillside that resembles Bakst's original design. The faun lays down his pipe and stretches in a luxuriously feline manner, moving fluidly through the space from one photographic pose to another. Whether reaching for a bunch of grapes and then throwing back his head as he opens his mouth to receive them, or stabbing in the direction of the chief nymph with his arms, Nureyev mimes Nijinsky's faun with picture-perfect accuracy. Yet somehow the faun's physical desire seems to have been dropped out of this picture, and I am surprised by the blankness of the whole experience. An immediate reaction might be to assume that this reconstruction, while choreographically accurate, was not completely authentic in that it did not fully embody the bound intensity of the original production. Or, as so many critics are wont to do, we could suggest that times have changed and that even the original production would not have fazed the sensibilities of a late twentieth-century audience. But I am not convinced that the ballet-going audiences have changed so dramatically; nor am I interested in pursuing an argument about the authenticity of the dancing. What I am interested in is thinking about reconstructions that do not simply try to copy the original, but rather are self-conscious about their approach to it—even if that means radically reinterpreting the original choreography.

In 1987, Marie Chouinard created a dance based on Baron de Meyer's photographs of Nijinsky's *L'après midi d'un faune*. Chouinard's production establishes a bas-relief motif of plastique poses similar to those in Nijinsky's dance. Working always in profile, Chouinard uses only a thin downstage slice of the space, traversing the stage laterally, back and forth, back and forth. She is dressed in a skin-colored unitard with extra padding in one thigh, and the other calf and her headpiece consists of two large ram-like horns. Still, poised with the attentiveness of a hunter, her gaze scans the horizon in a steady manner as a soundtrack of repetitive breathing gradually crescendos. Her steps are bulky and uneven, belying a fiercely bound sexual energy that explodes unexpectedly in thrusts and quivers of her pelvis. Time and time again, a contraction will grip her body, bringing her to her knees. As her breathing becomes louder, it takes on an industrial, almost menacing quality. What was once an internal accompaniment to Chouinard's movements becomes an external, oppressive sound, forcing her to continue. Images of an injured animal, a predator, a bacchant, even of Nijinsky himself dart across this tableau. Then Chouinard breaks off a section of her horn and attaches it to her crotch. What previously had been an image, a movement quality, crystalizes into a surreal moment as Chouinard, exhausted after an increasingly forceful series of pelvic thrusts, moves into Nijinsky's final pose.

Explaining her interest in experimenting with Nijinsky's dance, Chouinard emphasizes her impression of this great dancer's performing presence: "He could transform himself, become totally unrecognizable. I am inspired by his complex vocabulary of movements and am drawn physically as much as intellectually to his strength and the strangeness of his movements."[2] She connects her interpretation of *L'après midi d'un faune* to Mallarmé's pastoral poem in which he asks: "Did I dream that love?" Chouinard explains: "The Nymphs don't really interest me. It's the ambivalence of the object of desire that I find marvelous."[3] In translating this role onto her own body, Chouinard takes on the physical intensity of Nijinsky's desire, but she breaks up its erotic narrative by replacing the central object of that desire (first the nymph and then the scarf) with an evanescent sign—rays of light.

Chouinard's use of the lighting effects as a diaphanous stand-in for the nymph and her scarf further complicates this discourse of desire. At the same time that she seriously enacts this scene of male yearning (there is no sense of campiness during this solo), Chouinard frames it somewhat ironically. In order to take on the phallus, she has to first break it off her head—an action which, when taken out of context, suggests some rather humorous images. On a less comic level, her costume has dart-like projections attached to it and it is ambiguous whether they symbolize horns of the faun, the literal expression of the faun's sexuality, or the arrows of a hunter. In Chouinard's *Faune*, male desire, which is generally predicated on an object—an "other"— is given a vivid representation in the midst of an absence of the other.

Chouinard has reshaped Nijinsky's dance in two central and seemingly contradictory ways. By concentrating her focus on the intensity of the faun's desire, Chouinard at once affirms that desire and makes it strange. No matter how impressive Chouinard is in her intense, almost hungry physicality, the audience is always aware that she is a woman in the position of a man. Yet she does not seem awkward or out of place. The female body in the place of male desire does not negate the position or the movement. Somehow, there seems to be a physical reality in her representation of the faun's desire that also feeds the integrity of her own body. Becoming a "he" on stage does not erase the material sheness of Chouinard's body. It does, however, force us to question a number of assumptions about the polarity of male and female desire.

Intellectually, Chouinard's reconstruction and deconstruction of Nijinsky's dance is both witty and provocative. But it is also deeply compelling in a way that we have not yet developed a language to describe. The shifting triad of desire—Chouinard's desire to capture Nijinsky's physical presence, the faun's desire for the nymph who eludes him, and Chouinard's translation of that desire onto her body—flows in and around the choreography like a series of small waves, gently tugging the audience back and forth. Swept up in this co-motion, Chouinard embodies both the textual and the physical referents of Nijinsky's *L'après midi d'un faune*.

If Chouinard's *Faune* makes desire present, even as she problematizes its gendered narrative, Helmut Fricke-Gottschild's *Late, Late Afternoon of a Faun* humorously deconstructs the narrative of desire itself. The dance begins with Fricke-Gottschild casually walking onstage to greet the musician, Marshall Taylor. With a towel slung around his neck, he crosses the stage, pausing halfway to look out into the audience as if it were a mirror and adjust his profile, sucking in his stomach in a self-conscious manner. A chorus of nymphs and fauns rush onstage as he sits on a stool to watch their dancing. The lively group movement continues for quite some time with only very oblique references to Nijinsky's *Faune* until a series of frieze-like positions begin to materialize on the stage. A woman dancer (a nymph?) grabs the towel unceremoniously. Later, she returns it in an ironic reference to the scarf in Nijinsky's dance. This exchange prompts Fricke-Gottschild's faun solo, which is accompanied by a recording of Debussy's famous prelude.

With a few striking exceptions, the original choreography is replaced by a free-form interpretation of Nijinsky's faun characterized by a fluid, vibratto movement. At first this shimmery vibratto seems to symbolize the faun's beating heart—his desire for a nymph, for youth, for dancing—but Fricke-Gottschild interrupts this interpretation by stopping his dancing and coming downstage to talk with the audience: "Here the dance has a hole, or better, a seam has come apart and through it I step out of the dance into a gap, the inside of which is the outside of the dance." Slipping back into the dance, he allows the tiny vibratto to infect his whole body, and with the romantic swelling of the music, this faun becomes a swan-like creature, bourréing in a circle.

Yet once again the power of this image is interrupted by ironic commentaries from the younger dancers who dart onstage to mimic this aged faun. Taking his stool downstage, Fricke-Gottschild conceeds to the audience that "The faun is older, he tires more easily, occasionally he forgets . . . At any rate, fauns are not in demand anymore, but this one keeps insisting." Having admitted his limitations, this faun returns to the dance, shifting back and forth from a delicate sensuous quality of movement to humorously awkward positions, or comically insistent repetitions. Later he tells us, "And this was to be the solo with large space-taking movements, powerful leaps, sensuous drops, throbbing rhythms, suggestive poses . . . [Here he chuckles] Suggestive poses which turn out to be rests, shattering both fauns' and dancers' delusions." As he continues to dance, we see his own desire for youth, for dancing, struggle with the desire for the wisdom to let it go.

Now, how do we make sense of these two latter dances as reconstructions? Although they clearly refer to Nijinsky's *L'après-midi d'un faune*, they do not try to reproduce the choreography, set, costumes, or any other aspect of the original production in an authentic manner. In fact, they most extravagantly depart from what I have identified as a central impulse in

Nijinsky's dance, choosing to represent the faun's desire differently. I mean really—a faun in drag and a dragged-out faun. Talk about family values!

On a more serious note, I have placed these three dances together in order to touch upon some important issues of distance and closeness. Paradoxically, by pretending to be the closest, the most accurate reconstruction, the Joffrey Ballet's *Faune* can actually serve to pull our consciousness away from the original production. Sure, we realize that it is a *re*production of Nijinsky's masterpiece, but in this postmodern world of simulacra, it is all too easy to take the copy for the original, allowing them to merge into the same thing. By radically departing from the original choreography while at the same time constantly referring us back to it, Chouinard's and Fricke-Gottschild's *Faune* foregrounds both its existence and its absence. Because these two dances do not attempt to replace Nijinsky's *Faune,* they keep that production alive. In the eighty-year gap between these contemporary works and the original lies both a distance and a desire. In fact, it is the self-conscious acknowledgment of their difference that produces the desire to know more, pulling the spectators towards Nijinsky's dance without satisfying our curiosity about it. I think that is a healthy distance.

NOTES

1. Lynn Garafola, *Diaghilev's Ballet Russes* (New York: Oxford University Press, 1989), 56.

2. Chouinard, publicity materials, 1987.

3. Interview with the author, Montreal, October 15, 1988.

16

Embodying History

Epic Narrative and Cultural Identity in African-American Dance

From *Moving History/Dancing Cultures*, ed. Ann Dils and Ann Cooper Albright (2001).

What would it mean to reinscribe history through one's body? What would it mean to re-create the story of a life and the history of a people? How does one rewrite the history of slavery, the history of faith, the history of a past in order to project the story of our future? How can we reenvision the historical legacies of our time through the eyes of hope and human survival instead of rage and cynicism?

These questions guide my reflections on a genre of contemporary performance that I call the "New Epic Dance." Over the past seven years, I have witnessed full evening-length dance/dramas by choreographers as diverse as Garth Fagan, David Rousseve, Jawole Willa Jo Zollar, and Bill T. Jones. These works explore various facets of African-American cultural heritages, refiguring written history in order to embody a tale of the choreographer's own making. I am particularly interested in how these theatrical dances both enact and rework mythic and historical images of slavery, colonial power, and religious faith within a contemporary parable that allows individual dancers to infuse the story with their own histories and physicalities. Using dance as a metaphor for the physical desire to survive and the metaphysical need to fill that survival with hope, these choreographers have, with the help of their collaborators and companies, created theatrical spectacles that evoke the elegiac as well as the celebratory spirit of a people wedged in between two worlds. In many ways, these epic works remind me of the term that Audre Lorde used to describe her autobiographical work *Zami: A New Spelling of my Name*. Grounded in, but not limited to the historical facts of a people's existence, these epic dance narratives weave what Lorde calls a "biomythography," elaborating visionary sagas of social and personal survival.

The creation of an individual life narrative—the (auto)biography—is expanded in the New Epic Dance to include expressions of cultural identity which call upon mythic and archetypal, as well as historical, images of

African Americans. Works such as Garth Fagan's *Griot New York,* David Rouseve's *Urban Scenes/Creole Dreams,* Urban Bush Women's *Bones and Ash: A Gilda Story,* and Bill T. Jones's *Last Supper at Uncle Tom's Cabin/ The Promised Land* focus on the collective stories of history and survival of African peoples in America. Because of their narrative scope—which is to say their desire not only to remember the past and document the present but also to narrate future possibilities, as well as their ambitious integration of dance, song and theatrical text within a full evening-length performance, these works are clearly epic in scale. There is, of course, a crucial distinction between the traditional Western Homeric epic and these late twentieth-century revisitations of that densely layered form of narrative. Traditional epics tend, generally, to celebrate conquest and the lives of warrior statesmen. By contrast, these contemporary African-American epics celebrate and honor the legacy of a people who have survived conquest, locating heroism not in the defeater, but rather in the spirit of those who have refused to be defeated.

In order to be effectively and potently embodied in performance, history has to be recast, so to speak—situated in a different light and taken up by different bodies. The importance of history here is not the importance of historical fact or artifact. Such documents, having been authorized in the service of white dominance, are rightfully suspect. Rather, history for so many African-American peoples is located in the story—in the telling again and again. This retelling of ancestral blood memories is the compelling force behind much of the New Epic Dance. For stories to be historically meaningful, however, they need two things: a sense of truth (which, while it does not need to be static, must be galvanizing); and a sense of community between the speakers and the listeners—the realization of what is at stake in this exchange of the word. In her essay "The Site of Memory," Toni Morrison draws a distinction between "truth" and "fact":

> Therefore the crucial distinction for me is not the difference between fact and fiction, but the distinction between fact and truth. Because facts can exist without human intelligence, but truth cannot. So if I'm looking to find and expose a truth about the interior life of people who didn't write it (which doesn't mean that they didn't have it); if I'm trying to fill in the blanks that the slave narratives left—to part the veil that was so frequently drawn, to implement the stories that I heard—then the approach that's most productive and most trustworthy for me is the recollection that moves from the image to the text. Not from the text to the image.[1]

I believe that this distinction is vital in that it helps us to recognize the spiritual power of what Audre Lorde calls "biomythography"—that is, the re-creation of history as myth, as tales that embody common ideals. "Truth," as opposed to "fact," gives these (hi)stories an activating spiritual force that is so crucial, particularly in communities that are faced with the awesome task of rewriting their own subjectivity back into the prevailing historical narrative. It is not the primacy of the historical text that is so important for Morrison, but the potency of the embodied image. History is written about past events. Stories are told in order to connect the knowledge of the past and hopes for the future with one's experiences of present realities. In this way, history can be refigured as a living continuum rather than as chronologically dated events. This redeployment of history is predicated on a collective consciousness of cultural identity—a sense of self that is connected to a sense of one's peoples. (This is, needless to say, rarely a conflict-free connection.)

In her chapter on the power of storytelling at the end of *Woman, Native, Other,* Trinh T. Minh-ha begins her discussion of "Truth and fact: story and history" with "Let me tell you a story," and goes on to tell her readers a story about remembering, truth, and community. "The story depends upon every one of us to come into being. It needs us all, needs our remembering, understanding, and creating what we have heard together to keep on coming into being. The story of a people. Of us, peoples. Story, history, literature (or religion, philosophy, natural science, ethics)—all in one."[2] Although there are some people who, like my *American Heritage Dictionary,* still equate truth with fact and "fidelity to an original," many of us recognize that truths need to be creative rather than static. For truth must be the beginning of action, not simply its consequence or fate. Thus Minh-ha continues:

> Truth is when it is itself no longer. Diseuse, Thought-Woman, SpiderWoman, griotte, storytalker, fortune-teller, witch. If you have the patience to listen, she will delight in relating it to you. An entire history, an entire vision of the world, a lifetime story . . . To listen carefully is to preserve. But to preserve is to burn, for understanding means creating.[3]

It is this creative element in retelling the story that makes this history—the history of peoples and their stories rather than the history of facts—inherently performative. For the telling has a listener and the listener's reality affects the cadence and the "truth" of the telling. Of course, before the West became so enamored with writing history, epics were oral performances and so their "truths" necessarily evolved as they passed mouth-to-mouth through generation and region.

The genre of contemporary African-American performance that I define here as the New Epic Dance is staged in Jones's and Zollar's work as a collective biomythography. These dance/dramas combine music, dance, and text to present a revised history that plays with the tropes of ironic repetition, reenactment, and reinterpretation. While all the works I have mentioned deserve in-depth discussion, the limitations of time and space, as well as my desire not to treat these important works in a cursory fashion, have prompted me to confine my extended analysis to two works: Bill T. Jones and Arnie Zane Dance Company's *Last Supper at Uncle Tom's Cabin/The Promised Land* (1990), and Urban Bush Women's *Bones and Ash: A Gilda Story* (1995–96). I have chosen these two performative epics to compare because they provide a very different kind of theatrical experience for the audience, foregrounding the representation of race, memory, and historical experience in ways that ask the viewers to engage with their own historical memories. Although these two works look and feel very different from one another, they are both animated by a visionary sensibility that seeks to re-form the legendary evils of greed and the lust for power in order to create a new infrastructure of social interaction. Both works refuse our contemporary cynicism—meeting a fin-de-siècle hopelessness with a conviction that humanity can be reborn. And both works are, I believe, deeply feminist in spirit, if not always in detail. The complex interweaving of oral, danced, and theatrical texts in *Last Supper* and *Bones and Ash* documents our national legacy of interracial hate and gendered and ethnic inequalities. Yet this bleak history is enriched by personal narratives of love, religious faith, and spiritual transcendence. By reinterpreting classic stories and cultural stereotypes through contemporary dancing bodies, both Jones and Zollar refuse the static doneness of historical documentation—lifting the black-and-white print off the page and imbuing it with the ability to move, shift, and, finally, to transform itself.

> In this chain and continuum, I am but one link. The story is me, neither me nor mine. It does not really belong to me, and while I feel greatly responsible for it, I also enjoy the irresponsibility of the pleasure obtained through the process of transferring. Pleasure in the copy, pleasure in the reproduction. No repetition can ever be identical, but my story carries with it their stories, their history, and our story repeats itself endlessly despite our persistence in denying it.[4]

Minh-ha's words begin the story of my telling, my witnessing. For in the context of this essay, I am the conduit—the speaker who translates—these epic performances for the public. The dances I have seen have influenced how I think, how I see. Taken in and witnessed through my body, they come alive through my language and my ideas. Unfortunately, most people will not have had the opportunity to see these works for themselves and so my writing may be the only exposure they have to these epic dances. This is, indeed, a great responsibility. Thus I want to be clear about how I, a white, feminist dancer and writer negotiate the position of witness and critic here. My experiences with these works may well be different from other dance writers, particularly African-American dance critics. Yet while I acknowledge the potency of experiences of racism and my privilege in this regard, I do not believe that this difference invalidates my perception, nor do I believe that I cannot write about African-American performance in a way that is both cognizant of this difference and informed by knowledge of that cultural perspective. In other words, while I would never pretend to have an insider's viewpoint, neither will I be satisfied with claiming my outside status as a way of refusing responsibility for representing this very important work. Being white is no excuse for not making the effort to learn about and come to understand the complexities and multiple layers of meaning in contemporary African-American epic dance.[5]

In his inspiring book, *Negotiating Difference: Race, Gender and the Politics of Positionality,* Michael Awkward takes up the negotiations of power inherent in white critics' writing about black texts. Awkward is a professor of English and so his examples come mostly from literature, yet his careful delineation of a critical position that could both register the racial privilege inherent in white criticism and also recognize what he calls the possibility of "interpretive crossing-over" can provide an important example of conscious criticism for cultural critics involved with any form of cultural production. In his chapter, "Negotiations of Power: White Critics, Black Texts, and the Self-Referential Impulse," Awkward analyses various interpretive positions across the continuum of white criticism of African-American literature. While many white critics still approach African-American literature in purely formal Euro-aesthetic terms; as (using Houston Baker's term) "superordinate authorities," Awkward argues for the possibility of other kinds of readings. "I want to emphasize my belief that neither a view of an essential incompatibility between black literature and white critics nor of whites as always already dismissive and unsophisticated in their analyses of the products of the Afro-American imagination is still tenable."[6] Awkward later uses Larry Neal's discussions of white critical practices to suggest the possibility of a "thick" reading that reflects "some understanding of [black] cultural source."[7] For Awkward race is as much a political ideology and commitment as an essential or biological fact.

> For Neal, critical competence with respect to Afro-American expressivity is determined not by tribal connections into which one is born; rather, it is gained by academic activity—"by studying"—in the same way that one achieves comprehension of the cultural matrices that inform the work of writers like Joyce, Yeats, and e.e. cummings. Demystifying the process of acquiring an informed knowledge of Afro-American expressivity, Neal insists that the means of access for all critics, regardless, of race, is an energetic investigation of the cultural situation and the emerging critical tradition.[8]

My chapter on African-American epic performance is compelled by the conviction that this work is too important not to deal with, even if that means taking a risk by putting myself in a less comfortable critical position. Because I am a dancer and a theorist who is concerned about the fate of material bodies at the end of the twentieth century, I want to expand Neal's notion of "studying" to include not only book work, but also the physical situatedness of a culture—that is to say, investigating the ways African-American bodies live, move, perform, tell stories, walk, etc. Although issues of racial difference have greatly influenced academic discourse over the past two decades, too often these discussions of race or difference remain purely abstract—content to stay in the comfort of armchairs and ivory towers. I believe, however, that there is a crucial difference between merely talking about attention to diversity and actually committing oneself to a critical and personal engagement that recognizes and connects with the power and variety of African-American expressivity. I quoted Minh-ha earlier because I felt that the continuum and transmission of culture which she elaborates at once recognizes the differences between "I" and "they" ("No repetition can ever be identical"), but also sees the interconnectedness; the "our" ("but my story carries with it their stories, their history, and our story repeats itself"). It is with recognition of this difference, in tandem with the belief that this difference can produce a viable critical engagement, that I continue here.

*Re*writing, *re*inscribing, *re*-creating, *re*envisioning, *re*figuring, *re*framing, *re*incorporating, *re*interpreting, *re*presenting—the reader will no doubt have noticed the frequency with which I have used the prefix "re" so far. This is not merely a poststructuralist tic of mine. The act of going back to take up again—returning, reclaiming, repossessing—this is a strategy that is central to contemporary African-American performance. Adrienne Rich once described this process as "re-vision—the act of looking back, of seeing with fresh eyes, of entering an old text from a new critical direction."[9] Nowhere is this device more provocatively explored than in the first section of Jones's *Last Supper at Uncle Tom's Cabin/The Promised Land*. Here, Jones both re-enacts the sentimentalized Christian ethos of salvation embedded in Harriet Beecher Stowe's 1852 novel *Uncle Tom's Cabin*, and deconstructs the racist stereotypes connected to the popularized minstrel versions of that abolitionist story. At once fragmenting and reinventing the tropes of blackface, the family, religious faith, womanhood, slavery and "Uncle Toms," Jones outlines the ambivalent relationship that his dancers have with those historical characters. Employing theatrical devices to foreground the performance of racial and gendered stereotypes, Jones indicates the contradictory closeness and distance—the similarities and the differences—between then and now.

Prompted by the inhumanity of the Fugitive Slave Act of 1850, which required all U.S. citizens (both Northern and Southern) to return runaway slaves to their legal owners, as well as her sister-in-law's exhortations to use her literary talents in the service of abolitionism, Stowe wrote *Uncle Tom's Cabin* in serial installments for an antislavery newspaper, the *National Era*. In 1852, the novel was published by a small press in Boston, and it proceeded to sell more copies than any other book at that time, excepting the Bible. *Uncle Tom's Cabin* quickly entered the national discourse, as the character of Uncle Tom was taken up by both the North and the South—at once reified as a saint (indeed, a veritable black Christ), and vilified as a traitor to his race. In a capitalist marketing coup that would have made Disney proud, the figure of Uncle Tom proliferated within the growing industries of novelty consumerism and commodity culture—not to mention the wildfire of popular performance. Even before the novel was published in its final form, there was a theatrical version in repertory, and some historians speculate that for every one person who read the novel, fifty people saw the play in some form or another. The absence of copyright laws, in addition to the extensive network of small regional and traveling theater companies, paved the way for the hundreds of versions of Stowe's novel that dominated local and national stages over the next half-century. The ubiquity with which versions of *Uncle Tom's Cabin* saturated antebellum America is evoked by Richard Yarborough when he details how:

> Not only was a children's version of *Uncle Tom's Cabin* issued in 1853 . . . but within a year there also appeared "Uncle Tom and Little Eva," a parlor game "played with pawns that represented 'the continual separation and reunion of families.'" In fact, Stowe's best-seller inspired a veritable flood of Uncle Tom poems, songs, dioramas, plates, busts, embossed spoons, painted scarves, engravings, and other miscellaneous memorabilia, leading one wry commentator to observe [that Uncle Tom] became, in his various forms, the most frequently sold slave in American history.[10]

Tracing the various literary and performative histories of *Uncle Tom's Cabin* in antebellum America is a daunting task to say the least, and it is certainly not within the scope of this study to include an extensive analysis of how the character of Uncle Tom changed over the years. Nonetheless, it is important to note that unlike the folk images, which tend to picture Uncle Tom as an old, passive, Southern darkie, who is perfectly happy serving his white master, Stowe's Uncle Tom is a young, strong, vibrant man, who assumes a leadership role within whatever community he finds himself. Although his behavior toward his various masters is shaped by a Christian saintliness and maternal concern for these white souls, it is Tom's final act of resistance to white authority—his refusal to betray another slave—that gets him killed; beaten in body but not in spirit. Stowe has been faulted for valorizing Uncle Tom's refusal to betray his master's trust and flee slavery. But the Christian martyrdom of this character needs to be understood within the nineteenth-century economy of domesticity. As a black Christ figure, Stowe's character is male and heroic, but not masculine in the typical sense of that word. Rather than being simply a failure of Stowe's imagination to envision a defiant black man, this characterization can be seen as a deliberate attempt to reinstill traditionally feminine values into an increasingly industrialized and male public sphere. In her book *Sensational Designs: The*

Cultural Work of American Fiction 1790–1860, Jane Tompkins argues that: "the popular domestic novel of the nineteenth century represents a monumental effort to reorganize culture from the woman's point of view; that this body of work is remarkable for its intellectual complexity, ambition, and resourcefulness; and that, in certain cases it offers a critique of American society far more devastating than any delivered by better-known critics such as Hawthorn and Melville."[11] Although the legacy of Stowe's novel will continue to be debated (as it was at the time), there is no doubt that this story of social evils and private triumphs conquered the public imagination with a force unparalleled in American literature.

Within six months of the novel's publication, there were already several stage adaptations of Stowe's *Uncle Tom's Cabin,* including one by George Aiken that played in Troy, New York, before moving to the National Theater in New York City on July 18, 1853.[12] With its peculiar combination of dramatic plot and blackface, Aiken's production provides an interesting antecedent to Bill T. Jones's reenactment of Stowe's work. Even though it repeated the theatrical convention of having whites in blackface play African-American characters, Aiken's drama is one of the more politically progressive stage renditions of *Uncle Tom's Cabin.* Much like Stowe's novel, Aiken's version was a veritable nineteenth-century tearjerker—what one review called a "pièce de mouchoir," and its morally "uplifting" story was seen as theatrical fare suitable for families and women as well so that a whole new series of matinee performances were added to accommodate this new audience.[13] As family entertainment rather than vaudeville, the seriousness of dramatic intent of this play differed radically from other blackface melodramas. The Uncle Tom figure in this production was a white man in blackface, but the actor, G. C. Germon, reportedly struggled to maintain a sense of the theatrical power of the part. By refusing to indulge in the comic buffoonery that usually marked blackface roles, this actor was able to transcend the mode of performance in order to create a realistic persona onstage. One reviewer of the time spoke of Germon's very different performative presence (he was considered a "straight," as opposed to a comic actor). "His very first works, however, showed that a good hand had his part. The accent, a broad and guttural negro accent, but the voice deep and earnest—so earnest, that the first laugh at his nigger words, from the pit, died away into deep stillness."[14]

In his book *Love and Theft: Blackface Minstrelsy and the American Working Class,* Eric Lott argues that the largely Irish working-class audience was moved by this play because they associated their own struggles as new immigrants with a form of economic slavery. Indeed, the local Northern sentiment about the institution of slavery in the South radically changed at this time, as the working class became an ideological partner in the abolitionist movement. It is also important to realize that by September 1853, the National Theater, where Aiken's production of *Uncle Tom's Cabin* was playing, had begun to accommodate African-American spectators—a fact suggesting that somehow this staging of Stowe's story was able to cross over to a black audience as well.

Unfortunately, most other productions were less progressive. Indeed, several revised the play's themes so completely that they ended up supporting a proslavery stance. Replacing the anguish of an economic system based on the selling of black bodies and the cruelty of separating families with images of "contented darkies," these productions took the minstrel tradition to its logical racist conclusion, creating songs and dances that featured happy, carefree slaves. (In fact, one such burlesque turned Stowe's subtitle: *Life Among the Lowly*, into "Life Among the Happy.")[15] It was with the plethora of these comic, bastardized, versions of *Uncle Tom's Cabin* that the figure of Uncle Tom became increasingly comic, passive, and elderly, paving the way for the contemporary meanings surrounding the figure of Uncle Tom.

Given the cultural baggage that this particular character has acquired over the past 145 years, it seems reasonable to ask why an African-American male choreographer would want to re-create Stowe's narrative onstage. Is it in order to lend a more authentic voice to the story? Is it in order to rewrite the ending of Tom's life; to refuse his Christian martyrdom in favor of a more strident rebellion? Or perhaps to reanimate a figure who, although written into existence by a white Northern woman, has been repeatedly restaged by both black and white bodies throughout the histories of minstrelsy, regional theater, and Hollywood cinema? Fortunately, Bill T. Jones has been—not uncharacteristically—quite verbal and forthcoming about his artistic process. But the journey from a 1989 entry in his autobiography *Last Night on Earth*—"I read *Uncle Tom's Cabin*. I find it to be hokum, misinformation. I find it moving, infuriating, beautiful, embarrassing, and important"[16]—to the description one page later of *Last Supper at Uncle Tom's Cabin/The Promised Land*—"It would speak about being human. About how we are the places we have been, the people we have slept with. How we are what we have lost and what we dream for"[17]—requires more than a fleeting summary of Jones's artistic intentions; it requires a close analysis of the complex cycle of referentiality that gives his work such resonance for a contemporary audience.

The first section of Jones's *Last Supper* is staged as a frame within a frame. This scene is played within a two-dimensional backdrop created by hanging a checkered, gingham patchwork quilt that opens like a makeshift curtain to reveal a small stage. This "cabin" set simultaneously evokes both the influences of early Americana and the stylized replication of that period as folk art. It is on this stage within a stage that we witness a much-abbreviated version of Stowe's novel. Like many nineteenth-century theatrical renditions of *Uncle Tom's Cabin*, Jones's take is a series of allegorical vignettes and tableaux that punctuate Tom's narrative of redemptive faith with the equally uplifting and equally melodramatic stories of Eliza and Eva. With the notable exceptions of the narrator (played by Justice Allen), the authoress Stowe (played by Sage Cowles), and the character of Uncle Tom (played by Andrea Smith), most other dancers have on masks with highly exaggerated and often grotesque features. For example, the slave trader Haley's mask looks almost comically evil—a cross between a skeleton and a German Expressionist painting. The blackface masks are also cartoonish, especially the figure of "black Sam." However, to simply label these figures stereotypical caricatures, as many reviews of the *Last Supper* have done, is to misrepresent the repetition in Jones's staging. For Jones's reenactment of the iconographic features of the minstrel tradition does not simply repeat the racist stereotypes that underline Stowe's novel and run rampant throughout most of the minstrel versions of Uncle Tom's story. Rather, Jones ironically reframes these caricatures in order to create a perspective that at once distances and embraces this legacy of cultural reproductions.

Jones's work reflects the proliferation of meanings implicit in any reclaiming, reinscribing, or rewriting of one's history. Lott describes the strategy of reclamation in Martin Delany's black, nationalist novel *Blake* in terms that also reflect what I think Jones is doing in his version of *Uncle Tom's Cabin*. "*Blake* writes black agency back into history through blackface songs taken 'back' from those who had plundered black cultural practices. Rather than reject the cultural territory whites had occupied by way of minstrelsy, Delany recognizes that occupation as fact and occupies in turn."[18] Throughout his epic narrative of struggle and faith, Jones is employing repetition—but repetition with a crucial difference. Like Lott's description of Delany's work, Jones's redeployment of the minstrel tradition reflects that tradition's hybrid nature, while also claiming it as a vehicle through which to reassert his own historical voice.

For instance, the masks—a face on top of a face—foreground the performative nature of stereotypes, forcing the audience to recognize the clichéd sentimentality of those images. And yet these two-faced characters operate in a very postmodern fashion, for they split the actor and the character, refusing any essentialist notions about who should play whom. Indeed, Jones's use of masks allows him to cast across the performer's own racial, gender, or age groups. Aunt Chloe is played by a white man, Greg Hubbard, while Simon Legree—the monstrous slave owner described in the text as a mean man who prides himself on having a "fist of iron for hittin' niggers"—is portrayed by a black man, Justice Allen.

This kind of reframing, refiguring, and cross-referencing is most striking in the very first dance sequence when Harry, "a beautiful quadroon boy" is asked to entertain the slave trader by doing the "Jim Crow." Now the "Jim Crow" has a highly complicated history. The term first entered the national discourse in the 1820s with the arrival of T. D. "Daddy" Rice—a white Northern performer who popularized a parody of the "dancing darkie" by "blacking up" and performing a syncopated jig. To "jump Jim Crow" quickly became a main attraction in the minstrel shows, and even as African-American performers entered that tradition after the Civil War, the caricature remained a staple of minstrelsy. Played by black performers in blackface, the Jim Crow is a dance that simultaneously lampoons the white master and caricatures the black slave—at once portraying and ironically displacing racist notions of African Americans' inherent musicality and natural danceability.[19]

Although the Jim Crow first became known through white performances of black dancing on the minstrel stage, Harriet Beecher Stowe naturalizes this racist portrayal of the black body by placing it on the plantation. In Stowe's novel, the Jim Crow dance, performed by the young (and desirable) quadroon boy Harry, actually sets the dramatic action in play. The book begins with a conversation between the "kindly" (and paternalistic) slave owner, Mr. Shelby, who owes money to the not so kindly slave trader Mr. Haley. Their discussion is interrupted by Harry, who enters the scene and is requested by Shelby to entertain Haley by doing the Jim Crow. Stowe's description of the boy's dance reveals the racist views concerning the dancing black body so prevalent even among the abolitionists of her time. "The boy commenced one of those wild, grotesque songs common among the negroes, in a rich, clear voice, accompanying his singing with many comic evolutions of the hands, feet, and whole body, all in perfect time to the music."[20] It is after seeing Harry dance that Haley wants to buy him, underlining the connection between the performing body's public visibility (that it is always available for the spectator's gaze) and the slave's body's inevitable purchasability (that it is always for sale).

In the cabin section of Jones's *Last Supper,* the Jim Crow is performed by Sean Curran—a wonderfully accomplished white dancer whose roots in Irish step dancing give him the necessary skills to execute a very good Jim Crow. Despite its entertaining rhythms and virtuosic footwork, it is difficult to watch this divertissement without confronting the colonialist legacy of this dance. As Jacqueline Shea Murphy makes clear in her essay on Jones's epic, "Unrest and Uncle Tom," "The term 'Jim Crow' itself provides a clear instance of how tightly intertwined African American performance and violent oppression have been in this country. 'Jim Crow' originally named a minstrel song-and-dance act that today one understands to have stereotyped, parodied, and degraded African Americans; the term became synonymous, late in this century, with a system of (sometimes violently enforced) racial segregation."[21] The effect of this contemporary cross-racing of a historically racist image is both curiously disturbing and sensational. Jones's restaging of the Jim Crow takes place within Stowe's narrative, but the spectacular element of this scene is emphasized such that he provokes a double critique. In this scene, the audience witnesses the ambiguity of simultaneous entertainment and political confrontation. We see Curran, in blackface mask, aping a minstrel portrayal of Jim Crow, and yet we also see him doing a virtuosic solo that demands respect in its own right. By way of his directorial choices, Jones seems to be suggesting that there is absolutely nothing essential about the connection between the sign of Jim Crow and its referent in the black body—a move that allows Jones to both criticize the historically racist portrayals of Jim Crow and elaborate on the performative nature of any identity category.

The postmodern flickering in and out of history, race, and identity at play in much of this first section of *Last Supper* is grounded by the powerfully realistic representations of Eliza and Uncle Tom. The Eliza character is portrayed by a tall, lean, young African-American woman, Andrea Woods. Although the figure of the heroically maternal Eliza is masked in the cabin section, her brief appearance must be realistic enough to foreshadow her magnificent solo in the next scene of the dance. Eliza on the Ice is a complex theatrical meditation on the very brief but important moment in Stowe's book where Eliza escapes to freedom with her son by jumping on moving blocks of ice to cross the Ohio River. In his staging of this scene, Jones elaborates on the existential meanings implicit in Eliza's state of liminality—of being suspended between two shores—by creating multiple Elizas, variations on a central theme. This section is a good example of how Jones negotiates between deconstructing deterministic, essentialist, or racist notions about the inextricability of color and identity, and recognizing the historical legacies of such constructions. Jones knows that in order for history to be refigured, it must first be figured in such a way that powerfully evokes the real bodies at stake within the representation.

The Eliza section begins in darkness. As the lights rise slowly, they reveal a line of five different Elizas standing one behind the other. The first woman, Andrea Woods, holds the Eliza mask she wore in the first section of the dance. She removes the mask and turns to hand it to the woman behind her, who in turn hands it to the woman behind her. The mask passes through the hands of the four women until it ends up with the Stowe character. As she begins to recite Sojourner Truth's famous "Ain't I a Woman?" speech, the first Eliza (whom Jones has dubbed "the historical Eliza") begins to dance. To the stirring words of Truth's rhetorical questioning ("I have ploughed and planted and gathered into barns and no man could head me! And ain't I a woman?"), Woods delivers a physical evocation of generations of black women working, rejoicing, and confronting the world. Her movement is wide and strong as her torso loops down to the ground and then arches up to the sky, catapulting her long legs out into the space around her. Her arms can be powerfully direct—as in the moment when she shoots her arm straight to the audience in a defiant gesture, or wonderfully generous—as when she reaches out to embrace the possibilities of the world around her. Suddenly, the slow punctuated rhythm underlining Truth's speech switches gears and becomes upbeat and bouncy. Woods responds in kind until the final moment, which ends with a rolling strut off stage to Truth's declaration "And now I am here."

The next Eliza is a contemporary portrayal by Heidi Latsky—a short, Jewish woman whose fierce dancing provides a tangible accompaniment to the story of abuse and betrayal she recites. In this section, we move from the archetypal figure of Eliza as an African-American woman struggling with crossing over from slavery to freedom to a contemporary portrait of Eliza as a survivor. Her text (which she speaks into a microphone held by the Stowe character as she moves across the stage) is potently embodied in Latsky's movement eruptions. "I believe . . . My father told me turn the other cheek . . . My mother told me not to expect much," contextualizes her dancing, marked by the contrast created as she alternately clenches her body to herself or strikes out at the forces around her. As she pulls at her own body, it seems as if Latsky wants to tear off her own skin. The lyrical movement of the historical Eliza changes here into the tight, explosive movement of a woman who desperately wants to resist society's admonishments to be good. This Eliza is also caught between the shores of expectation and freedom, but the terms of her struggle have changed.

The next two Elizas similarly embody archetypal situations for women, but because their solos have no direct textual accompaniment, they are much less specific in narrative detail. The third Eliza is danced by Betsy Mc-Cracken, a tall, white dancer whose legs shoot out with military precision as she wields her staff around the stage. Her character is like a powerful Greek goddess, perhaps Athena, who directs the male corps de ballet into parade-like formations. Jones speaks of this Eliza as the one "who commands men—part Joan of Arc, part dominatrix, and part martial arts master."[22] This power, of course, is tenuous. It is exhausting to watch McCracken always on her guard; never able to release the tension in her body. Eventually she decides that this power is not worth the stakes involved and, throwing her staff away, she runs offstage—free at last.

The fourth Eliza is Maya Saffrin, whom Jones describes in his autobiography as "exotically pretty," and whose dance is a metaphoric struggle between the various men who lift and pass her among themselves and the first Eliza, who tries to rescue her from their control. This Eliza is clearly the most disempowered. Zombielike, her passive physical presence makes it seem as if she has no will of her own. Even when she dances a duet with the first Eliza, she is dancing her partner's movement, always looking at her friend for guidance. Although she is not floppy like a rag doll (which in some ways would be a sort of resistance, making it hard for anyone to lift or carry her), her energy is so contained that one wonders whether this Eliza would have even left the first shore, let alone have the strength of purpose to actually make it across to the promised land.

As this fourth Eliza exits, a fifth and final Eliza—one that the audience has not previously seen—enters. This Eliza is danced by a very tall, African-American man, Greg Hubbard. He is wearing only a bright white miniskirt and white pumps. Perhaps the most contemporary of all, this Eliza is figured as a gay man in drag. Standing awkwardly on these heels, his almost naked body giving him a childlike innocence, he executes a series of gestural movements that are very much like Jones's signature gestures where the arms continually circle the upper body like an elaborate frame. Tracing his hands over his head and down the front of his body, Hubbard stops to grab his crotch in a sudden gesture. Is he meant to surprise us or reassure himself? This brief moment of doubt changes into a work-it attitude as he turns and walks off the stage with a body wave slyly snaking from his head down to his toes.

In the *Alive From Off Center* television special focusing on the making of *Last Supper* (aired in 1992), Jones details the process of creating these various Elizas. He speaks eloquently about the importance of the dancers involved in the making of these solos, especially with regard to the first two Elizas, whose own personas were so deeply embedded into their characters. Then Jones shifts to a discussion of the final Eliza and talks about this figure's own struggles between a different kind of slavery and freedom. Speaking as a gay man about this final Eliza, Jones declares: "Our sexuality exists on neither shore, that of femininity and that of masculinity. It is its own thing, but because of the strictures of our society, we are left suspended, doubtful, fearful even, of where we belong."

Jones clearly identifies the Eliza on the Ice section as a feminist statement of sorts. Certainly the progression from the "historical Eliza" to that of Hubbard's gay Eliza thoroughly deconstructs the static concept of woman so embedded in Western representation. Woman as a universal term actually meaning white, feminine, defined by her relationships to men, or even as suggesting a biological femaleness is fractured by the different and contradictory embodiments of Eliza. Although Jones is playing here with the historical/fictionalized character of Eliza, he is also intent on underlining the universal dimensions of a liminal state—the way in which many people find themselves existentially between two shores. The final Eliza could be problematic for feminists who are hesitant to fully deconstruct the category of women altogether (for as Hubbard's crotch-grabbing gesture makes clear, a man in a skirt really has not given up his social power; it is merely hidden, available to be reerected, so to speak, at a moment's notice). Yet, for me, the crucial question is whether "her" appearance actually adds another dimension to this investigation of gender in our culture, or whether it serves to dismiss the earlier images of women's struggles. I believe that Jones consciously left Hubbard's Eliza out of the original lineup in order to give these female Elizas their own voices. Indeed, the autobiographical as well as historical character of their stories allows Jones to make the ideological connection—that gay men's sexualities are also suspended between two shores—without usurping the material and political realities of women's lives. Jones thus problematizes, even deconstructs, gender without rendering it a vacant category. This balance of realism and performative spectacle is absolutely critical to the genre of epic dance. The potency of this form lies precisely in the witnessing of people's stories, as well as the reconstructing of their historical legacies. And too, there is the issue of merged identities here, for Jones has often declared the powerful influence that black women have had in his life—most notably his mother (who appears onstage in this piece) and his sisters. If we take the Hubbard character as Jones himself, one might argue that he is, in fact, trying to bring out the female embedded in the male persona.[23]

Nonetheless, Hubbard's appearance at the end of the Eliza section serves to return the focus of the narrative to men. For, like the majority of Jones's work, most of *Last Supper* concentrates on the telling of his/story. This story starts with that of Uncle Tom and is told and retold in various form throughout the dance. This is the story of black men in a white man's world—the history of racism and tales of its (and their) survival. This authorial voice is evident from the beginning of the cabin section, embodied in the onstage figure of the narrator by Justice Allen. Much like a master of ceremonies, Allen welcomes the audience to *Uncle Tom's Cabin* and introduces the figure of Harriet Beecher Stowe, played by Sage Cowles. Allen and Cowles take turns telling the story of *Uncle Tom's Cabin* until the figure of Uncle Tom is introduced into the scenario. Uncle Tom is played by Andrea Smith—a strapping young man who infuses this character with a riveting stage presence. His powerful voice is first heard in sermon. Up until this moment, no one within the staged drama has spoken; all the other characters' thoughts, feelings, and actions have either been mimed or narrated by someone else. The fact that Uncle Tom controls his own voice gives him an immediate dignity within this minstrel setting. In *Last Night on Earth*, Jones mentions the combination of optimism, gentleness, and sensuality that he thought Smith could embody in his portrayal of Uncle Tom. "André was young in many senses of the word, and the openness and curiosity implied by his youth were necessary in re-creating such a worn, misunderstood icon as Uncle Tom."[24]

Re-created by Jones's directorial vision, this Uncle Tom is vulnerable yet strong; young but wise. Interestingly, Smith's presence onstage immediately stands out in contrast to the minstrel icons surrounding him. Whereas their movements are often puppet-like, repetitive, and spatially truncated, his physical presence is grounded but graceful, with his arms arching to the heavens. Working in unison with his voice, his movement commands attention. Preaching, he stands above the others like a magnificent old tree whose branches dance in the wind all the while being rooted deeply to the earth. Uncle Tom's spiritual and inspirational leadership is foregrounded by Jones's use of theatrical retrograde. After Uncle Tom is killed by Simon Legree and ascends to heaven, Stowe asks what is there for those who are left behind. The cast faces out and together shouts "Freedom!" Refusing closure in order to rewrite the possibilities of another kind of resistance back into the story, Jones stops the play and all the characters backtrack through their movements until the scene where Legree tries to "break Tom's Spirit." Here, Jones reproduces, with a crucial difference, the stylized whipping of slaves by Legree. Instead of one or two characters, the whole cast comes back out without masks and one by one lines up to confront Legree. Shaking their heads "NO!" and circling their arms in front of their bodies in a defiantly martial gesture, these people—black, white, young, old, male, female—refuse Legree's domination, even as he whips them. They line up again and again such that Legree has a constant group of protesters in his face. Their perseverance, and their refusal to become submissive (like Tom's refusal to be beaten down even as he is beaten up), makes Legree's relentless whipping gesture look increasingly ridiculous.

In this section, Jones set up a narrative logic that he will pursue throughout *Last Supper at Uncle Tom's Cabin/The Promised Land*. Scene after scene, Jones highlights the importance of African-American men's experience and then connects that experience to issues of power, exclusion, pain, and survival that affect us all. Allen, Smith, Hubbard, and Arthur Aviles are spotlighted as the central figures, as various embodiments of Christ in the Last Supper. In the documentary on the making of this dance, Jones tells us "this dance is a dance about differences—race, sexual, class. About how we can work through those differences and move to another place." The desire to balance a sense of specific history with a sense of global harmony serves as the impetus for the following sections of the dance (the Supper and the Promised Land), in which Uncle Tom becomes Bill T. Jones; becomes Justice Allen; becomes Christ; becomes naked; becomes us all.

After an interlude in which Bill T. Jones improvises to his mother's singing and praying, the Supper begins with a live depiction of Leonardo da Vinci's famous painting. Standing in front of the allegorical tableau is Justice Allen, holding an imaginary basketball and dribbling in slow motion. He then joins the tableau that metamorphoses into a group dance, leaving Smith and Allen standing facing one another on the table. Inching closer to one another, seemingly arguing, it then becomes clear that their old-fashioned-sounding language is not medieval English or even Shakespeare, but rather Martin Luther King Jr.'s "I Have a Dream" speech recited backwards. All of a sudden, this long table is a meeting place where King's speech becomes the connective tissue that draws Uncle Tom—an antebellum fictional character, as well as a layered iconic image that must be grappled with, to Justice Allen—an example of the complex and conflicted life situations in which many African-American men find themselves. As these two men stand side by side, their attention (and the audience's) shifts to Arthur Aviles, who is dancing onstage in front of them. The physical strength and fluidity of Aviles's dancing, the kinesthetic dynamism of his body, offers a palatable release from the angst of their spoken words.

Eventually, Allen comes forward and sits down to tell us a rap version of his own life story. He begins the tale with "Young, gifted, and black was my identity." Caught up in a racist system, he goes to war and then to jail, describing himself as "just another nigger in a cracker box." At this point there is a chorus in which the company joins him, echoing the first words of each line.

> SLAVE—three fifths of a man
> BIAS—it's the law of the land
> DEATH—better fight if you can, 'cause clubs is trumps in the corporal plan
> TIME—the master of illusion
> PAIN—the core of this confusion
> LOVE—an emotional intrusion, survival tools were my only solution

The last two verses, which bring Allen's story up to the present performance, reveal a self-empowerment and a decision to take responsibility for his own future, ending with "now I'm rockin' 'round the world with Bill T. Jones."[25] A stunning tale of survival, Allen's autobiographical rap transforms Uncle Tom's faith in God and King's faith in humanity into a reconstructed faith in his own self. Allen's story is powerful not only because we believe its truthfulness and are activated by its rhythms, but also because it stands as part of the epic chain of black men's histories resurrected in Jones's work.

Resurrection in the sense of rebirth—even in the more literal sense of arising from the dead with a new knowledge—is one of the central themes in Urban Bush Women's *Bones and Ash: A Gilda Story*. In this her/story, choreographer Jawole Willa Jo Zollar and her company are joined by the writer Jewelle Gomez, the composer Toshi Reagon, and codirector Steven Kent in a dance/theater collaboration that re-creates another nineteenth-century literary genre—that of the vampire story. Jewelle Gomez's lesbian vampire novel *The Gilda Stories* serves as the textual basis for *Bones and Ash*, although some features of the novel were dropped and others were added to make this story into a performance. In this reinvention of the gothic genre, the self-indulgent, obsessive vampire figure is transformed into a caring, maternal angel-cum-lover; a spiritual guide for humanity. In the context of the

African-American tradition, sharing blood is an aspect of mutual exchange, marking a respect for balance based on African ideologies of ritual sacrifice. Gomez's work is much more surreal than Stowe's domestic novel. It chronicles the evolution of the character Girl, from her rescue as a runaway slave in 1850 and her conversion into the vampire Gilda (what is called somewhat euphemistically the "long life"), through the twentieth century, right into the future in a chapter entitled "Land of Enchantment 2050." Although the need for theatrical coherence has limited the time frames of *Bones and Ash,* the performance still highlights a sense of history as a continuum of people—a literal bloodline that, interestingly enough, has little to do with biological family and more to do with generations of communities. Epic in scale and mythic in genre, *Bones and Ash* traces historical change through the life of one body—one body, that is, that will live for hundreds of years.

Like Gomez's novel, *Bones and Ash* has two central vampire characters: Gilda (originally played by Deborah Thomas in 1995 and later played by Pat Hall-Smith) and Bird (played by Emerald Trinket Monsod, a guest artist). These two women's historical knowledge gives them both the wisdom and the responsibility to guide their surrogate daughter—the runaway slave Girl (played by company member Christine King). Gilda, who lived in Brazil several hundred years ago, runs a bordello with her lover, Bird—a Filipino woman who lived with the Lakota tribe before starting this life. It is the coming of yet another war—the Civil War—that compels Gilda to give up her eternal life. But before Gilda can cross over into the Promised Land, she and Bird must teach Girl how to understand her terrifying nightly dreams, which mix images of past fears and present realities. They must teach her how to fully understand her history so that she can begin to envision her future. These lessons take the form of a dancing apprenticeship in which Bird helps Girl to remember her own body by leading her through a series of martial dance forms. These dances give Girl a renewed sense of agency and pride, and it is only after the dancing has taught her to be physically present that Girl can begin to remember and embrace her own history: "Of her home their mother spoke about, the girl was less certain. It was always a dream place—distant, unreal. Except the talk of dancing . . . Talking of it now, her body rocked slightly as if she had been rewoven into that old circle of dancers. She poured out the images and names, proud of her own ability to weave a story. Bird smiled at her pupil who claimed her past, reassuring her silently."[26]

Once Girl has reclaimed her past, once she has found the voice with which she can tell her own history, Gilda can move on, bequeathing her spirit and her name to Girl. Because Gilda is a vampire, her "gift of long life" takes place as an "exchange of blood," where the two individuals involved in the exchange suck blood (not from the neck, as one might expect, but from a space just below the breast). This motif of exchange—of blood, life, and body—reverberates throughout the individual biomythography of Jewell Gomez. In her collection of writings, *Forty-Three Septembers,* Gomez has a piece entitled "Transubstantiation: This is my Body, This is my Blood." She begins this essay with a simple summation of the contradictions which defined her childhood religious experience: "I was raised a Black Catholic in a white Catholic town."[27] Although Gomez has since revised her spirituality to accommodate more fully her life choices, the passion and the physical vitality of that early training has never really left her. Thus, the blood of communion becomes the blood of social action and a belief in the interconnectedness of people and their histories.

> The key is in the sea change: the place where the small incident is transformed into the belief, the daily wine into the blood. In that change I am learning to treasure the things of my past without being limited by them. [. . .] To make the past a dimension of my life, but not the only perspective from which I view it. In that way my youth is not more important than my middle years; . . . my knowledge is not better or truer than anyone else's, its value comes when it is made useful to others."[28]

For Gomez, blood becomes the bond becomes the body that can change, through the redemptive power of love, the ordinary into the spiritual, life into history, and words into a dance.

In *Bones and Ash,* however, the exchange of blood is not the central event that it is in Gomez's novel. Rather, it is the exchange of movement, of energy, of dancing between the company that signals the physical and spiritual interconnectedness of the women onstage. This is most striking in the dancing sections, which serve as metaphoric frames to the narrative action of the first act. The opening scene of *Bones and Ash* is a prologue spoken from the present about the past. The light comes up slowly to reveal a lone figure, moving through the shadows of the stage's dim lighting. An offstage voice is heard speaking memories about a life that has lasted many centuries. The woman onstage begins a solo that will parallel many of the emotional states called forth by the poetic prose. At times she lifts her arms slowly, fluidly, stretching her body luxuriously. Other times she skips lightheartedly, and yet other times she seems agitated. Although she is silent, it is clear that we are hearing her memories, her thoughts, her story. Images of cotton and blood are woven into a tapestry of reflection that speaks of slavery and a historical memory that is an ongoing puzzle. For the past, like the vampires at the center of this story, refuses to "lie down and die."

> The shape of my life is motion through fields, through time, through blood. Each decade is woven into the next, embroidered centuries draped across my shoulders, a rainbow of lives, everyone my own. Behind me—one hundred and

fifty years of those I've loved, those I've lost. All taking or giving blood. Dangerous, Reviving, Vital. The thin red line I follow down one row, up the next. A rhythmic dance draws the attention of the gods—Yemeya, Yellow Woman and many others. I am enamored of motion.

Someone said to me once: It must be hard in this world being black, descended from slaves, 'buked and scorned, benign neglect. I said no . . . actually it's being two hundred years old that pulls my patience. To live forever is a puzzle. Each piece snapping into place beside the next, but the picture is never fully seen.[29]

This sense of life and history as movement is triply reflected in the figures of the Irissas who soon enter upstage. In the program for *Bones and Ash,* these characters are described as the oldest teachers—the wise elders who guide their vampire family through the ages.[30] Danced by Gacirah Diagne, Beverley Prentice, and Christine Wright, these dancing sages often appear behind the scrim or sheer curtains, as if they are protecting, by the mere fact of their presence and attention, those onstage. In the prologue, they haunt the upstage space, emerging from the shadows to follow Girl's journey across the space. Quick and light-footed, breathy yet grounded and forceful, their dancing can shift unexpectedly from a slow, steady bowing and rising motion to a whirling dervish-like spinning that sweeps across the stage, sending energy out in every direction. Their breathing is often audible, and sometimes they whisper or sing advice to the central characters. Half Greek chorus, half African shaman, the Irissas embody archetypal spirits whose presence underlines the fact of life's continuity.[31]

The Irissas's presence in *Bones and Ash* provides a historical metanarrative to the specific action going on downstage, for they embody the past as well as the future. In many ways, their otherworldly presence has an angel-like quality. The main characters may sense the Irissas as they move with or surround them, but they never seem to see these dancing spirits. Like the vampires in Gomez's novel, the Irissas can hear other people's thoughts, and entering their minds, make them more positive. They remind me of the trench-coated angel figures in Wim Wenders's film *Wings of Desire,* whose very presence next to someone on a subway can alter the most cynical and disheartened thoughts, bestowing the gift of hope. In the middle of the first act, the Irissas chant the mantra of life-enriching vampires: "We take blood not life. Leave something in exchange." Indeed, the difference between good vampires—embodied by Gilda and Bird, and bad ones—embodied in the figure of Fox, is clearly demonstrated in the first act. When Gilda and Bird come upon a distressed figure flailing around the stage, obviously confused, they surround him with sympathy; embracing him more like sisters than vampires, even as they take the blood they need. When they leave him, his sense of purpose is restored. In contrast, Fox seduces a woman with a courtly dance, and then leaves her dead.

In her study of vampires in nineteenth- and twentieth-century literature, wittily entitled *Our Vampires, Ourselves,* Nina Auerbach expresses her frustration with what she calls the "anestheticizing virtue" of these good fairy vampires in Gomez's novel:

> Instead of killing mortals, Gilda and her friends bestow on them edifying dreams after taking fortifying sips of blood. Vampirism is not bloodsucking or feeding or the dark gift; it becomes "the exchange," an act of empathy, not power, whose first principle is, "feel what they are needing, not what you are hungering for" (p.50). Like the construction of lesbianism *The Gilda Stories* celebrates, vampirism is purged of aggression.[32]

Although they do not fit into Auerbach's own definition of power as domination, the vampires in both *The Gilda Stories* and *Bones and Ash* provide what I consider a radical new vision of humanity. It is certainly true that these vampires do not excite that frisson of dangerous seductivity that seems a mainstay of traditional vampire novels. Yet their commitment to a sense of common bond with others, even those very different from themselves (i.e., mortals), presents an intriguing reconfiguration of identity, desire, and love within this gothic genre. The vampire figure rewritten as storyteller, as griotte, as spiritual guide, is a compelling example of how *Bones and Ash* weaves an Afrocentric belief in the interconnectedness of the world into a European literary genre. Drawing on performative traditions that include ritual possession, as well as West African and disaporan dance cultures, Urban Bush Women's collaborative epic builds on these influences to create the climatic ending of act 1, where Gilda "crosses over" to her final death. Once Gilda has decided to leave this world, she first initiates Girl into the vampire life. At this moment, the theatrical action or "plot" is temporarily suspended as Gilda and Girl are joined by the Irissas in a ritual exchange of identity.

As Gilda's farewell letter is read by an offstage voice, Gilda begins her journey back to the earth. Alone onstage, Gilda emerges from the shadows with movements that suggest she is struggling to find the right pathway back. Her dancing becomes more convulsive as she continues; flinging her long sandy blond dreadlocks first in one direction and then in another. Turning here and then there, bending down and arching up, twisting one way and then another, she seems to be fighting with her own choice, dissatisfied with every available position. Slowly, the background fills with the rest of the company, newly dressed in African robes. They line up at the back of the stage as if they are protecting her from what lies beyond. Drawn to their presence, Gilda moves back and forth across their space, trying to find the right fit—the right rhythm, the right pathway, the right expression for her death. A drummer enters the space, accompanying her movement with ambient sound. Soon, however, the company's breaths take on a rhythm of their own as they speak and then sing to Gilda. The drummer joins their rhythm and then starts to intensify it as Gilda works herself into a state of divine possession. Suddenly, this energy quiets down as she opens her body to the voyage over. Two women help her to disrobe, and a priestess figure (played by Valerie Winborne) begins to sing "Coming Home Through the Morning Light," metaphorically washing Gilda down with her powerful voice. A slide of a river delta, then a close-up of the river are projected on the back scrim as Gilda opens the curtains and disappears into the water.

The exchange of energy between the company and Gilda in this last scene is paradigmatic of much of Urban Bush Women's work in which an individual transformation is assisted by the energy of the group. This sense of interconnectedness between self and community is reflective of both the present moment and a historical continuity—defining who your community is at present and who your community was several hundred years ago. As their name suggests, Urban Bush Women bring their ancestral roots into the twentieth century. In commenting on the diversity of African-American women within the company, Veta Goler describes what she calls the "stunning mosaic of black womanhood." Despite the clear celebration of individuality, Urban Bush Women's work usually focuses on the sense of community between women. Goler describes this legacy of collective experience:

> Historically, black women have always established ways of coming together
> for mutual benefit. From the female networks in the family compounds of
> traditional African societies to the club movement and extended families of the
> New World, black women have supported and affirmed each other. Urban Bush
> Women's name evokes images of women assisting each other in maneuvering
> for their survival within challenging environments.[33]

Most of Zollar's choreography for Urban Bush Women centers on the cultural experiences of African-American women, creating what Goler calls a "cultural autobiography."

In many ways, the trope of the vampire allows Zollar to trace that cultural autobiography through different bodies. In this vein, vampires can help us to create a new sense of family, subverting the notion of bloodlines to fit different styles of familiar relationships. This is clearly a theme within Gomez's novel, which focuses on the vampire as lesbian more than *Bones and Ash* does. The lesbian perspective of Gomez's novel (which has several steamy passages) is replaced by a less sexual and more womanist perspective in Zollar's choreography. What gets exchanged through the dancing in *Bones and Ash* is not so much desire, but memory and history. Urban Bush Women is the only professional African-American women's dance company, and Zollar and the company members are committed to making manifest that legacy of challenge, survival, and hope. In an essay entitled "The New Moderns: the Paradox of Eclecticism and Singularity," Halifu Osumare describes Zollar in terms that echo her sense of legacy: "In Jawole Willa Jo Zollar one sees Katherine Dunham's and Pearl Primus' fierce passion for roots, their bold adventurousness in walking the urban back alleys and the rural dirt villages to research their subject matter, and their ingenious artistic transformation of cultural information."[34]

Given her very conscious representations of African-American women's cultural experiences in her choreography, I was surprised to find out that Zollar does not see herself as directly addressing issues of race or gender in her work. This is not to say that Zollar is not acutely aware of racism or misogyny within representations of African-American women. Anyone who was present at her plenary talk at the 1990 Dance Critics Association conference in Los Angeles cannot doubt her commitment to these issues.[35] However, she does not foreground the categories of race and gender in quite the way that Jones does. Instead, she builds on a specific cultural experience right from the start, never framing race as a topic within the performance, but rather speaking right away in an Afrocentric idiom. This strategy allows Zollar to claim a black female voice while also refusing the problematic assumption that by claiming that culturally rooted voice, you are speaking only to people with knowledge of that specific experience. Rather, Zollar believes, as does Jones, that ultimately, many experiences of exclusion and oppression, as well as inclusion and community, are shared across cultural differences.

Although Jones's work originates within the historical perspective of an African-American gay man, his work continually interrogates these identities, even while claiming them. In the Cabin and Eliza on the Ice sections of his dance discussed earlier, Jones questions the constructions of race and gender. In almost every scene, the audience is confronted with the issues surrounding how we come to see blackness, maleness, and femaleness. But what is also clear is that we are never allowed to see these performers, even when they are in blackface or drag, as statically defined objects of our gaze. In this work, performers claim and embody identities in ways that resist pat or simplistic constructions of race, gender, or sexuality. Thus when Justice Allen tells his life story, he both fulfills a stereotype of the black criminal on drugs, but at the same time refuses its deterministic rigormortis by also claiming an identity as a writer and performer who is "rockin' 'round the world with Bill T. Jones."

Jones is a deconstructionist at heart and rarely gives his audience any answers to the questions he insistently asks. What he does give us is a through line of spectacular dancing. This is undeniably the role that Arthur Aviles (a self-described New York-rican, who is one of the company's most virtuosic dancers) takes on throughout *Last Supper*. Although he does not have a speaking role, and is never placed in a specific identity (such as Greg Hubbard's drag scene at the end of Eliza on the Ice), his dancing serves as a sort of physical antidote to the existential quandaries implied by the text. This is true of the scene in which he is dancing downstage while "Uncle Tom" and Allen are speaking on the table. It is also Aviles's dancing that precipitates the final section of the dance, the Promised Land, in which the stage is flooded with fifty-two naked people of all sizes and shapes, who stand and face the audience.

I see Aviles's dancing as the physical metaphor for faith—the other focus of Jones's epic dance. Even as Jones doggedly deconstructs our assumptions about race, gender, life choices, family, he relies on a leap of faith to take his audience to the Promised Land. His improvisational questioning (maybe grilling is a more apt word) of a member of the clergy chosen from whichever community he is performing in is relentless. On the video of the premiere at the Brooklyn Academy of Music, he is talking with Paul Abel, a gay minister. After asking him a series of questions: "What is faith? Is Christianity a slave religion? What is evil? Is AIDS punishment from God?" Jones probes Abel's feelings about serving a religion that does not recognize his own life choices. Yet this line of questioning takes place after two scenes in which faith is reclaimed: Jones's improvising to his mother's praying, and his dancing to the story of Job as narrated by the clergy. In both instances, Jones's dancing, like Aviles's, fills an existential void with a potent physical reality. Even though Jones questions faith in the midst of loss, he can still choreograph dances in which being present in the world with others takes on a healing spirituality. This is certainly the message of the final scene. In his autobiography, Jones sums it up this way:

> The Promised Land, with its hordes of naked flesh coming wave after wave into the footlights, pubic patches, pert breasts, sagging breasts, wrinkled knees, blissful eyes, furtive expressions of shame, is a visual manifestation of my profound sense of belonging. This was my portrait of us. All of us. And this is who I am too. One of us. It was my battle to disavow any identity as a dying outcast and to affirm our commonality. In it, some one thousand people from thirty cities stood naked, took a bow, and said, "We are not afraid."[36]

This mass of naked humanity is meant to place the very real bodily differences of race, age, ability, and gender in the midst of a symbolic embodiment of vulnerability and sameness. One wonders, however, how different things really are once the euphoric final moments have subsided and everyone is clothed again. Although he began *Uncle Tom's Cabin/The Promised Land* with a searing critique of race, mimesis, and representation, Jones ends this epic dance rather blandly, bringing his audience through a potentially uncomfortable confrontation with histories of domination and survival to a present-day *communitas*. Is community really that easy? Didn't the 1960s teach us that politics are harder to change than one's clothes?

Like Jones's piece, *Bones and Ash* draws on African-American memory and spirituality to stage the history of black women's bodies. Registering both the abuse and resistance of these women's lives, *Bones and Ash* celebrates a spirituality based on the interconnectedness of past, present, and future. In Gomez's and Urban Bush Women's vision, the exchange of self and other is considered an intersubjective act—not one of domination and subordination. This exchange of life force that does not destroy one partner (be it another person or the environment) but rather creates a mutual energy, is, of course, a wonderful model of performer/audience interaction—a model of responsiveness that is also grounded in African aesthetics and spirituality. Watching this piece, I came to appreciate the interconnectedness between the women onstage without feeling a need to identify their experience as my own. Unlike the final scenes in *The Promised Land* where difference is multiplied to the point of losing its meaning in a mass of humanity, *Bones and Ash* holds onto its own cultural moorings. I do not think that this differentiation is necessarily a problem. Indeed, it might be a very healthy distinction, one that recognizes the interconnectedness of our histories without erasing the importance of difference in choreographing the body's identity.

NOTES

1. Toni Morrison, "The Site of Memory," in *Out There: Marginalization and Contemporary Cultures,* ed. Russell Ferguson, Martha Gever, Trinh T. Minh-ha, Cornel West (New York: The New Museum of Contemporary Art, and Cambridge MA: MIT Press, 1990), 303.

2. Trinh T. Minh-ha, *Woman, Native, Other: Writing Postcoloniality and Feminism* (Bloomington: Indiana University Press, 1989), 119.

3. Ibid., 121.

4. Ibid., 122.

5. This is the excuse that Sue-Ellen Case uses in her simultaneous recognition and dismissal of theater by women of color at the end of her book *Feminism and Theater.* For an interesting analysis of her critical position see Michael Awkward, *Negotiating Difference: Race, Gender, and the Politics of Positionality* (Chicago: University of Chicago Press, 1995), 87–90.

6. Awkward, *Negotiating Difference,* 60.

7. Ibid.

8. Ibid., 61.

9. Adrienne Rich quoted in Awkward, 1995, 41.

10. Richard Yarborough, "Strategies of Black Characterization in *Uncle Tom's*

Cabin and the Early Afro-American Novel," in *New Essays on Uncle Tom's Cabin*, ed. Eric J. Sundquist (New York: Cambridge University Press, 1986), 63.

11. Jane Tompkins, *Sensational Designs: The Cultural Work of American Fiction 1790–1860* (New York: Oxford University Press, 1985), 124.

12. Eric Lott, *Love and Theft: Blackface Minstrelsy and the American Working Class* (New York: Oxford University Press, 1993), 214.

13. Ibid., 221.

14. *New York Daily Times*, July 27, 1853, quoted in Lott, 216. For more on Germon's acting see Thomas Gossett, *Uncle Tom's Cabin and American Culture* (Dallas: Southern Methodist University Press, 1985), 278–79.

15. Lott, 228.

16. Bill T. Jones, *Last Night on Earth* (New York: Pantheon Books, 1995), 205.

17. Ibid., 206.

18. Lott, 236.

19. In his book *Love and Theft*, Eric Lott elaborates the multiple and complex layers of meaning and subversion in the American minstrel tradition, complicating the analysis of blackface that only points out its racist stereotypes by asking what kinds of unconscious desires and conscious class connections are also negotiated in blacking up.

20. Harriet Beecher Stowe, *Uncle Tom's Cabin or, Life Among the Lowly* (New York: Penguin, 1987), 44.

21. Jacqueline Shea Murphy, "Unrest and Uncle Tom: Bill T. Jones/Arnie Zane Dance Company's *Last Supper at Uncle Tom's Cabin/The Promised Land*," in *Bodies of the Text: Dance as Theory, Literature as Dance*, ed. Ellen W. Goellner and Jacqueline Shea Murphy (New Brunswick, NJ: Rutgers University Press, 1995), 82.

22. Jones, 214.

23. I thank Caroline Jackson-Smith for pointing out this reading to me.

24. Jones, 207.

25. Allen's text is printed in the program for the world premiere of *Last Supper at Uncle Tom's Cabin/The Promised Land*.

26. Jewelle Gomez, *The Gilda Stories* (Ithaca, NY: Firebrand Books, 1991), 39.

27. Jenelle Gomez, *Forty-Three Septembers* (Ithaca, NY: Firebrand Books, 1993), 69.

28. Ibid., 78–79.

29. This quotation is a transcription of the narrator's voiceover during this section of the piece.

30. I saw a performance of *Bones and Ash* in Columbus, Ohio, on September 23, 1995, and another one in New York City in November 1996. I am grateful to the company for providing me with an early video of their performance in Iowa City (September 15, 1995). These are the sources for my movement descriptions in the piece. As with any performance work, the dancing and even the text can go through various and multiple revisions. Recently, Pat Hall-Smith has replaced Deborah Thomas as Gilda in the first act.

31. Although the Irissas are not featured in Gomez's *The Gilda Stories* per se, there are teacher characters like them in the novel, particularly Sorel and Anthony.

32. Nina Auerbach, *Our Vampires, Ourselves* (Chicago: University of Chicago Press, 1995), 185.

33. Veta Goler, "Dancing Herself: Choreography, Autobiography, and the Expression of the Black Woman Self in the Work of Dianne McIntyre, Blondell Cummings and Jawole Willa Jo Zollar," PhD diss., Emory University, 1994, 167.

34. Halifu Osumare, "The New Moderns: the Paradox of Eclecticism and Singularity," in *African American Genius in Modern Dance,* ed. Gerald E. Myers, American Dance Festival, 1993.

35. See the printed version of Zollar's talk in David Gere, ed., *Looking Out: Perspectives on Dance and Criticism in a Multicultural World* (New York: Schirmer Books, 1995).

36. Jones, 223.

17

Matters of Tact

Writing History from the Inside Out

Dance Research Journal 35 no. 2; 36, no. 1, 2003–2004.

Long before I became a committed academic, long before I was a college professor teaching dance history, long before terminal degrees and professional titles, I chanced upon an exhibition of early dance photographs at the Rodin Museum in Paris. I bought the small catalogue, and from time to time I would page through the striking black-and-white images searching for dancing inspiration. I always paused at a certain one of Loïe Fuller. There she is, radiant in the sunlight of Rodin's garden; chest open, arms spread like great wings, running full force toward the camera. It is an image of a strong, mature woman—one who exudes a joyful, earthy energy. A copy of this photograph taken in 1900 by Eugène Druet currently hangs above my desk.

Let's begin with traces. Traces of the past. Traces of a dance. Traces of light . . . and color and fabric. Traces of a body, animating all these sources of movement. Traces of a life, spent spinning across nations, across centuries, across identities. How do we trace the past? Reconfigure what is lost? Are traces always even visible?

With a nod to the meanings embedded in historical study, Walter Benjamin once wrote: "To dwell means to leave traces."[1] Indeed, traces are the material artifacts that constitute the stuff of historical inquiry—the bits and pieces of a life that scholars follow, gather up, and survey. The word itself suggests the actual imprint of a figure who has passed—the footprint, mark, or impression of a person or event. These kinds of traces are omnipresent in the case of Loïe Fuller. Some traces are more visible than others; some more easily located. But all traces—once noticed—draw us into another reality.

Someone passed this way before.

I had been thinking about writing a book on Loïe Fuller for some time, but it took me awhile to come to terms with how I wanted to respond to the less visible traces of her work. My book project began with a question: why do so many critics and historians dismiss the bodily experience of her dancing in their discussions of Fuller's theatrical work? The question grew into a dance. The dance, in turn, taught me how to write history from inside the vibrations of its ongoing motion. This is the story of an intellectual approach to the past that not only recognizes the corporeal effects of the historian's vantage point, but also mobilizes her body within the process of research and writing. This is the story of a dance shared across a century of time and two continents, a dance that takes place at the meeting point of physical empathy and historical difference.

Perhaps we should lose the noun, which renders us nostalgic, maybe even melancholic at the extreme. Replace our ambition to find out what happened with a curiosity about how it came to be that it was happening. Replace traces with tracing—the past with the passion. Tracing the contours of fabric which spiral upward and outward, we spill over beyond any one historical or aesthetic discourse. This act of tracing can help us become aware not only of what's visible, but also what is, has been, will always be, less clearly visible. Beyond the image into the motion.

I am engaged in writing on Fuller. I use this term "engaged" very consciously, for I want to highlight both the sense of binding oneself to another person and its etymological meaning as "interlocking"—a literal as well as a figurative meshing with someone or something. I have chosen to work on this project in a way that integrates conceptual and somatic knowledge, engaging my physical as well as my intellectual and analytic facilities. Dancing amidst clouds of fabric in elaborate lighting effects, I try to understand something of Fuller's experience from the inside out. I also dance with words; moving with my writing to see how ideas resonate in my body. Then too, as I weave my way through archival materials and historical accounts of cultural milieus, I practice staying attentive to what I have learned through that dancing experience. This research process challenges traditional separations between academic scholarship and artistic creation, between criticism and autobiography—in short, between dancing and writing. More than just another layer of historical excavation, my dancing creates a strand of physical thinking that weaves back and forth between the presence of historical artifacts (posters, reviews, photos, memoirs, and paintings) and the absence of Fuller's physical motion.

This essay is an attempt to articulate the theoretical implications of my rather quixotic methodology; an attempt to understand the very conditions of its possibilities. In what follows, I identify two strategies—two practices, if you will—that guide my scholarship on Fuller. While one is primarily intellectual and the other is based in physical study, both practices refuse the conventional separation of scholarship and the studio, folding themselves into a mix of dancing and writing that houses a certain physical receptiveness at its core. These strands of embodied study create a textured fabric in which aspects of Fuller's work are made visible through my body, as well as my writing.

Tracing the past—the past in light of the present. Present tense, the tension produced by the conjunction of light and dance—the subjunctive mode—the connection of her and me. She. Aware of my desire to trace history through choreography, to write with my body, I meet another's dancing with my own.

> In all writing, a body is traced, is the tracing and the trace—is the letter, yet never the letter; a literality, or rather, a lettericity, that is no longer legible. A body is what cannot be read in writing. (Or one has to understand reading as something other than decipherment.) Rather, as touching, as being touched. Writing, reading: matters of tact.)[2]

Despite its linguistic unwieldiness (an effect, no doubt, of the difficulties of translation), this quotation from Jean-Luc Nancy's "Corpus" signals what is for me a profound difference in my current approach to historical work. Moving from traces to tracing incorporates the tactile, and thereby refuses the traditional separation of object from subject. Reaching across time and space to touch Fuller's dancing means that I allow myself, in turn, to be touched, for it is impossible to touch anything in a way that does not also implicate one's own body. Touching, then, becomes the space of our interaction, a mutual engagement. As I touch Fuller through my historical research, both textual and physical, I am touched in return.

Spinning in this vortex of historical representation and kinesthetic legibility, I read the exchange, rewrite the communication because in my time the core dynamic remains the same, but the periphery changes. My skin is the silk is the cloth which extends her dancing into light and my dancing in and among the folds of others. Did you get it? Skin is my silk, my way of dancing beyond myself and losing the dancer in the dance. Contact. As the context changes, the contact changes, but the passion remains the same, for contact is the way I connect across, through, by way of, with, for, and among her desires to know the other; to know God or love. This exchange powers me for it holds the passion, the weight, the grit, and the friction that sent her whirling among clouds of fabric and sends me turning into the bodies of those around me.

This metaphysical conundrum (How is one touched by history?) has, in my case, a very physical complement. Much of my dance experience over the past two decades has been generated by a form of contemporary dance called contact improvisation. In contact improvisation, the actual point of contact (defined, most usually, in terms of physical touching, although it can be rhythmic, visual, or kinesthetic) creates an improvisational space in which assumptions as to what the dance will be like (future tense) are eschewed in favor of a curiosity about what is happening now (present tense). The meeting point of contact improvisation creates an interconnectedness of weight, momentum, and energy that channels a common physical destiny. The partnering in contact improvisation is not simply an addition of one movement to another, but rather a realization that both movements will change in the midst of the improvisational duet. In addition to learning how to meet others in a dance, contact improvisation dancers train in extreme spatial disorientation. Releasing the uprightness of the body and learning how to be comfortable upside down, rolling, and spiraling in and out of the floor, falling without fear—these are all aspects of a training that redirects visual orientation into a kinesthetic grounding.

I think of the physical aspects of my research on Fuller in terms of a contact improvisation duet. My body is influenced by her dancing as I imagine how she must have used her spine, her head, her chest. Spinning with my arms raised high and my head thrown back, historical descriptions of Fuller laid up in bed with excruciating pain and ice packs on her upper back begin to make sense. I realize that Fuller may have slipped a disc in her cervical spine. These kinds of biographical details resonate in my body as I incorporate some aspects of the physical tolls her nightly performances must have incurred. Even on an intellectual or metaphysical level, I think of our interaction as a contact improvisation duet—a somatic meeting set up by the traces of history. I believe that envisioning this relation in terms of an improvisational duet usefully redefines the traditional separation of a historical subject (treated as the "object" of study) and the omniscient writer of history. When, for instance, I review the enormous variety of images of La Loïe—the posters, photographs, paintings, prints, and program covers—I try not only to analyze the visual representation of her work, but also to imagine the kind of dancing that inspired such visions. That is to say that I allow myself to be touched (these "matters of tact") by what remains only partially visible.

In her introduction to *Choreographing History,* Susan Foster also sees the interaction of historian and the bodies of history as a dynamic tango between traces and tracing—artifacts and the language that reanimates their cultural significance. Her notion of "bodily theorics" engages with similar metaphors of writing history as a tactile duet—an improvisational connection between past and present bodies. But, she reminds us:

> This affiliation, based on a kind of kinesthetic empathy between living and
> dead but imagined bodies, enjoys no primal status outside the world of writing.
> It possesses no organic authority; it offers no ultimate validation for sentiment.
> But it is redolent with physical vitality and embraces a concern for beings that
> live and have lived. Once the historian's body recognizes value and meaning in
> kinesthesia, it cannot dis-animate the physical action of past bodies it has begun
> to sense.[3]

Like so many before me, I am seduced by the snake, caught up in her serpentine motion. That sign of a journey that never ends, never finds a destination. The movement of her silks suspended in the air; the figure eight traced by my arms as I spin beneath the shower of fabric, interpreting what my motion says about her history. Hungry to know more, to feel the power that generates her waves of motion, I study the place of this motif in Art Nouveau, read about late nineteenth-century Orientalism, dismiss as overly deterministic the lesbian reading of this figure as sexual insignia. I claim all of the above; none of the above.

Loïe Fuller is one of the most interesting and paradoxical figures in early modern dance. Born in 1862 in Chicago, Fuller began performing in her teens—first as a temperance speaker and later as a member of the Buffalo Bill troupe, touring America on the vaudeville circuit. Her various dramatic roles included cross-dressed ones, such as the lead in the fast-paced melodrama *Little Jack Sheppard,* but it is as a Serpentine, or skirt dancer, that she became well-known. In the 1890s, Fuller created an extraordinary sensation in Paris with her manipulations of hundreds of yards of silk, swirling high above her and lit dramatically from below. She embodied the fin-de-siècle images of woman as flower, woman as bird, woman as fire, woman as nature. One of the most famous dancers of her time, Fuller starred as the main act at the Folies Bergère, inspiring a host of contemporary fashions and imitators. Fuller's serpentine motif is also visible in much of the decorative imagery of Art Nouveau, and she was the subject of many works by renowned artists like Rodin, Toulouse-Lautrec, and Mallarmé. Yet despite the importance of her artistic legacy, Fuller's theatrical work fits uneasily within the dominant narratives of early modern dance. Most historians do not see Fuller in light of the development of expressive movement, but rather relegate her to discussions concerning dance and lighting, or dance and technology.

Fuller's work embodies a central paradox of dance as a representation of both abstract movement and a physical body. Her dancing epitomizes the intriguing insubstantiality of movement caught in the process of tracing itself. Surrounded by a funnel of swirling fabric spiraling upwards into the space around her and bathed in colored lights of her own invention, Fuller's body seems to evaporate in the midst of her spectacle. Nonetheless, her body is undeniably present, and discussions of Fuller's sartorial style and physical girth break through these romantic representations of her ethereality and femininity in interesting ways. Splayed across history and geography, Fuller's dancing takes place at the crossroads of diverse languages, two centuries, and many cultural changes.

Intellectually, the material is fascinating. But there is something even more compelling for me in this subject. It is a gut thing. I feel that many scholars cover over the kinesthetic and material experience of her body in favor of the image, rather than reading that image as an extension of her dancing. Descriptions of Fuller's work get so entangled with artistic images or poetic renderings that they easily forget the physical labor involved. Then too, there are all those apologies and side notes about how Loïe Fuller did not have a dancer's body, or any dance training really; as if the movement images were solely dependent on the lighting; as if it were all technologically rendered. (One typical example: "The influence of Loïe Fuller upon the theater will always be felt, particularly in the lighting of the scene and in the disposition of draperies. *But she was never a great dancer. She was an apparition*" (emphasis added).[4] There is an odd urgency in my responses to these commentaries; my whole body revolts with the kinesthetic knowledge that something else was going on. *My body tells me this.*

Ten years ago, I made a dance called *Traces of Light*. It was the first time I incorporated light as a source of movement and stillness within the choreography. The first time I experienced what it was like to dance in, with, through, and next to light. The following year, I traced another dance that used light as a partner for movement. I re-created Fuller's *Lily* dance (1895), or, at least something approximating it. It was part of an evening-length choreography and although we meticulously reconstructed Fuller's patented design for costume and curved wands, I did not think about this dance as a historical reconstruction, but rather as more of an interesting effect plundered from the abundant resources of early modern dance. Because of budget constraints, we used parachute material, not silk. Purple, not white.

I remember the first time I danced in her costume. It felt odd to be cloaked in yards of fabric—me—who was so used to dancing in pants and a top, with nothing in my way; every movement and each direction easily accessible. Her costume obliges me to prepare each step in order not to trip on the extra fabric. Twisting to one side, then to the other, I gather my strength and then launch the spiral, catching the air underneath the fabric, opening my arms and reaching towards the sky. Two minutes later, I collapse, exhausted and dizzy. I am awed by the upper-body strength and aerobic stamina Fuller must have had to keep the fabric aloft and swirling for upwards of forty-five minutes a night. How odd that some historians insist that she was not a dancer?[5] Was it that she did not look like a dancer? That she did not act the way they thought a dancer should? Clearly she had a trained body and specific movement techniques in her body. In order to make a mere twelve-minute solo with much less fabric than she used, I had to intensively train my upper body for several months. *In motion, my body talks back to historical representation and teaches me to look again, to read beyond the visual evidence and into its source.* Ironically, then, where others savored the image of her disappearance (into the dark, into the folds of cloth, into the ideal symbol), I have come to appreciate the dynamic of her vital presence, those moments of becoming, and becoming again.

I was bitten by the spider. Caught up in the tarantella; the pleasure of spinning, of turning continuously, sending waves of fabric higher. Swirling and twisting. Spinning and running. I felt nauseous at first; my arms ached for weeks. Bitten by what used to be called the devil and what contemporary feminists would reclaim as creative hysteria, I danced possessed—possessed by a body that was not mine and not, not mine. Spinning in lights that dramatically shifted intensity, I lost my spatial bearings and felt history from another place. I knew very little about Loïe Fuller, but I felt that somehow I understood quite a bit more. It was this bodily curiosity, this physical desire to understand her swirling from the inside out that motivated my decision many years later, to engage with this material—to dance with Loïe Fuller once again.

In the ensuing decade, I would return to the costume and her dancing each time I taught early twentieth-century dance history. Taking history from the classroom to the studio, my students would try on Fuller's costume. But nothing happens until you begin to move and spin. Some students would get caught up in Fuller's whirl; the mystique of her dancing. Their enthusiasm inspired me. So did the increasingly sophisticated scholarly work being done on her by scholars such as Felicia McCarren, Rhonda Garelick, and Amy Koritz. Eventually, I became aware of a need to write about Fuller. Part physical, part intellectual, this desire was fueled by the intriguing complexities of a cultural moment in which a short, stocky lesbian from Chicago arrives in Paris to inspire a famous poet's evocation of the dancer as at once feminized and yet also decorporealized into a vision of pure movement.

In the introduction to their collection of essays, *Acting on the Past,* Mark Franko and Annette Richards describe this process of culling many different kinds of historical sources when they write: "Absent performative events have conceptual, imaginary, and evidential, as well as actively reproductive bases. They are especially characterized by movement between present and past, one in which archive and act, fragment and body, text and sounding, subject and practice, work in provocative interaction . . ."[6]

I see my work as taking place in the midst of this "provocative interaction," right at the imaginative intersection of the past and the present. I visualize this (double) crossing spatially, marked in the center of a vast, cavernous space—much like the old wooden dance studio where I teach and work. At one end is the stage of the Folies Bergère. My view is from backstage, with all the workings of its magical effects revealed. Programs, posters, images of Loïe Fuller, as well as pages from her autobiography and countless other articles about her, dot the floor, creating a historical landscape and defining various pathways through the space. Improvising my way through these artifacts, I come to the opposite end where I also envision a backstage. This time, however, it is backstage of the theater where I work. There is a new plexiglass floor in the middle, underneath which we will project lights in multiple colors, reinventing Fuller's lighting designs within a contemporary context. It is the motion between these two backstage spaces (one in the past, one in the present) as well as the dancing pathways I construct from source to source that inform my research methodology.

As a major attraction in Paris at the end of the nineteenth century, Fuller left her mark on the imaginations of many poets and artists of her time. My scholar's cubicle in the library is filled with images of Fuller's dancing: posters, sculptures, photographs, articles about her. How do I respond to these traces? Looking at the reproductions, reading texts, I am fascinated—and moved. What would happen if I took these images, these ideas, into the studio? *I grab my notebook and sprint out of the library.* Inspired to move as well as to write, I take the plunge back into the physical, using my body as both a point of departure and a vehicle that transports me into history.

In an early essay entitled "Rereading as a Woman: The Body in Practice," feminist scholar Nancy Miller discusses the ways in which readings of literary texts are very much affected by the cultural experience of the reader. She writes: "To reread as a woman is at least to imagine the lady's place; to imagine while reading the place of a woman's body; to read reminded that her identity is also re-membered in stories of the body."[7] My studies in feminist theory, inspired by the work of scholars such as Miller, have taught me to be aware of the double reading I produce as a scholar and a woman. These days, I am challenging myself to push the implications of Miller's essay even further—that is, to read (and, by extension, to write) as a dancer, allowing my body to be present, even in the midst of a scholarly project.

Because I have decided to posit my dancing body as a research tool or guide (perhaps assistant is a more apt expression, for my body certainly has a mind of its own and it does not always follow my instructions), I feel compelled to grapple with the relationship of my body to history. In the dance field, there often seems to be a split between researchers who focus primarily on reconstructing a dance from the past on bodies from the present, and those scholars who use dance as the hook into a broader cultural study of modes of production, representation, and reception of artistic endeavors. Now, of course, we all might quickly assert that we do both, but it is rare that I read an essay in which I feel that the writer's bodily knowledge was a crucial part of the scholarly process. Indeed, although we might be interested and excited by the possibilities of a dialogue between the dancing body of the researcher and that of the subject they are researching, we are rarely willing to confront that methodologically murky territory for ourselves. With this work on Fuller, I am asking what it would mean to research a historical body, a dancing body, a desiring body precisely through the intertext of an "other" body: my own. How can I use my embodied knowledge to move beyond the traces of artistic and literary representations of Fuller's dancing into the physicality at their core?

The dance begins in a dim light with a simple arm gesture. Looking down to my right, I scoop the space next to me and reach up, as if making an offering. Releasing the suspension with a breath, I twist behind me to find another cone of light. This light intensifies as I walk into its center. Surrounded by the light, shrouded by the light, I can see it, feel it, touch it, dance through it, but I cannot hold onto it.

Over the past two years, I have developed a series of solo performances inspired by my work on Fuller. These dances take place at the intersection of historical research and choreographic expression. Although they do delineate a movement vocabulary that references Fuller's work, these choreographies are not reconstructions of her works. Spinning, spirals circling out of the upper body, and large expansive gestures of the arms with an upward gaze of the face: these motifs constitute much of the dancing. My first solo, *Searching for Loïe,* was a structured improvisation that used my earliest writings on Fuller as a sound score. Playing with the juxtaposition of poetic and expository prose, the voice-over text created an open field (semi-serious, semi-playful) in which to explore my physical response to Fuller's historical legacy. Later, the dance morphed into a performative lecture entitled "Acts of Passion: Tracing History through Desire." In this more recent incarnation, I interrupt an academic discussion with dancing that pairs my movement with slide images of Fuller's dancing. Moving back and forth across the stage, my body interrupts the projections, flashing my shadow onto the screen. In these moments, Fuller's image is joined by my image, creating a complex duet involving interpretation, interconnection, and reflection. Bringing myself into the dancing in this manner forces me to reflect on my own intellectual position and physical experience, as I ask myself: "So, what does this embodied experience tell me about history?" My answers to this question encompass both specific details as to her movement, staging, and lighting techniques, as well as a more general sense of her performance energy and the role light played within Fuller's own personal cosmology.

Fuller thought of her theater spaces as laboratories in which to combine lights and movement in increasingly sophisticated ways. Fortunately, I have a wonderful collaborator and lighting designer who is also interested in Fuller's work and legacy. We were able to spend a significant amount of time experimenting with lighting in the theater. Our university situation gave us the luxury of time to create the lights and movement both simultaneously and interactively. Although we were not attempting to reconstruct her dances per se, we did use Fuller's original design patents and depictions of her staging (with live lighting technicians above, below and to the sides of her specially raised platform) to inform our updated use of her lighting inventions. We created a floor out of plexiglass, with intelligent lights revolving above and below its surface. The result was a twelve-minute performance entitled *Dancing with Light*.

Collaborating with a lighting designer for days on end brought me closer, I believe, to the reality of Fuller's working environment. Not only did I begin to understand the physical labor involved, I understood why she is always pictured wearing shoes (the stage floors of the variety theaters were notoriously dirty and riddled with nails and bits of this and that). I also realized that the reason she never mentions using haze to intensify the rays of light (an effect every critic comments on) was because the theaters were already so dusty and smoky, one did not need any additional stuff in the air. It seems so simple and obvious, but the physical experience of making a dance in the middle of a busy theater jerked me out of the modern dance paradigm of solo artiste working alone in the studio, waiting for inspiration, and brought me headlong into the gritty realities of popular theater. While it is true that at the beginning of her career Loïe Fuller was best known as a soloist, she never performed anything without the committed assistance of a whole crew of technicians. Both an artist and a craftsperson in the theater, she transcended a deep and still omnipresent division between artists and technicians, directors and staging hands, dancers and electricians.

Dancing with Light left me with a new appreciation for the experience of moving in strongly defined light. Unlike lighting created simply to illuminate the dancers, the lighting we designed was an equal partner in the dance. Sometimes the light obscured me, sometimes it revealed my dancing, and sometimes I was simply a screen onto which a variety of moving lights were projected. At various times, I felt sheltered and enclosed, inspired, even disoriented (especially when dancing on clear glass with lights shining from underneath). The palpable presence of these lights reminded me of otherworldly spirits.

Returning to my study, I began to understand more concretely the spiritual role that light played for Fuller. I believe that she experienced a certain kind of euphoria when dancing that was intensified by her dramatic approach to lighting. Her dances generally followed a classic creation narrative. They began in a total blackout (which was highly unusual for that time), with the first strands of music calling forth a dim illumination of the small motions of her hands and fabric. The lights, movements, and music would generally crescendo into a final frenzy of color and motion that faded abruptly back into a primordial darkness. Fuller's writings—her published autobiography, unpublished letters, and fragments of a book she was writing later in her life—indicate that for her, light held spiritual overtones. In an excerpt from a series of unpublished accounts of her life, Fuller describes the first moment she met Queen Marie of Romania: a woman with whom

Fuller was to develop an intimate (albeit complicated) friendship. Under the sensationalized title of "The World Asks: The Truth About Loïe Fuller and the Queen of Romania," Fuller writes:

> There, coming toward me from the other end of a marvelous golden fairy-like room, was what appeared to be a spirit of light gliding along as if swept by the wind with the ends of its flowing garments, transparent in the sun that fell upon her as she approached . . . All was white, gold and blue around her. A smile such as I had never seen illuminated her countenance and permeated the atmosphere with joy and happiness.[8]

Clearly, Fuller saw Marie as a saintlike figure—the physical embodiment of an enlightened being. Indeed, this is just one example of the many times Fuller uses light metaphors for spiritual goodness. I do not yet know what I will make of this visionary aspect of Fuller's work and life, but I do know that I would never have understood its significance without having danced in a light so defined I could pierce it with my body.

In her essay "The Concept of Intertextuality and Its Application in Dance Research," Janet Ashead-Lansdale identifies the imaginative possibilities of an approach to dance research that resonates with my own. She writes: "These methodological shifts of position are sometimes in harmony and often not, but they can be tolerated and made to function by seeing that it is in the spaces created between a multiplicity of texts and traces [that] there is the opportunity, indeed, more strongly, the demand, that each reader should engage in this process of constructing meaning by unraveling what seems to be implied by the work, or the method, or the discipline, while simultaneously creating their own threads from their own experience."[9]

This layering of texts forms a web of signifying practices that merge and emerge depending upon the historical or methodological lens one chooses to use. Yet these intertexts can also produce a misleading sense that we have captured the thing itself—the presence of a dancing body. I want to introduce the concept of intertextuality, not just to add another historical layer or methodological option, but rather to point out the space between these texts. While this space may figure as an absence, it is not necessarily a loss. Rather, I see it as a distance (both historical and cultural) across which desire always pulls interpretation. At once opportunity and demand (which I sometimes experience as an internal command; an urgency that compels action or speaks to a particular direction of thought), this intertextuality marks the space of improvisation possible within historical work. It recognizes the gap between myself and the subject of my inquiry—that historical distance—while foregrounding the desire to close that gap, to build bridges and cross over from one period to another. Not every subject would necessarily elicit such mobile strategies. But given the elusive quality of Fuller's work and reception in combination with the unpredictable edge of my physical commitment to exploring her dances, this methodological fluidity seems right at the moment.

I need to replace the act of history with an act of love—an act of rebellion against the pressure to separate in the name of academic integrity. Scholarly objectivity. Believe in the union, our unity, a trinity, with light casting its third shadow from there to here. Ripping through the conventions of textual analysis I enter the dance. She calls me, invites me to come, to penetrate the obvious with my kinesthetic imagination, to pierce her flesh with a language that writes its way into her body and mine. My mind mines hers, and mine too. Underneath her skin, I feel the rush of writing, the ecstasy of pouring my sweat, my blood, my need into her. Our juices blend, and blended they whirl into an aquatic tornado of signification. You cannot capture water, but you can feel it—feel its force as it forces you to acknowledge the pressure, the pleasure of being wet, soaked to the bone with another's reality.

Writing an academic book on Loïe Fuller while making a series of dances incorporating aspects of her oeuvre opens up an intertextual space, which can become the site of a negotiation between past and present bodies, between history and desire. More than a poststructuralist ploy (one in which movement is simply a slippery strategy of evasive criticism), however, this approach presses beyond the seams of traditional historical inquiry. Researching with my body brings me face to face (or body to body, so to speak) with my own physical predilections, intellectual interests, artistic agendas, and writerly desires. Certainly, I would never claim, as Giovanni Lista does in the introduction to his extensively researched book on Fuller, that nothing is fictionalized; that everything is "exact" fact. On the contrary, I have no desire to erase my voice within a critical project. I do, however, want to be self-conscious about my own connections to Fuller.

As I gaze once again at the photo above my desk (the one I described at the beginning of this essay), I begin to understand what it is about Loïe Fuller that I find so compelling. Fuller was never only a dancer. This photo, along with so many other pieces of evidence (including the fact that she performed almost every day for years—even when she could have easily substituted a younger dancer in her stead) confirm her deep need to dance. Yet she was most often seen not as a dancer, but rather as a lighting designer—a "Magician of Light," to quote one biography. I, too, have a split identity—that of dancer and academic. Most people are more familiar with my writing than with my choreography. I point this out not to lament cultural prejudices about which bodies get represented as dancers (are you thin enough, young enough, nonverbal enough, etc.), but rather to highlight that my books, like Fuller's lighting, were composed from inside the vortex of motion. This co-motion fuels my interpretation as I trace the sources of her work.

She. Me. We meet in a third space—a third mind provided by the light which stretches across time to warm my hands, to bake my heart, to infuse me with a desire to reach back, back into another world to find myself. The light comes from her smile, spirals out through my chest. Open, open-hearted, I embrace her experience and I realize that this project is more than an academic exercise, more that a history book. I am writing about her, but I am writing myself into her dancing.

NOTES

1. Walter Benjamin, *The Arcades Project* (Cambridge, MA: Harvard University Press, 1999), 9.

2. Jean-Luc Nancy, "Corpus," in *Thinking Bodies,* ed. Juliet Flower MacConnell and Laura Zakarin (Stanford, CA: Stanford University Press, 1994), 24.

3. Susan Foster, "Choreographing History," in *Choreographing History,* ed. Susan Foster (Bloomington: Indiana University Press, 1995), 7.

4. J. E. Crawford Flitch, *Modern Dancing and Dancers* (London: Grant Richards, Ltd., 1913), 88.

5. This is true of early writers such as Flitch (1913), as well as more recent work such as Richard Nelson Current and Marcia Ewing Current's *Loïe Fuller: Goddess of Light* (1997) and Giovanni Lista's *Loïe Fuller: Danseuse de la Belle Époque* (1994).

6. Mark Franko and Annette Richards, eds., *Acting on the Past* (Middletown, CT: Wesleyan University Press, 2000), 1.

7. Nancy Miller, "Rereading as a Woman: The Body in Practice," in *French Dressing* (New York and London: Routledge, 1995), 47.

8. Loïe Fuller, *The Loïe Fuller Collection,* Lincoln Center Dance Collection, New York Public Library, n.d., folder 215, 15.

9. Janet Ashead-Lansdale, "The Concept of Intertextuality and Its Application in Dance Research," *Proceedings of the 22nd Annual Conference, Society of Dance History Scholars,* 1999, 111.

18

The Tanagra Effect

Wrapping the Modern Body in the Folds of Ancient Greece

From *The Ancient Dancer in the Modern World*, ed. Fiona Macintosh (2010).

At the turn of the twentieth century, to put one's body on display as a spectacle and still claim subjectivity onstage was a difficult and complex balancing act for a female performer. Equally difficult for a woman was claiming authority as "writer," particularly if she had been known as a performer.[1] Resisting the societal strictures of "appropriate" behavior for women, Colette, Loïe Fuller, Isadora Duncan, and Eva Palmer found unique ways to negotiate their specific social and economic circumstances, not only to stage their bodies consciously, but also to produce written manifestos that articulated the artistic vision that inspired their work. Whether they began in dance, pantomime, or theater, these women all started with a corporeal practice, producing a physical language that focused on breath rhythms, the dynamic use of the torso, and the articulation of gestures that galvanized space in new and important ways. Then they articulated the cultural potency of that physical work while describing the meanings of their life missions. Their writings give us their ideas. The photographic images help us to infer their movement vocabulary and the stylistic aspects of the staging of their work. But these visual and written traces are necessarily fragmentary, and rarely do they directly address the implications of this physical engagement with the world—what we might call their corpo-realities. In this essay, I propose to read through the historical evidence with an attention to the physical practices (these practices were often inspired by a conception of antiquity as a holistic trinity combining body, mind, and soul) that created a somatic foundation for these women's courageous and ambitious interventions in the performance culture of their time.

Performance and autobiography are genres of representation that foreground the problematic relationship of body to signature and of gender to power. Of course, at the beginning of the twentieth century, performing and writing were highly gendered occupations. With few exceptions, women performed onstage, and men wrote about them. This historical fact was reinforced by a cultural alignment of bodily display as feminized (whether the performer was a man or a woman), and the writer's signature as masculine (the pen as the phallus). In the nineteenth-century bourgeois culture that still reigned in Paris society at the beginning of the twentieth, these activities were imbued with class values. Refusing to be passive instruments of another's vision, Isadora Duncan, Loïe Fuller, Eva Palmer, and Colette all took responsibility for shaping both the larger theatrical frame and the expressive nuances of their (self-)representations.

While these women—three American and one French—all lived emancipated lives in Paris at the beginning of the twentieth century, and while they even sometimes shared a stage (or lawn, to be more precise) and a passion for performance as an ethical, life-affirming force, they developed radically different interests and aesthetics. Before she became a journalist and full-time writer, Colette worked on the stages of music halls for seven years, traveling all over France with a small pantomime company. Loïe Fuller, who was at the height of her career as the century turned, began to choreograph for her own group of dancers, as well as serving as an impresario for two Japanese theater companies, and (very briefly) for Isadora Duncan, among others. Expounding a rhetoric of dance as art, Duncan, in turn, shunned the music-hall stage and danced exclusively in the concert halls, opera houses, and salons of upper-class European society, launching a career of mythic proportions. Eva Palmer, who once shared a couple of afternoon performances with Colette at Natalie Barney's, and who would later marry the brother of Raymond Duncan's wife, recast an early infatuation with Sappho and Hellenism into an ambitious project to revive ancient Greek drama, producing at Delphi two of the biggest theatrical festivals in modern Greece.

There are, of course, overlapping spheres of influence among these women. Some of these have been routinely charted, including Fuller and Duncan's brief and mutually unsatisfactory professional relationship, or Colette and Eva Palmer's appearances at Natalie Barney's home. Others that, to my knowledge, have never been explored, include Colette's invocation of Fuller's dancing and her short portrait of Duncan in *Paysages et Portraits*. In this essay, I hope to map out the unique performance trajectories of these four women, and sketch in some of their commonalities. For, despite the quite different looks of their performances—these women were connected by the fact that, at some point in their careers, they all conjured a vision of ancient Greece to enhance the representation of their bodies as agents of self-expression. This, then, is what I refer to as the Tanagra Effect.

Tanagra dresses, Tanagra scarves, Tanagra corsets that go from the armpits
to the knees and don't allow one to sit, to eat, to bend over, or anything! This
corset contains everything, holds everything back . . . Poor little "Tanagras"
of Paris, what can we make of this cruel fashion which places women, snake-

like, sitting on their tails! Their dimpled backsides, restless and aggressive, their . . . expressive hips—all these are sacrificed to the Tanagra corset, a hard master who crushes their bodies . . . Their impatient bodies shake, fettered by this "Tanagra" dress, which emphasizes their rumps and constrains their feet.[2]

These comments by Colette—the famed novelist, journalist, and woman-about-town in Paris—were occasioned by a review of a performance by Isadora Duncan at the beginning of the twentieth century. As always, Colette was watching the audience as much as the stage, and while she notes that Duncan danced with great expression and with her whole body engaged, Colette remarks on the contrast between Duncan's Greek tunics, which were loosely fitted and lightweight, and those "Tanagra" dresses of the women applauding her. Colette also registers the irony that her audience was filled with women who were physically (not to mention psychically) bound by bourgeois conventions and idiotic fashions such as Fortuny's famous "Tanagra" dresses. "Let us not fool ourselves," she writes, "[these women] acclaim her but they don't envy her. They salute her at a distance, and they contemplate her, but as an escapee—not as a liberator."[3]

When I originally titled this essay "The Tanagra Effect," I was thinking, of course, of the Tanagra sculptures of ancient Greece—those carved figurines whose draping clothes and folded scarves brilliantly capture the underlying movement of their bodies. I wanted to compare the implications of the uses of this kind of Greek costume and humanist references to ancient civilization in performances by Isadora Duncan, Loïe Fuller, and Eva Palmer. But when I found the aforementioned quote, I realized that it was important to first foreground the extraordinary and often amusing range of popular interpretations of "Tanagra" at the cusp of a new century. Although modeled on ancient costumes, the Tanagra style of dress most often symbolized a modern woman, one whose lifestyle incorporated choices—about career, leisure activities, dress, and family—with a mobility unheard of twenty years earlier. Yet this mobility was also partially suspect, and a looseness of clothing could also suggest a loose morality as well. This is certainly true of women dancers who wore Grecian-style tunics onstage (Isadora Duncan being the most famous example), which is why most of the women in their audiences were still bound by the paradoxical fashion of wearing a long corset underneath the mobile dress. In the publicity and press concerning performances by women dancers at this time, claims of "aesthetic," "intelligent," and "chaste" dancing, or an appeal to the idealism of ancient Greek culture, all constitute various strategies to subvert this overdetermined social discourse.

In 1911, Colette appeared on the cover of *La Culture Physique*—a bimonthly journal that calls itself the "organe de l'Énergie française" (organ of French energy), thus invoking a provocative slippage between body and industry. In this issue, Colette is profiled as a fervent advocate of physical culture. Ironically, although Colette exercised in a sleeveless knit body suit on assorted gymnastic equipment, the cover shot has her posing like a Grecian statue, standing in profile with one arm stretched up holding the white cloth that is artistically draped around her torso. This French voguing of Hellenism vacillates between an image of the middle-class aesthetic postures à la Delsarte and the more lowbrow titillation implied by the fact that underneath the graceful folds of the fabric, she is naked.

By the time she posed as the cover girl for *La Culture Physique,* Colette had been seriously working out for about nine years, and her letters to her friends reveal how proud she was of her hard-earned muscles.[4] As a young girl, Colette was outdoorsy and a tomboy. Until arthritis crippled her in her old age, Colette prided herself on being robust and physically active. When in 1902, Colette moved to larger (and lighter) quarters on the Rue de Courcelles with her husband, Willy, Colette claimed the artist's studio on the top floor. She outfitted this bachelorette pad with gymnastic equipment; she exercised and entertained her friends there to distract herself from her faltering marriage. In *My Apprenticeships,* Colette describes this austere, but inspiring, space of her own:

> Mine had no ornaments beyond the fittings of a gymnasium, the horizontal bar, trapeze, rings, and knotted rope. I used to swing and turn over the bar, suppling my muscles half secretly, without any particular zeal or brilliance. Yet when I reflected on it later, it seemed to me that I was exercising my body in much the same way that prisoners, although they have no clear idea of flight, nevertheless tear up their sheets and plait the strands together, sew gold coins into their coat-linings, hide chocolate under the mattress.[5]

Whether she was conscious of it or not at the time, Colette was crafting a modern woman's body—exploring through her exercise routine the psychosomatic experience of muscular stability and strength. Colette had begun to emerge from the bourgeois cocoon of domesticity, and the photographs of her in her gym reveal a self-possession that contrasts markedly with earlier images. Natalie Barney describes the change in Colette at this time: "At the beginning of the century, when I saw Colette for the first time, she was no longer the thin, long-braided adolescent cradled in a hammock which a photograph shows us. She was a young woman firmly fixed on solid legs, with the small of her back arching down to a full behind; with manners as frank as her speech."[6] In her biography of Colette, Judith Thurman affirms Barney's portrayal, connecting the literal to the metaphoric as she emphasizes the sociological implications of Colette's actions:

> In the process of becoming fit, she discovered that exercise strengthens one's moral . . . She was also, consciously or not, training herself for the profession [as

a dancer and a mime, that] she would take up when her marriage ended. Colette had understood, precociously, that the true beauty of a woman's muscles is identical with their purpose, and that's self-support.[7]

First came the focus on fitness, then the flight. By the time Colette was ready to leave the domestic hearth that had charred her provincial innocence, she had trained with the well-known mime Georges Wague. Eventually, she would join him and his partner on the professional stage. In *The Vagabond,* she describes the satisfactions of this new career: "Solitude, freedom, my pleasant and painful work as mime and dancer, tired and happy muscles, and, by way of a change from all that, the new anxiety about earning my meals, my clothes, and my rent—such, all of a sudden, was my lot."[8]

At the end of April 1907, Colette penned her response to socialites who considered that she was "a woman of letters who has turned out badly" for *La Vie Parisienne.* Entitled "Toby-Chien Parle," this ironic dialogue between her dog and cat contains the defiant language of a manifesto:

I want to do what I want. I want to play pantomime and also comedy. I want to dance nude if the leotard constrains me and humiliates my figure. I want to cherish who loves me and give him whatever is mine in the world: my body resists sharing my gentle heart and my independence![9]

In the midst of this fierce declamation, Colette describes in the future tense the kind of dancing that she envisions for herself:

I will dance nude or dressed for the sole pleasure of dancing, to time my movements to the rhythm of music . . . I will dance, I will invent slow beautiful dances where at times the veil will cover me, at times will surround me like a spiral of smoke, at times will stretch behind me like the sail of a boat.[10]

Colette's language here—her "invented" dance with fabric that surrounds her like a spiral of smoke, or billows behind her like a sail, so closely resembles published descriptions of Loïe Fuller that it begs the question of influence. Did Colette ever see Fuller perform? I have not found any mention of Fuller in the abundant scholarship on Colette's life and writings. Yet Colette must have been aware of Fuller's artistic legacy, as well as her reputation as an independent and enterprising woman, if only through her husband's circle of friends, which included some of the most influential fin-de-siècle music and theater critics. We know, for instance, that Colette and Willy frequented the 1900 Paris Exposition Universelle, which opened several months after the publication of *Claudine at School.*[11] It is likely that during this time Colette passed by (if she did not attend) Fuller's theater on the Rue de Paris. Although I am not really concerned with proving that Fuller had a direct influence on Colette, I find most intriguing a short review by Louis Delluc published in *Comoedia illustré* in January 1913 in which he describes Colette in a series of *poses plastiques:* "She plays with a great white veil, in which she surrounds, drapes, and sculpts herself."[12]

Playing with her veil, Colette seems to incorporate Fuller's hieroglyphs in motion. In the aforementioned description of her dancing, Colette abandons the classic narrative and static gestures of pantomime for the improvisational challenge of moving with a large piece of fabric. Reading Delluc, I can imagine Colette tracing Fuller's figures. Yet the reflexive tone of the French verb *se sculpter* shifts the emphasis from the object (what she sculpts) back to the subject (who is doing the sculpting). Using this "great white sail," Colette sculpts herself. In *My Apprenticeships,* Colette recalls her growing awareness at this time of the interconnected poetics of gesture, rhythm, and language: "The melodic and the written phrase both spring from the same elusive and immortal pair—sound and rhythm."[13] As the rhythm becomes the word, my image of Colette doing Fuller dissolves, and I imagine, in turn, the white sail morphing into a blank page—the possibilities of which Colette has learned to explore through reclaiming her body. Moving from the stage back to the page (she would give up performing regularly with the birth of her daughter in 1913), Colette renders, as Nancy Miller notes, "the rhythms of performance *in writing.*"[14]

Like Colette, Isadora Duncan also staged the psychosomatic implications of physical autonomy and then wrote about them in her manifestos. At the beginning of her book on Duncan, *Done Into Dance,* Ann Daly describes Duncan's amazing ability to make visible what she calls a "narrative of force":

> The general components of force are also those of Duncan's dancing: interaction, motion, directionality, and intensity. Duncan's solos—a single body struggling against, shrinking from, floating on, and thrusting into space—were enactments of agency, the self in the process of engagement with the external world, whether that meant love or fate, oppression or death.[15]

It is this concentrated unity of focus (her presence) that Abraham Walkowitz has captured so compellingly in his many drawings of Duncan's dancing. Reflecting Colette's remark that "son corps parle plus que son visage" (her body speaks more than her face), Walkowitz leaves Duncan's face blank, allowing the viewer to focus instead on how her head follows the expressive motion of her torso. More importantly, Walkowitz's sketches and watercolors help us to comprehend how Duncan was able to transform her ideas about nature into a fleshy, weighty corporeality. In his work, Walkowitz blends watercolors (or shading) with ink lines to represent the hallmarks of Duncan's fame: the poetic tension of her stillness, her luxurious open reach to the sky, the lively skipping of her incarnation as a Bacchant, and the contracted anguish of loss. More than specific movements or gestures, however, Walkowitz's drawings evoke the vital spontaneity of Duncan's pleasure in dancing. For Duncan, the source of this pleasure was the interplay of forces, that "central spring of movement" in the solar plexus, and its inspiration was Nature.

The first paragraph of Duncan's essay on "The Dancer and Nature" establishes the marriage of beauty and wisdom through which nature reveals herself as a woman dancing. Later in the same essay, Duncan declares:

> Woman is not a thing part and separate from all other life organic and
> inorganic. She is but a link in the chain, and her movement must be one
> with the great movement which runs through the universe; and therefore the
> fountain-head for the art of the dance will be the study of the movements
> of Nature.[16]

As Ann Daly makes clear: "'Nature' was Duncan's metaphorical shorthand for a loose package of aesthetic and social ideals: nudity, childhood, the idyllic past, flowing lines, health, nobility, ease, freedom, simplicity, order and harmony."[17] Duncan's take on "Nature" was connected to a nostalgic return to Greece. It was essentially an antimodern impulse—one that shunned many technological advances of the early twentieth century. Even though she certainly took advantage of her historical position as a modern woman, Isadora Duncan fetishized Greek culture. In her hybrid Hellenism, she wedded her notion of an eternal and inspiring "Nature" to Platonic ideals of "Beauty":

> In no country is the soul made so sensible of Beauty and of Wisdom as in
> Greece. Gazing at the sky one knows why Athene, the Goddess of Wisdom, was
> called "the Blue-Eyed One," and why learning and beauty are always joined in
> her service. And one feels also why Greece has been the land of great philos-
> ophers, lovers of wisdom, and why the greatest of these has called the highest
> beauty, the highest wisdom . . . [18]

Eventually, of course, Duncan evolved choreographically from her early renditions of a sweet and gentle nature in her *La Primavera* days, in which she enacted a number of figures in Botticelli's painting (complete with flowers circling the neck and waist), to representations of "Nature," which included fierce and destructive energies as well as harmonious ones. Certainly by the time she was dancing her Greek vignettes such as *Orpheus* or *Iphigenia in Tauris,* Duncan's expressive palette had expanded to include both Apollonian and Dionysiac themes:

> My idea of dancing is to leave my body free to the sunshine, to feel my san-
> daled feet on the earth, to be near and love the olive trees of Greece. These are
> my present ideas of dancing. Two thousand years ago a people lived here who
> had perfect sympathy and comprehension of the beautiful in Nature, and this
> knowledge and sympathy were perfectly expressed in their own forms and

movement . . . I came to Greece to study these forms of ancient art, but above all, I came to live in the land which produced these wonders, and when I say "to live" I mean to dance.[19]

Isadora Duncan spent much of 1903 in Greece with the whole Duncan clan. Led by Raymond Duncan's fierce desire to reinvent an archaic Greece (one not sullied by modern equipment or politics), the family crossed the Ionian Sea in a small fishing boat to make their first pilgrimage to this ancient land. The chapter in her autobiography, *My Life,* documenting this odyssey is filled with poetic quotations from Byron and Homer, as well as depictions of Isadora and Raymond gamboling about the Greek countryside, drunk with Plato.[20] Its euphoric tone is also inflected with wry comments about bedbugs, hard wooden planks for sleeping, the assorted perils of the countryside, not to mention the astonishment of the modern Greeks to this band of foreigners who looked like ancient sculptures come alive. The rest of the story is well known—a testimony to the odd myopia of a radical American fundamentalism. Dressed in tunics and shod in sandals, the Duncans bought some land with a view of the Acropolis and proceeded to build their house, Kopanos. Eventually, it dawned on them that there was no water to be had in the area, and although Raymond would have deeper wells dug (at Isadora's expense), eventually they would give up the fantasy of living in Greece permanently, and Raymond would return to Paris to start a theater school there.

While in Greece, the Duncans met the Sikelianos family: Philadelpheus, an archeologist; Angelos, who would become a renowned poet and later marry Eva Palmer; and Penelope, a singer, who became Raymond's wife. The alchemy between the Sikelianos family and the Americans was very interesting. Both Penelope and Angelos helped Raymond Duncan actualize his dreams of living like the ancients. But then again, the impulsive utopianism of the Americans (not to mention their financial assistance which, in the case of Eva Palmer, was considerable), also helped the Sikelianos family to dream of reaching back past the modern Greek state to reconstruct the simplicity of peasant life, as well as the humanitarian power of an ancient, popular theater.

In 1927, and again in 1930, Angelos and Eva Palmer-Sikelianos produced two theatrical festivals at the ancient theater in Delphi, which included athletic games and exhibitions of folk art, and featured Eva Palmer's stagings of Aeschylus' *Prometheus Bound*—the first time in modern Greece that anyone had attempted to mount ancient Greek tragedy in an outdoor setting of that scale. Through her directorial work, Palmer managed to accomplish what Isadora Duncan loftily envisioned when she wrote her short essay on "The Greek Theater":

Greek Tragedy sprang from the dancing and singing of the Greek Chorus. Dancing has gone a long way astray. She must return to her original place— hand in hand with the Muses encircling Apollo. She must become again the primitive Chorus, and the drama will be reborn from her inspiration.[21]

Born in 1874 to a well-to-do and well-placed New York City family, Palmer had all the advantages of money, connections, and liberal-thinking parents. Her father introduced her to some of the most radical thinkers of the late nineteenth century, Robert Ingersoll among them. Her mother developed both her fine musical sensibility and her interest in the arts, as well as sponsoring an awareness of social injustice and modeling a fervent belief in the cause of women's suffrage.[22] As she grew up, Palmer went to schools in America, France, and Germany, giving her a patchwork education that was long on English literature and short on mathematics.

Precocious, but undisciplined, Palmer took up the challenge posed by M. Carey Thomas, the legendary president of Bryn Mawr College, who flatly told Palmer it was unlikely she could pass the entrance exams. She studied hard ("eighteen hours a day for six months") and managed to gain admission to this bastion of women's education and classical studies, where she spent the next two years studying Greek for the first time and immersing herself in English literature. She also directed the annual class plays, and was pleased when Thomas suggested she direct *Hamlet* the following year. In her memoirs, Palmer writes that Thomas "had also a knack of sensing and encouraging one toward one's own strong but still unexpressed leanings."[23] I suspect that it was her pleasure in the more practical, hands-on nature of theater that compelled Palmer to abandon the scholarly cloistered setting of Bryn Mawr for the freedom of Europe, where she spent a year in Rome with her brother before settling in Paris, in a pavilion near Natalie Barney's place in Neuilly.

From the time she was first sent to school, Eva Palmer evinced a passion for recitation. Her autobiography recounts numerous occasions of standing on a chair performing Shakespeare, Swinburne, or Poe to a spellbound group of her schoolmates. They were witnesses to some of Palmer's first attempts to merge language and rhythm, and although she was told by a teacher to stop, as these events were considered "too exciting" for the girls, Palmer's passion for "melody in words" was ignited. In a chapter on "The First Delphic Festival," Palmer connects these early experiences to her later work:

So this impetus toward the singing of words was for long obscured; and Mrs. Dowe's negative imperative was perhaps still working, while entirely new conceptions of Greek Choruses were building in my consciousness. But then I no longer was interested in either reciting or acting myself. I had come to long for many voices, for many women, or preferably many men, expressing in perfect individual freedom, and in perfect composite unity, the complete inner meaning of the word.[24]

In Paris, Palmer studied acting and performed in amateur theatricals such as those with Colette in Natalie Barney's garden. Her striking long red hair and beautiful eyes led both Sarah Bernhardt and Mrs. Patrick Campbell (well-known actresses of the day) to invite her to play *Pélléas and Mélisande* with them. In both cases, her professional aspirations were thwarted; one because of Bernhardt's fear of being upstaged, and the other because Palmer refused to give up her friendship with Natalie Barney—an association Mrs. Campbell claimed was bad for her protégée's reputation. In any case, Palmer recounts: "I had seen by that time a good deal of back-stage politics and meanness, and my ambition to go on the French stage, or any other stage, was not so ardent as it had been."[25]

During the spring of 1905, while Palmer was trying to decide what to do with her life, she met Raymond Duncan and his wife, Penelope Sikelianos, and their baby. Upon hearing Penelope sing Greek ecclesiastical melodies, Palmer had an epiphany. "I felt that I had heard music for the first time; heard a human voice for the first time."[26] Because of worker strikes that threatened to become violent on the first of May, Palmer invited the Raymond Duncan family to move out to Neuilly with her. Soon the house was in the midst of a mini Greek revival, with Raymond painting friezes on the walls, and the women sewing their own apparel. Presently, they built a loom and decided to try to weave a cloth that draped and folded just like the fabric on ancient statues. One afternoon, while resting, Penelope explained the shifts in tone that Palmer found so compelling in her singing:

> A mode . . . is not a scale; it has nothing to do with the piano. Each mode has special intervals of its own, which do not exist on the piano. A mode is a mood; and a Greek song uses the mode which suits its content: one mode if the words are gay, another if they are melancholy, another if they are martial, and so forth. We have many musical modes. We therefore have infinite melodic variety.[27]

Inspired by the sound and rhythm of the language and intrigued by a lifestyle that sought to capture the essence of ancient life, Palmer went to Greece with Raymond and Penelope, and there met Angelos Sikelianos, with whom she would find the focus for her life's work in the theater.

Galvanized by Nietzsche's *Birth of Tragedy,* her husband's epic poetry, as well as her studies of Greek culture, Eva Palmer-Sikelianos set out in the mid-1920s to stage *Prometheus Bound* at Delphi. As her guiding mantra, she kept two lines in mind. The first was from Plato's *Republic* and the second one was from Aristotle's *Poetics:* "The tragic chorus is the union of poetry, music and gymnastics," and "the tragic chorus expresses in movement the character, the sufferings, and the actions of the actors."[28] What helped her transform these lofty ideas into a living, breathing, moving, theatrical unit, however, was her extraordinary facility at movement analysis.

It is unclear to me whether Palmer-Sikelianos ever had any specific movement training, either in some kind of Delsartesque living tableau during her youth in New York City (which is a good probability), or as part of her studies in acting in France. Maybe she was just naturally perceptive at distinguishing the physical dynamic of stance and gesture, both on and off the stage. In any case, her autobiography, *Upward Panic,* contains a number of compelling descriptions of people's physical personalities. One of her most perceptive movement descriptions comes in her chapter on Isadora Duncan. Even before Palmer met Raymond Duncan, she had seen Isadora dance several times: "We all felt that the shackles of the world were loosened, that liberation was ahead of us."[29] Indeed, at the beginning of her chapter on Duncan, Palmer-Sikelianos recalls how everyone originally thought of Isadora as the embodiment of Greece: "What she did was always connected with Greek vases and Greek bas-reliefs; and only gradually, after a number of years of unquestioning gratitude for what she brought us, one began to date the vases which were evoked by her dancing."[30] Palmer-Sikelianos's search for the movement forms of an ancient, archaic Greece led her to recognize the inconsistencies in Isadora's gloss on Greece, ones that Duncan herself points out in the end of *My Life* when she claims that: "It has often made me smile—but somewhat ironically—when people have called my dancing Greek, for I myself count its origin in the stories which my Irish grandmother often told of crossing the plains with grandfather . . ."[31] Nonetheless, Palmer-Sikelianos's articulation of Duncan's movement style is evocative:

> Her arms were beautiful, and the soft undulations were infinitely charming
> to a world that knew only the tiresome stiffness of the ballet; but there is not
> a single example of any work of Greek art before the fourth century which
> resembles Isadora's dancing. It was always flowing. Even in powerful dances
> like her "Marche Slave" and her Chopin "Polonaise," the lines of her body went
> into curves. She always faced her audience frankly, head and chest in the same
> direction. There was never the powerful accent of a strong angle, and never the
> isolating effect of keeping the head in profile with the chest "en face" which is
> characteristic of archaic Greek art. Even in moving around the outside circle
> of the stage, it was always straight ahead, more like a child running, with none
> of the pause and power which are added by what I have called the Apollonian
> movement in the dance.[32]

As we know, Isadora used her classical connections to legitimize her own dancing and distinguish her work as art. Eva Palmer-Sikelianos, on the other hand, was interested in using a more archaic movement vocabulary, not because she was dedicated to being strictly authentic (she was not), but because she thought that this Apollonian style best carried the dramatic power of the tragic chorus. In his portrait of Eva Palmer-Sikelianos in *The Splendor of Greece,* Robert Payne recounts the comments of a modern Greek actress which reveal how Palmer-Sikelianos's skills at movement analysis created a foundation for her uncanny ability to animate history:

> She was the only ancient Greek I ever knew . . . She had a strange power of entering the minds of the ancients and bringing them to life again. She knew everything about them—how they walked and talked in the marketplace, how they latched their shoes, how they arranged the folds of their gowns when they arose from the table, and what songs they sang, and how they danced, and how they went to bed. I don't know how she knew these things, but she did![33]

One of the tools available to Eva Palmer-Sikelianos in her search for the appropriate gestures and movements in reconstructing the role of the chorus in ancient Greek drama was a book called *The Antique Greek Dance* (English translation, 1916), written by Maurice Emmanuel and originally published in French in 1896. In this massive tome, the author meticulously cross-referenced gestures and positions of the body found in Greek sculpture, bas-reliefs, and vase paintings with passages from poetry and drama. He categorizes these designs into three basic groups: (a) gestures that are ritualized and symbolic, (b) gestures of everyday life, and (c) mostly decorative gestures. Moving from poetic rhythms to music rhythms to dance rhythms, Emmanuel reconnects the visual and the written evidence, creating an encyclopedic documentation of ancient Greek movement styles.

It is unclear whether Eva Palmer-Sikelianos ever consulted this exhaustive reference. In her autobiography, she speaks of going to museums to look for visual evidence and consulting archeological texts, but never directly mentions Emmanuel's book. There are, of course, some obvious similarities. For instance, in the group of ritual and symbolic gestures is a gesture of worship referenced in a sculpture from the Berlin Museum and described as a boy "holding the arms out with the palms up."[34] This is exactly the position that the Oceanids chorus takes in *Prometheus Bound.* In a photograph by the Greek artist Nelley of the 1930 production, we see a semicircle of women facing Prometheus in this supplicating pose.

Later in Emmanuel's book there is a section on the "Chorus of the Dance," in which he analyzes women's groups' movement, including the folk dance that Palmer-Sikelianos used in her choreography, as well as the Pyrrhic or warrior dances, which were also included in the Delphi festivals. In this section, Eva Palmer-Sikelianos would have found clear justification for her belief that the chorus moved as a rhythmical unit in circular patterns, using their whole bodies to create a wave-like ripple across the stage space. In any case, Palmer-Sikelianos was pointedly less interested in historical accuracy than in reviving the spiritual aspects of Greek drama. In response to a compliment by a Mr. Buschor, the director of the German School of Archaeology concerning the "archaeological correctness" of her 1927 production, Palmer-Sikelianos declares:

> The performance was bristling with archaeological mistakes; but even you did not detect them, and you are not conscious of them even now. And that is because the play was moving around its own pivot; it was emotionally true, or almost true—and that was sufficient to make even you feel that it was correct archaeologically. But there is not such thing as archaeological correctness. There is nothing in Greek drama except the emotional truth and consistency of the performers, and the immense responding emotion of those who are present. The faculties of the actors, the chorus and the audience in the great circular theatre become one and form an overwhelming magnetic force. It is a tidal wave which nothing can resist; not even archaeological conscientiousness.[35]

The one place where Palmer-Sikelianos worked assiduously for historically accurate reproductions was in the area of costumes, weaving all the fabrics she used. Early on in their collaboration, Raymond and Eva had found that by combining a heavy warp with a thin weft, they could create a cloth that draped with the same kinds of folds they admired on ancient sculptures. Indeed, Palmer-Sikelianos was quite proud of the fact that later archeologists found evidence that her method was exactly the same one used in ancient times. Although she used silk—which the Greeks did not use—for the chorus dresses, Palmer-Sikelianos believed that this artistic liberty was justified on the grounds that the silk "would look like the folds on a Greek bas-relief,"[36] and would create the image of waves rippling across the ocean. In her autobiography, Palmer-Sikelianos devotes a whole chapter to weaving. Clearly weaving gave her a great deal of pleasure. It was the physical enactment of her creativity—one that merged individuality and sociability. She writes: "There is something about the loom, something eminently sociable on one hand, because of the different stages in setting up a warp where several usually work together, and something restful and rhythmical in loneliness when the swift shuttle seems to clarify one's thoughts . . ."[37]

Eva Palmer-Sikelianos's theatrical genius lay in how she used the elements of costume, gesture, and movement to galvanize the theatrical space. Unlike the proscenium frame of most indoor theaters, the outdoor arena at Delphi emphasized the three-dimensionality of space, which Palmer-Sikelianos further animated through her choreography. This sense of moving with and through space is a mark of American modern dance. Eva Palmer-Sikelianos brought this sensibility with her to Greece, using it to help her reinvent the epic sensibility of Greek drama. In *Upward Panic,* she recalls how her chorus of young Athenian women had practiced for two years, finally becoming "word-perfect, melody-perfect, move-perfect." But something was missing. They had not yet learned to animate the space. Then, they went out to the ancient theater. "It was a revelation. The thing that none of us had been able to do in Athens happened by itself on the great mountain. Their voices were free and strong, their movements beautiful and powerful. They were inspired."[38]

For Palmer-Sikelianos, the physical space was also a metaphysical arena—the orchestra (literally meaning a "dancing-place") held a spiritual energy—the potent possibility of creating a *communitas* among all those present. The chorus moved in the central circle, which was ringed by an ascending and expanding circle of seats for the spectators. Like the ripples from a pebble thrown in the water, the lines of energy in the ancient theater radiated outwards from the chorus and actors toward the audience. In her essay "What is Great Theater?" Palmer-Sikelianos articulates how space and rhythm can create a spiritual connection. Palmer-Sikelianos's four physical "laws" delineate how "the attention of actors, chorus, and audience was centered on a point, the orchestra, and formed circling waves of power which increased in intensity as the drama unfolded."[39] She describes this moment as the "thrill" of great performances—the moment when the audience and actors experience a mutual sense of belonging—an awareness of their shared humanity. In an essay titled, "The World's a Circular Stage: Aeschylan Tragedy through the Eyes of Eva Palmer-Sikelioanos," Gonda Van Steen connects this focus in her directing to the Sikelianoi's larger project of creating a university:

> Her choice of circular and centripetal choreographic movement within this "sacred" setting of nature and ruins expressed her belief that a simple, primitive form could help to transmit the Delphic Idea. The Sikelianoi's ideal was to create a universal center of centers, a univers-ity [*sic*], at Delphi, which would unite peoples around spirituality and Art.[40]

This ideal university proved to be elusive. After depleting her own fortune and after many attempts to secure state institutional support for the Delphi Festivals, Palmer-Sikelianos returned to the United States to try and interest Americans in her ideas and raise money. While in the states, she worked with Ted Shawn and his men's group at their dance retreat at Jacob's Pillow, and also staged *The Bacchae* at Bryn Mawr and Smith. Eventually, she returned to Greece, where she died after suffering a stroke at a performance held in her honor. As I am writing this, there are still a lot of gaps in Eva Palmer-Sikelianos's biography. I wonder, for instance, how much she was aware of the American dancers appearing in Greece in the 1910s and 1920s. In February 1914, Loïe Fuller and her troupe gave an outdoor performance at the Athens Stadium. It is possible that Palmer-Sikelianos saw or heard of Fuller's performances, but so far as I can tell, there is no documentation about any interaction between these two women artists.

Interestingly enough, the last line of Anatole France's introduction to Loïe Fuller's autobiography, which was first published in French in 1908, reads:

There you have to the life this Loïe Fuller . . . who reanimates within herself and restores to us the lost wonders of Greek mimicry, the art of those motions, at once voluptuous and mystical, which interpret the phenomena of nature and the life history of living beings.[41]

For someone who was seen as the living embodiment of Art Nouveau, a woman who was acclaimed at the Paris Universal Exposition of 1900 as "La Fée Électricité" and who played Salomé as recently as 1907, the rhetorical shift evident in France's language is rather remarkable. Indeed, this idealization of an eternal nature and universal humanity, with nods to Greek antiquity, attests to Fuller's amazing ability to reinvent herself. This last section takes up Loïe Fuller's work with her troupe to analyze how she incorporated the contemporary cultural evocations of nature and the Greek in her stagings of what were, essentially, modernist theatrical landscapes.

Of course, it is important to remember that early on in her career Fuller had invoked the "origins" of dancing in ancient cultures to distinguish her movement inspiration from the music-hall dancing that framed her first appearances in Paris. While she disassociated her movement style from that of academic dancing, Fuller had long connected her work to the ancient Greeks, who "danced with their whole bodies—with their head and arms and trunk and feet."[42] By 1908, however, the term "Greek dancing" clearly referenced Duncan's dancing and that of her imitators. Fuller was thus careful to distinguish her school of dance from that of her early protégée:

By no means is my kind of dancing like Isadora Duncan's, although there are one or two points in common. The two kinds are as different as night and day. Miss Duncan's dancing is essentially a cultivated art—a learned kind of dancing that takes much practice—whereas mine is natural, inspirational, and spontaneous. Miss Duncan imitates the movements of dancers as represented on Greek vases and her pupils copy her. I and my pupils give the original natural expression and movements which inspired the Greeks when they made their vases . . . [43]

What Fuller meant by "natural" dancing can be seen in the photographs taken by Harry C. Ellis of Fuller's young students rehearsing outdoors. This extraordinary series of action shots shows the group of long-limbed girls with turbans and tunics, skipping, swinging, and generally cavorting in a chaotic manner. They are usually leaping in the air—sometimes with their faces open to the sky, sometimes curled over, with their arms continuing the C curve of their body. While they may be all doing the same thing (skipping, for instance), they are not all doing it in the same manner, or at the same time. This makes for a random visual field, but also gives their movement a sense of spontaneity and individuality—two qualities that Fuller wanted to cultivate in her group. Unlike similar photographs of Duncan's pupils that portray young girls moving as a unit, all with the same leg forward and the same lifted chest, Fuller's students exude a sense of the wilder, less tamed side of nature. Rather than cultivating her dancers, Fuller seems to have simply let them loose.

Despite her strategic differences from Duncan, Fuller's "Muses," as they were often called, wore the stylized tunics and bare legs made famous by Duncan. Although her movement vocabulary differed substantially from Duncan's, Fuller was savvy enough to cash in on the trend for "aesthetic" or "natural" dancing that was sweeping her home country at the time. Thus, on her 1909–1910 North American tour, one of Fuller's troupe, a young German woman named Gertrud Von Axen, performed solos—both on Fuller's programs and separately—that apparently were remarkably similar to Duncan's early work.[44] In the Fuller collection at Lincoln Center, there is a program for a concert of solos by Von Axen to the music of Beethoven and Shubert given, the heading notes, "By Special Arrangement with Loïe Fuller." The cover photo shows Von Axen with her arms outstretched in front of her, her upper body leaning away, with the end of her wrapped tunic draped gracefully down her back. The inside carries Fuller's endorsement: "Miss Fuller considers Gerturd Von Axen the most perfect and real Greek dancer before the public today," and the back excerpts press comments from Fuller's recent tour. Von Axen's performance was predictably acclaimed as "graceful," "charming," and "spontaneous"—exactly the descriptions used when Duncan was first dancing.

Alternately billed as "Loïe Fuller's Ballet of Light," "Loïe Fuller and her School of Dance," or "Loïe Fuller and her Muses," the company usually presented an evening of dances that ranged from *Midsummer Night's Dream* set to Mendelssohn's music, or Scriabin's *Prometheus* (basically Fuller's *Fire Dance* en masse), to more abstract works set to modern, impressionistic music, such as selections from Debussy's *Nocturnes,* Stravinsky's *Feu d'Artifice,* or *Orchestrations de Couleurs sur Deux Préludes* by Armande de Polignac: a piece that was composed expressly for Fuller's company. Works such as *Midsummer Night's Dream* sketched out a vague narrative—"In a forest, a Shepard sleeps and dreams of fairies, gnomes, and elves . . . "—onto which Fuller would hang a series of atmospheric events that swept, like waves, cross the stage. There is a photograph of the company in a bucolic setting, perfectly arranged like a picture, with Loïe Fuller on the far right, draped in flowing fabric. Although it is more staid than the frolicking, action shots by Ellis, one can imagine the curtain rising on the tableau, with the lighting gradually growing brighter, like a rising sun, as the stage action begins.

The more abstract works were essentially music visualizations, in which Fuller's exquisite lighting effects were further enhanced by the manipulations of fabric (often with little mirrors sewn on it to reflect the lights) by the girls onstage. No longer a solo figure evoking fleeting images of a lily, clouds, or fire, Fuller was now working with a larger palette, allowing her to create an impressive series of theatrical landscapes. In the same way that Duncan's dancing realized "a narrative of force," Fuller's choreography now depicted the forces of nature. Giovanni Lista describes Fuller's work at this time in terms that echo Emerson's notions of the transcendence of nature. "She thinks, like Emerson, that human beings, to truly communicate with the universal aspects of nature, need to downplay their unique position in the world."[45] Unfortunately, most of the visual documentation of these works by Fuller are still studio shots, with the young girls of her company posed in formal tableau. There are two outdoor photos, however, taken at dusk, which give us an idea of the kinds of atmospheric play of light and shadow that would become a trademark of her later work.

Fuller thought of her music visualizations as a "new form of art." In a 1914 interview, she describes her efforts to merge "pictorial orchestration" with "magical lighting":

> Specialists of the dance do not understand that I aim only to give an harmonious impression trying to express the spirit of the music. I intend to continue it, in some way, to continue it as the waves unfurling on the shore continue to obey the breath of the wind. I try to follow thus the musical waves in the movements of the body and in colors; I am trying to create a harmony between sound, light, and movement.[46]

While some music critics disparaged Fuller's dances for betraying the music, others claimed she had unified the different genres, creating a fusion of sound, movement, and light. Léo Clarétie calls her work a "transposition." Clearly refuting a previous commentary, he writes: "Music is a joy for our ears, she gives us again a joy for our eyes. She renders the music pictorial. Claude Debussy is translated, he is not betrayed."[47] Distinguishing Fuller's efforts from either ballet or what he dubs decorative spectacle, Lista also suggests that Fuller was onto something new. "In fact, it was really about creating a new form of expression, neither ballet nor decorative spectacle, but rather a sort of tableau vivant which unfolded like a pure music visualization."[48] I find his phrase, "a living tableau unfolding through time" intriguing, for it points not only to the influence of Muybridge's and Marey's experiments in chronophotography but also to the future of cinema. Ironically, these works also recall the earlier nineteenth-century magic lantern shows that depicted landscapes changing dramatically from dawn to dusk, or with the arrival of a storm. Once again, Fuller was harnessing a variety of technologies to produce exquisite images of nature.

Occasionally, Fuller participated in these creations (playing in *Prometheus,* for instance), but mostly she served as choreographer/director for the company. One exception was her *La Danse des Mains*. This solo, inspired by Rodin's sculptures of hands and his observation that the soul can express itself through any part of the body, was performed in total darkness, with only her hands illuminated. Several of Fuller's programs for 1914 contain a sketch entitled *La Danse des Mains,* which portrays four sets of hands in different expressive gestures: clawing the air, commanding attention, holding something, or simply reaching towards the sky. Writing in *Le Théâtre,* Jean D'Orliac echoes Rodin's aesthetic sensibility by claiming: "The entire human being, with all his multiple emotions is evoked by these expressive fingers whose rhythms move her supple hands."[49] If Fuller's music visualizations were changing landscapes that indicated her future directions in cinema, her *La Danse des Mains* pointed towards the expressive montage of light, shadow, and close-up that would mark her signature on this new medium of film.

In response to a question from an interviewer for the *Dramatic Mirror,* Fuller once declared: "It is an American monopoly to combine stage dancing with self-respect."[50] This essay has explored very briefly the theatrical work of Colette, Eva Palmer, Isadora Duncan, and Loïe Fuller, and its invocations of ancient Greece, with an eye to understanding how self-respect was cultivated in the bodily practices of these women, and how they learned to stage that experience of physical subjectivity for the world to see. Through their embodied training, these women learned how to mobilize the space and enact force, creating a dynamic in which their bodies could affect change. True feminists as well as humanists, they were encouraged at the beginning of a new century by the potential for their own personal and professional realization, and they shared the fervent desire to communicate those possibilities to the world.

NOTES

1. Throughout her life, Colette's past career as a music-hall entertainer caused various protests by an older generation whenever her name was suggested as the possible recipient of a literary prize. See Judith Thurman's introduction to *Secrets of the Flesh* (New York: Alfred A. Knopf, 1999), xiii.

2. Colette, *Paysage et Portraits* (Paris: Flamarion Editeur, 1958), 153.

3. Ibid., 153–54.

4. Thurman, 210.

5. Colette, *My Apprenticeships and Music-Hall Sidelights* (New York: Penguin, 1957), 104.

6. Robert Phelps, *Belle Saisons: A Colette Scrapbook* (New York: Farrar, Straus and Giroux, 1978), 62.

7. Thurman, 133.

8. Colette, *The Vagabond,* trans. Enid McLeod (New York: Farrar, Straus and Giroux, 1955), 32.

9. Colette, *Oeuvres,* vol. 1 (Paris: Éditions Gallimard, 1984), 994.

10. Ibid., 997.

11. Thurman, 109.

12. Claude et Vincenette, ed., *Album Colette* (Paris: Éditions Gallimard, 1984), 114.

13. Colette, *My Apprenticeships,* 110.

14. Nancy Miller, *Subject to Change* (New York: Columbia University Press, 1988), 232.

15. Ann Daly, *Done Into Dance* (Bloomington: Indiana University Press, 1995), 6–7.

16. Isadora Duncan, "The Dancer and Nature," in *The Art of the Dance*, ed. Sheldon Cheney (New York: Theatre Art Books, 1969), 68.

17. Ibid., 89.

18. Ibid., 66.

19. Duncan, quoted in Daly, 1995, 101.

20. Isadora Duncan, *My Life* (New York: Liveright, 1927), 116–35.

21. Duncan, *The Art of the Dance,* 87.

22. Eva Palmer-Sikelianos, *Upward Panic: The Autobiography of Eva Palmer-Sikelianos,* ed. John Anton (Philadelphia: Harwood Academic, 1993), 32.

23. Ibid., 25–26.

24. Ibid., 105–6.

25. Ibid., 57.

26. Ibid., 46.

27. Ibid., 50.

28. Ibid., 106.

29. Ibid., 181.

30. Ibid., 181–82.

31. Duncan, *My Life,* 340.

32. Palmer Sikelianos, 182.

33. Robert Payne, *The Splendor of Greece* (New York: Harper and Row, 1960), 102.

34. Maurice Emmanuel, *The Antique Greek Dance,* trans. Harriet Jean Beauley (New York: John Lane Company, 1916), 25.

35. Palmer-Sikelianos, *Upward Panic,* 113–14.

36. Ibid., 109.

37. Ibid., 78.

38. Ibid., 114–15.

39. Eva Palmer-Sikelianos, "What is Great Theater?" *Eos* 103, no. 7 (1967): 301.

40. Gonda Van Steen, "The World's a Circular Stage: Aeschylan Tragedy through the Eyes of Eva Palmer-Sikelioanos," *International Journal of Classical Tradition* 8, no. 3 (Winter 2002): 379.

41. Loïe Fuller, *Fifteen Years of a Dancer's Life* (Boston: Small, Maynard, 1913), x.

42. J. E. Crawford Flitch, *Modern Dancing and Dancers* (Philadelphia: J. B. Lippincott, 1912), 88.

43. Fuller, quoted in Richard and Marcia Current, *Loïe Fuller: Goddess of Light* (Boston: Northeastern University Press, 1997), 196.

44. Ibid., 202.

45. Giovanni Lista, *Loïe Fuller: Danseuse de la belle époque* (Paris: Editions Stock, 1994), 468.

46. Margaret Haile Harris, *Loïe Fuller: Magician of Light* (Richmond: The Virginia Museum, 1979), 28.

47. Quoted in the program for "Loïe Fuller et son école de danse," Théâtre Municipal du Chatelet, May 1914.

48. Lista, 489.

49. Jean D'Orliac, "Madame Loïe Fuller et Son École de Danse," *Le Théâtre,* September 1914.

50. Fuller quoted in Clare de Morinni, "Loïe Fuller: The Fairy of Light," in *Chronicles of the American Dance,* ed. Paul Magriel (New York: DaCapo Press, 1978), 216.

IV

CONTACT IMPROVISATION

Contact improvisation is one of the main reasons I devoted my life to dancing. I took a series of contact classes during my college days and was immediately hooked. The range of physical possibilities combined with the improvisational impulse in this form of kinesthetic partnering spoke to my desire for feisty, anything goes, movement. In addition, the life lessons concerning the relationship between one's self and another as they are negotiated through the subtle exchanges of weight and momentum, leading and following, kept me engaged in a form that evolved as my interests also changed. Contact improvisation trains for disorientation in its many guises (including spatial and emotional), and I appreciate the form's insistence that we cultivate a willingness to experience awkward moments and suspend expectations about what constitutes a successful duet. The somatic work that informs contact improvisation has been crucial to keeping me dancing throughout my middle years and I often talk about my approach to dance history as a kind of contact duet. Paradoxically, it was precisely my closeness to this dance form that initially kept me from engaging with it critically or theoretically. That changed when I moved to Oberlin and began to teach contact improvisation in the same beautiful wooden studio that sponsored one of contact's seminal explorations—Steve Paxton's 1972 dance for twelve men entitled *Magnesium*.

This section begins with "A Particular History," the first conference presentation I gave on teaching contact improvisation at Oberlin College. The palpable sense of contact improvisation's history is imbued in the beautiful wood floor of Warner Main Space—the big old gymnasium where Steve Paxton taught movement skills during January 1972 and where Nancy Stark Smith danced first as a student. By the time I wrote this essay, I had been teaching contact improvisation at Oberlin for almost a decade, and I had developed a quasi-religious reverence for that space and its floor that I imparted to my students. This feeling is wonderfully articulated in the concluding paragraph of that short talk, which quotes a former student's description of that floor as a sort of ancient grail reserved for the ritual of dance. I do not know whether it is the importance of Oberlin in contact improvisation's early history, whether the floor is indeed magical, or whether there is a special affinity between Oberlin students and contact improvisation, but I feel really lucky to have found a job in a place that can generate so much energy for this form, year after year. Precisely because contact improvisation is not a static practice, I never get tired of teaching it, and I am deeply appreciative that each fall season a new crop of students learn to share my enthusiasm for its physical and psychic lessons, inspiring, in turn, my continued engagement with the form.

How ironic, then, that when I spent a year living in Strasbourg, France, and had anticipated dancing a lot of contact improvisation, I found myself instead doing a weekly capoeira class and *roda,* mixing it up with a variety of teenage boys (who could all do backflips). Needless to say, that experience was a weekly lesson in humiliation for my forty-year-old self, but I stuck it out because there was a palpable sense of community and respect for all our differences that I had found missing from the local contact improvisation jam. Our teacher was African French—a former professional volleyball player who moved his long limbs with an extraordinary fluidity and grace. Inspired by my time practicing capoeira in France and later back in the United States, "Open Bodies," is a comparison of contact improvisation and capoeira, two forms of physical engagement with an increasingly global influence.

This essay was originally written for *Protée*—a French-language publication—and in it I try to articulate the ways in which these two forms encourage a meeting of the "other" in oneself within a circle of witnesses. I was intrigued with how contact improvisation and capoeira, although they come from very different historical and cultural roots, are hybrid improvisational forms that encourage an experience of vulnerability, disorientation, as well as a certain feisty resistance to being challenged. And both forms can sponsor gorgeous moments of kinesthetic collaboration, providing a physical model for engaging across cultural difference. Several months ago while I was in Porto Alegre, Brazil, I had the opportunity to witness a class and *roda* at the studio of Contramestre Guto. Even though I was dressed up and had just given an academic talk, I could tell that there was no way I would be allowed to leave that space without participating. My host and I entered the circle, shifting between capoeira and contact improvisation in an attempt to demonstrate the affinities and differences between the two forms. Later, Mestre Guto, who had never heard of contact improvisation before, told us that he felt he had witnessed a ritual that had created a "sacred space between two people," confirming once again my sense that these forms share much in common.

The next essay, "Present Tense: Contact Improvisation at 25," discusses the twenty-fifth anniversary celebration of contact improvisation that was held at Oberlin College during the summer of 1997. The organization and structure of that event revealed several of the underlying tensions of a form that has expanded and influenced so many aspects of contemporary dance practice. In this anniversary essay I describe the friction between the beginning three days of intensive training that focused on the cultivation of highly virtuosic technique and the following mixed-ability weekend that sought to include a wide diversity of bodies within the core definition of the dance form. This very short discussion of contact improvisation and questions of ability is expanded in an essay entitled "Strategic Abilities," which is featured in the Occasional Pieces section at the end of this collection.

The final piece here, "Feeling In and Out: Contact Improvisation and the Politics of Empathy," was written as a presentation for the Kinesthesia and Empathy in Dance conference held in Berlin during the summer of 2011. In this talk, I propose that contact improvisation affords us a new approach to feeling and empathy. Instead of categorizing feeling as a psychological affect, I suggest that contact improvisation encourages us to approach feeling as a process—a verb, rather than a noun. Framed as an ongoing practice instead of an emotional state, this sense of "feeling" can keep us from getting stuck in personal psychology where feelings, once articulated as "mine," can get in the way of really feeling what is going on between two people. Drawing on Susan Foster's genealogy of the term empathy, I argue that keeping the gerund in play in feel*ing* can help us escape either pigeonholing emotion or the rigid pathology of psychoanalysis, connecting us to the more open corporeal realm of sensation within our interpersonal exchanges.

19

A Particular History

Contact Improvisation at Oberlin College

Given as a talk at the Society of Dance History Scholars conference, June 1999

As I write this, I am sitting in the middle of an empty wooden space, the smell of which is intensified by the heat on this summer afternoon. Today the space feels like a big attic—old, woody, slightly airless—one whose contents have evaporated over time so that only the dust, memories, and ghosts remain. This large, brown, hollow gymnasium has at times reminded me of a ship, an old swimming pool, a Roman amphitheater, and a huge, but comfy, womb. The space I am describing is Warner Main Space, unquestionably one of the most beautiful dance studios in the world. I have danced in this space at sunrise and at sunset. I have danced here throughout all the seasons of the year; in storms and in fair weather. I know the magical effects of the sun at different times of the day, and I have personally rolled over almost every inch of the wonderfully responsive floor (which is like a trampoline). I have danced in this space alone and with over 300 people. Two months ago, during Oberlin's twenty-four-hour contact jam, I climbed the fire escape at 3:30 in the morning and entered the space, expecting to dance a short good-night turn, and ended up being lured by an ecstatic pianist into a thirty-minute solo that did everything but put me to sleep.

This is just one example of the kind of energy that reverberates in the space. These days, I consider it home—a place of dwelling in which I feel most fully present. It is also the home of one of the most vibrant contact improvisation communities in any university setting. In her introduction to the collection of essays entitled *Choreographing History*, Susan Foster describes a similar shift when the historical subject materializes to take on a body of its own, moving in partnership with the dancer/writer:

> When this transformation in the nature of the inquiry occurs, a corresponding redefinition of authorial function also takes place: the author loses identity as the guiding authority and finds him or herself immersed in the process of the project getting made. *This is not mystical; it's really quite bodily. Rather than a transcendence of the body, it's an awareness of moving with as well as in and through the body as one moves alongside other bodies.*[1]

Foster is describing here an ideal contact duet, where the dancing occurs with both creative inspiration and critical awareness—a space in which she is neither leading nor following. Wrapped up in the particular history of contact improvisation at Oberlin College is also a personal history of my body's engagement with that form. How these separate histories intersect to create a dance pedagogy based on past legacies, an enduring sense of place, as well as new visions of community, is the subject of this essay.

It was in Warner Main Space twenty-seven years ago that Steve Paxton created *Magnesium:* the dance that is cited by most historians as the seminal work of contact improvisation. While he was in residence, Paxton came to know two Oberlin students—Curt Siddall and Nancy Stark Smith—who joined him later that summer for a series of dance events at the John Weber gallery in New York City. Unlike Curt Siddall, who eventually stopped dancing and entered the business world, Nancy Stark Smith has continued to teach and perform contact improvisation throughout the world. In addition, she has been instrumental in creating and editing the journal *Contact Quarterly,* an ongoing forum for discussions about contact improvisation and related disciplines. Smith's connection to Oberlin has led to several high-profile events, including the 1997 summer event—CI25—a two-week celebration of contact improvisation, which brought some 250 dancers from all over the world to dance together in Warner Main Space. Just two weeks ago, Nancy returned for her twenty-fifth reunion, spawning Oberlin's first annual commencement/reunion jam. That occasion also marked the first alumni reunion where students whom I had trained in contact came back to dance, thus bringing four generations of contact dancers together in Warner Main. For anyone as addicted to contact improvisation as I am, it was a supremely satisfying event. It was also the perfect time to reflect on Oberlin as an institution that provided the environment not only for Paxton's early investigations, but also for an extraordinary flourishing of the form over the past decade.

In the early 1970s, Oberlin College, like many other small liberalarts colleges, was experiencing a variety of revolutions both on and off campus. The president, Robert Fuller, was the youngest and perhaps one of the most radical college presidents at the time. His desire to include not only faculty, but also students in the administrative decision-making processes galvanized the students into realizing the college's motto of "Learning and Labor." One of the most interesting curricular experiments at this time was the Inter Arts program, which combined the art department, the composition program in the Conservatory of Music, and the theater and dance programs into a single interdisciplinary performance program facilitated by Herbert Blau. Building on connections with the experimental theater and dance scene in California and New York City, Oberlin's program was a mini-performance oasis in the middle of Ohio. Money from the National Endowment for the

Arts was available for bringing New York City artists out to the Midwest in order to set new work on the students, and over the course of two years Oberlin's dance program was host to extended residencies by Twyla Tharp, Yvonne Rainer, the Grand Union, and, of course, Steve Paxton.

In January 1972, Paxton came to Oberlin to teach a winter-term workshop. Each day began with a sunrise movement class opened to anyone willing to get up that early. The emphasis of that class was the "stand," or "small dance." As Paxton explains it: "It's a fairly easy perception: all you have to do is stand up and then relax, and at a certain point you realize that you've relaxed everything that you can relax but you're still standing and in that standing is quite a lot of minute movement."[2] Later in the day, Paxton worked with a group of eleven other men, teaching them the improvisational structure that would later become *Magnesium*. Although there was, as yet, no official name for the form, Paxton's teaching focused on the physical investigations of stillness and falling that quickly became the foundations of contact improvisation training. At its inception, contact improvisation embodied issues of self, independence, community, and change that were emblematic of the 1960s. Beginning with a state of shared responsibility for one another's weight (a state which contactors describe as being "mutually weight dependent," that is, leaning on one another so that neither individual is fully holding her own weight or that of her partner), the dancers follow a common point as it revolves around their bodies and travels through space. Influenced by Asian martial arts and contemporary release techniques, the movement training of the dance form is meant to equip the dancers with the skills necessary to follow this point of contact as it moves across the chest, down the stomach, across the thigh, up the back to the top of the head. The physical techniques of rolling, learning when and when not to give weight, and how to accept another's weight, as well as learning how to fall safely, enable the improvisation—that common choice to explore an unforeseen moment—that is the creative basis for the dancers' engagement in the duet. In her book on contact improvisation and American culture, *Sharing the Dance*, Cynthia Jean Cohen Bull describes the videotape that Steve Christiansen took of *Magnesium*:

> The tape shows an event obviously set in the 1960s (taken as a cultural period). The assorted loosely fitting pants and shirt and the long hair provide obvious signs, but the quality of movement—the loose, awkward, wild abandon, the earnest directness—are immediately apprehended kinesthetic markers of this historical moment. Performing on several wrestling mats, the men stagger about, crash into each other, fall, roll, and get up only to lurch around again. A lot of hand clasping and pulling or dragging occurs, so that the dance looks like drunken wrestling at times. The performers have no orientation towards the audience, pursuing their falling with a task-like attitude.[3]

Good dance historians that we are, we can certainly recognize in Cynthia's movement description the classic elements of postmodern dance, particularly the casual, task-oriented attitude of the movers. What Cynthia does not discuss, but what is present in most students' minds when they watch this video, are the other cultural markers of that historical moment—the implicated metaphors of death and war, especially given the soundtrack. Ironically, there was no actual soundtrack. The sounds you hear on the video are the highly amplified sounds of the floor, the men's breathing, and the audience's applause and cackle. Whenever Paxton or those present at the original performance of *Magnesium* hear that my students see the piece as a cultural commentary on the Vietnam War, they seem surprised, maybe even a bit suspicious that I, a dance historian and academic who tends to spend too much time talking about cultural meanings, have fed them that line. In any case, they hasten to point out that the dance was not intended as a political statement. These shifts in perception between then and now—between veteran contactors and my students—create what I consider to be interesting historical disjunctions, the negotiation of which provides extraordinary opportunities for teaching about history and dancing bodies.

As a committed dancer as well as a dance critic, I teach contact as a physical discipline that has greatly influenced styles of contemporary dance, as a historical adventure that began in the very studio we dance in, and as a form of cultural representation that can both reflect and create values in American society. So that while we are learning how to fall softly, roll over one another, and loft, I encourage the students to ask questions about the cultural ideologies implied in the dancing—but not all at once. Although I am currently fascinated by how contact improvisation helps me think through the body in ways that problematize contemporary debates about bodies, identities, and cultural theory, I choose to start the semester without directly addressing this intellectual material. Instead, I begin with physical skills, for the movement training in contact improvisation builds an important sense of trust within the class—a physical grounding from which we can take those kinds of intellectual risks.

One of the most disorienting aspects of contact improvisation, especially for people who are new to the dance form, is the whole issue of bodily contact—of physical touch. Physical contact, of course, is societally determined. One of my most difficult tasks, then, is to create a dancing environment in which everyone feels safe enough to push their focus beyond the mere fact of touching and being touched to the how of that interaction. In order to build this trust, I begin with simple exercises, choosing the more neutral points of bodily contact such as the wrists, forearms, and backs to begin with. Often, I will have the class work on the same exercise with different partners so that everyone gets a sense of how different bodies hold weight and how the various combinations of bodies negotiate the physical tasks I set up for them.

As soon as the students start to grasp these basic physical skills, I introduce one of the most difficult and fundamental concepts of contact improvisation: replace ambition with curiosity. This is a mantra that I picked up from Nancy Stark Smith and by locating this core concept within the history of Warner Main Space—that is, within the history of the studio in which we all dance—I give the students the possibility of entering the form from whatever direction they choose. Indeed, the focus on refusing any notion of "mastery," even as I encourage increasing physical awareness, seems to be the key to Oberlin students' wholehearted embracing of this particular form of dancing. As one student wrote:

> Contact Improvisation is the greatest life metaphor. There is no mastery, only practice.
>
> There aren't enough hours in an eon to master a form like contact. Andrew Harwood never mastered it, Nancy Stark Smith never mastered it, Danny Lepkoff never mastered it, Ann Cooper Albright never mastered it, Isadora Duncan never even knew about it, Lisa Nelson never mastered it, Steve Paxton never mastered it, you never mastered it, you don't know anyone who has mastered it, and the story you heard about someone mastering it was a myth, so Lord knows I'll be eat'in some fine puddin' if I ever master it. (Joey Rizzolo, 1997)

In the first half of the semester, issues of power, trust, desire, sexuality, as well as cultural norms and biases about what constitutes an able body surface intermittently through discussions of our physical experience in contact improvisation. Later, the class begins to address these issues explicitly, bringing them into our dancing on a much more conscious level. For example, we explore the dramatic possibilities of social hierarchy in contact improvisation duets, as well as the various ways to "make contact" that do not require touch, such as kinesthetic synchronicity, and visual, vocal, and rhythmic connections with one another. Similarly, we might question the assumption of "following" the point of contact, and look instead for the possibilities which lie in willful resistance. Interestingly enough, I have found that by recognizing the cultural meanings implied by bodies in contact with one another, my students have become increasingly interested in the history of contact improvisation and the experience of various generations of dancing bodies. During the spring of 1997, as part of the preparations for CI25, Steve Paxton came to Oberlin for a three-week residency, ostensibly to remount *Magnesium*. When he arrived, however, Steve decided not to reconstruct the piece on the grounds that he thought it would be too dangerous, especially for female students. Although they were respectful of his decision, the students still desired to revisit that seminal moment in Warner Main Space's history, and this past spring they conceived of a "history" performance as part of a lecture/demonstration in which aspects of *Magnesium* were re-created.

The students' avid interest in the history of contact improvisation fascinates me. I recognize, of course, my own role in sponsoring this vital inquiry, and the various ways that I have helped to create a sense of contact improvisation's legacy at Oberlin College. But the magic of their curiosity—that kind of spiritual partnering with the ghosts of the historical bodies that danced in Warner Main Space—does not come from me. Rather, it seeps up through the floorboards and into our skin as we stand or lie at the beginning of class, tuning into the subtle shifts of weight that mark our entry into the small dance.

> We were on our backs on the floor doing the imagery exercise. Ann started to embrace the history of contact in Warner Main and explain how she feels that the experience of each dance coats the floors and walls of the space. I started to feel for the first time how loaded that room is, thinking of *Magnesium* being in the floor beneath me, of the injuries, of the joy, and of all the classes that have experienced the expansion I have been feeling all semester. I started to envision Warner Main as an ancient wooden cup or grail that is only used during its specific ritual and ceremony of dance. We are, and they have been, the wine of the nectar that swirls in the cup, and after it is emptied, its essence and flavor remains, shaded into the grain of the wood, so that it can never be washed away. (Nick Thompson, 1999)

NOTES

1. Susan Foster, *Choreographing History* (Bloomington: Indiana University Press 1995), 10.
2. *Contact Quarterly* 3, no. 1 (Fall 1977): 11.
3. Cynthia Novack, *Sharing the Dance: Contact Improvisation and American Culture* (Madison: University of Wisconsin Press, 1990), 60–61.

20

Open Bodies

(X)changes of Identity in Capoeira and Contact Improvisation

From *Protée* 29, no.2, 2001.

A lone dancer enters the circle, first crawling, then rolling and finally waltzing toward the center. He almost trips, turns and then stops, looking around and catching someone's—anyone's—eye. Another dancer accepts this silent invitation and enters the dance, bursting in like a meteor spinning through a galaxy. He launches his body into a furious series of movements. Some kind of gravity (or maybe just exhaustion) pulls him into the other dancer's orbit and as they turn, their hands meet in a tentative balance. Fueled by that joining of forces, they trace a pathway that follows its own logic through the space. They are driven by the exchange of momentum, weight, and breath, moving through shapes and space so quickly they must release any desire to make decisions and simply be content to observe their journey as it unfolds. Eventually, their exchanges become slower and more subdued, arriving in a fragile balance—one dancer's head nestled into the other dancer's back.

They crouch expectantly, surrounded by the syncopated rhythms and the voices of the people on either side. Their hands meet only briefly, but their eyes lock, maintaining contact even as they flip over onto their hands. On their feet once again, they shift back and forth in unison, keeping their joints loose and their imaginations supple. The fluid mirroring shifts dynamic as one gestures and the other takes up the challenge. This engagement sparks a playful responsiveness as they explore the possibilities of a movement exchange that flirts with—but never involves—physical contact.

These two descriptions of movement duets—that meeting an "other" in motion—map out the genres of physical encounters I discuss in this essay. The first passage is a moment within contact improvisation. The second is a moment within capoeira. On the surface, these forms represent disparate cultural histories and very different dynamics of physical interaction. After all, one is about merging into a physical union; the other is about emerging (safely) from physical combat. Yet both forms have taken hold of the kinetic imaginations of contemporary dancers and influenced movement vocabularies throughout the world. Both forms are increasingly global phenomena. Contact improvisation and capoeira emerged from moments of historical and cultural confusion and combustion, and both forms still have elements of those resistive and rebellious moments embedded in their physical strategies. And yet, both forms have also continued to reinvent themselves—incorporating contemporary concerns into their movement vocabularies. Most importantly, both forms have helped to revise conventional notions of identity and geography, creating in their stead a somatic experience that reconstructs our notions of alterity from the inside out. As I argue over the course of this essay, both capoeira and contact improvisation have shaped a physical and metaphysical practice that can help us survive—even thrive—in our ever-changing, challenging, intercultural world.

This essay is an attempt to articulate a powerful, gut-felt conviction that something truly important is going on here. That in the midst of these improvisational exchanges of attention, gesture, sweat, and energy, one is trained to confront an "other" in such a way as to confound the usual distinctions between self and "other." This is my first try at translating my physical involvement with these movement forms into a theoretical language. The evangelistic tone of the writing emerges from a belief that the experience of dancing and performing contact improvisation for most of my adult life and training in capoeira over the past few years has given me an interesting perspective on the increasingly specific delineation of subjectivity and alterity. As I have become alternately confused, elated, depressed, or just plain bogged down by the seemingly endless contestations over identity politics in both academic circles and artistic communities, I have found myself seeking refuge in the body-to-body interactions of the studios where I move. This is not to suggest that these physical relations are necessarily easier, less complex, or unproblematic. But it seems to me that while issues of diversity are never confined to the physical body—they are always implicated in social contexts and representational structures—they are made present through our bodies. As a feminist, I realize that bodies are deeply constructed by cultural attitudes and economic conditions. As a dancer, I am aware that bodies can also be physically retrained and consciously retheorized; that nonverbal behavior plays a significant role in negotiating identity politics. How we approach, walk, talk, and dance with one another means a lot.

As we know, difference is about power. This is to say that cultural difference is written (most often) onto the physical body in ways that are then read in terms of social identities. Race, gender, class, ethnicity, sexuality, age, and ability are all (still) crucial markers of difference at the beginning of the twenty-first century. All these differences, however, are manifestations of a binary structure of difference basic to Western epistemology. The mind is separated from the body, and the two are then figured in terms of self

(Descartes's famous line "I think, therefore I am") and otherness—where the self is an internalized mind and the "other" is inextricably tied to the body (which we understand scientifically, not intuitively). In the last two decades, feminists have provided us with a litany of examples documenting just how pervasive the separation of body and mind is in our culture. As they have aptly demonstrated, the foundational philosophies and religious ideologies of Western civilization first constructed, and then sought to naturalize, a dualistic paradigm that divided the world into oppositional categories—body/mind, nature/culture, private/public, spirituality/corporeality, and experience/knowledge. These schematic polarizations created, in turn, unavoidable hierarchies, which positioned the body as the material "other" to the transcendence of the mind.

These bodily categories of difference—racial difference, class difference, ethnic difference, as well as differences in physical ability and sexuality—have radically altered both popular imaginations and academic discourses. Yet after several decades of brilliant and detailed cataloguing of social oppressions, we need to ask: what difference has difference made?

I do not mean to be facetious here—quite the contrary. I am deeply committed to the liberatory possibilities, both individual and communal, of these cultural analyses. What I am indicating, however, is the direction of the next step; for there must certainly be a next step. The problem with an encyclopedic detailing of differences is that they run the risk of reifying the binary, reducing difference to a static, monolithic fact of difference. Rather than seeing difference as one set position, I am arguing for a positioning (and, by extension, a *re*positioning) that is always in motion. In this sense, then, I offer capoeira and contact improvisation as examples of movement forms that incorporate that physical confrontation with the other—in which difference can be acknowledged and still moved through, with, toward, under, beyond, in accordance with, etc. These forms represent physical exchanges across difference in which the bodily fact of difference is celebrated and mobile.

The last two decades have ruptured a certain complacency with the world that is truly important and I believe that the hesitancy we all feel—that moment of awareness that makes us stop and think when we talk or write—is critical for a reorganization of the dynamics of privilege and power. I am deeply aware that all these liberatory struggles must continue, that they are, in fact, more important than ever. But I am also sensible of how a hyper-awareness of difference brings people to a self-consciousness that can be completely debilitating. The result is that everyone retreats into their respective corners; so nervous about offending or being offended that the gulf between us all widens. How do we train ourselves to launch across that divide? How do we encourage a willingness to engage with difference? How do we move from the idea into the practice? I believe that we must take the risk of failure, risk the embarrassments and the awkwardness, risk feeling uncomfortable and having our toes stepped on, in order to launch ourselves across that metaphysical slash between self/other. The first moves of any new partnership are rarely smooth, but we must take that chance and ask an "other" to dance.

Contact improvisation is a dance form developed in the early 1970s by a group of people who were interested in exploring the dancing produced by the exchange of weight between two (or more) people. The movement in contact improvisation is structured by the specific physics of this exchange of bodies—the changing dynamics of weight, space, momentum, and force. Of course, how we experience this combination of physical elements is ideologically and historically determined, and the cultural ramifications of this dancing can shift from moment to moment, dance to dance, and year to year. At its inception, contact improvisation embodied many of the issues about self, independence, community, and change that were emblematic of the 1960s.[1] Beginning with a state of shared responsibility for one another's weight (a state that contactors describe as being "mutually weight dependent," that is, leaning on one another so that neither individual is fully holding her own weight or that of her partner), the dancers follow that common point as it revolves around their bodies and travels through space. Influenced by Asian martial arts and contemporary release techniques, the movement training of the dance form is meant to equip the dancers with the skills necessary to follow this point of contact as it moves across the chest, down the stomach, across the thigh, up the back to the top of the head. The physical techniques of rolling, learning when and when not to give weight, and how to accept another's weight, as well as learning how to fall safely, enable the improvisation—that common choice to explore an unforeseen moment—that is the creative basis for the dancers' engagement in the duet.

The history of capoeira is longer and more contested than that of contact improvisation and which his/story you get depends a lot on whom you ask or read. Still, most people agree that capoeira is an Afro-Brazilian martial dance form that started in the colonial days when European landowners had all but depleted the indigenous supply of manual labor and began importing slaves from Africa, particularly the Kongo-Angola regions. Under the surveillance of the European masters, the traditional warrior training evolved into a combat form for two based on a rhythmic exchange of attacks and defenses. This martial pas de deux was done in a protective circle (the *roda*), whose rhythms would change to signal the danger of surveillance. Quickly, the dynamics of the combat would shift into a nonthreatening movements (a simple dance). Later, after abolition and with increasing urbanization, capoeira shifted once again into more of a street-fighting mode, and began its long association with a global urban youth culture. This link, in fact, is still evident today with the various mixes of capoeira and hip-hop performed on plazas and street corners all over the Americas, Africa, Asia, and Europe.

Eventually, in the mid-twentieth century, capoeira became increasingly codified and structured in Brazil, with capoeira academies opening in order to train young players in the "game" of capoeira. At once fighting and dancing, capoeira has been used throughout its history as a form of improvised resistance, not only in terms of the colonial institution of slavery, but also within other, more local, dynamics of racialized and economic power. This "resistance" is not simply a question of how capoeira was deployed within Brazilian history, but how a certain subversiveness is actually embedded within the physical experience of the form.

Contact improvisation's ongoing connections to a variety of "alternative" practices—tai chi, body-mind centering, authentic movement, aikido, etc.—and capoeira's associations with street life and youth culture place these forms on the margins of institutional spaces: governmental, academic, artistic lieus. With few exceptions, contact improvisation is generally taught by a shifting, migrant population of teachers/performers. Like worker bees traveling from city to city to pollinate dance scenes all over the world, these dancers share their expertise with dancers trained in whatever styles of dance are favored in their own culture at the moment. These bouts of teaching can take the form of an intensive weekend workshop, or a two-week-long retreat. Unlike many forms of dance, contact is rarely taught on a continuing basis. Capoeira also has a similar pattern of globally roving master teachers. Although it has been institutionalized in certain areas—especially in Brazil and New York City—much of the body-to-body transmission of the form takes place through informal exchanges and local networks. The contact improvisation jam, like the capoeira *roda,* is a space of experimentation for both amateur and professional movers.

While the training can seem (superficially) more casual than say ballet or karate, and while these forms embody aspects of their egalitarian, counter-hegemonic histories, both contact improvisation and capoeira have refined precise skills that are taught worldwide. These exercises constitute a foundational somatic experience that remains consistent despite individual priorities and regional differences. Although contact improvisation and capoeira train for different outcomes, the core physical discipline is remarkably similar in several ways. Both forms work (especially in the early stages) to build physical endurance, including an emphasis on upper-body strength and the ability to support one's weight on unusual combinations of body parts (hands, head, elbows, etc.). While this strength gives the dancer a refreshing sense of fierceness and energy, it is never allowed to harden into a tight, resistant, or bound use of muscles. In contact improvisation, this strength is used with momentum to lift one's partner or to support them in such a way that keeps the point of contact moving through space. The partnering in contact is circular; rarely do any "straight" lifts occur. In capoeira, strength is used to continue the motion of one's partner's moves, and hard, direct blocks (as in some forms of martial arts) are rare. Usually, one tries to evade the attack (to duck or move away from a foot or head) in order to turn around and reenter the fight at a more advantageous point. This kind of strength is strategic—connected to realizing the patterns of resistance and flow between the two figures in motion. In both forms, strength is used to create an aesthetic synchrony of energies in which one move evokes a fluid response from the "other."

This sense of fluidity in the midst of strength is one of the provocative contradictions that link capoeira and contact improvisation. In her compelling discussion of capoeira in "Headspin: Capoeira's Ironic Inversions," Barbara Browning refers to these contradictions as a kind of irony: "the no in the yes, the big in the little, the earth in the sky, the fight in the dance."[2] And, we might add, the fluidity inside the strength. Training for an awareness of this flexibility gives practitioners of contact improvisation and capoeira insight into the changes and exchanges of identity possible without sacrificing one's own experience of physical groundedness.

In his fascinating paper linking the thinking of Levinas to the practice of contact improvisation, aptly titled "(In) the In-Between," David Williams explains this meeting as an "in-between or go-between, [it] is another space in which the 'I' is both implicated and (re)conceived; it is the articulation of meeting-in-difference."[3] Williams continues to stake out the existential possibilities of the form when he claims that:

> For each of the partners, Contact constitutes the possible coexistence of form and spontaneity, rules-of-the-game and dance, cause and effect, center and margin, proximity and distance. It is the "play" within the obdurate fixity of corporeal identities, its "give," its supple-ment, its différance: the unstable borderlands where an ethics of alterity occurs.[4]

Behind this tall existential order lies a physical practice based on disorientation, curiosity, and a willingness to confront the "other" both internally and externally. Williams's words describe the effects of a somatic experience in which the usual boundaries between bodies, that sense of fixed identities, is suspended. For instance, one of the first themes one introduces to beginning students is the point of contact. Facing one's partner, one presses one's forefinger against theirs. Attending to how the energy of one's partner's whole body can move through their spine out their arm and into their finger, one waits and listens to that point of contact that will eventually begin to move. The point made by the joining of two energies—sometimes referred to as a "third mind"—becomes the focus of the partner's mutual attention as they endeavor to follow its spatial and rhythmic journey. At first, it may seem clear who is leading and who is following, but eventually, with time and practice, the shifting back and forth evolves into such a rapid and subtle exchange that those categories of leader and follower begin to lose their meaning. The binary is subverted as the attention shifts onto the play of space and touch between the two movers. Williams describes this intellectual idea in terms that easily translate into the dynamic of this partnership in contact improvisation: "The crucial factor here is not how many ways two different units can relate to each other, but recognition that this 'third element' is not a unit but an axis, not an entity but a state of being, *less a relationship than an act of relating*."[5]

The very real pleasures of sophisticated contact dancing are found in the moments of mutual suspension or falls; in the seeming magic with which complicated movements are spontaneously executed. This connectedness is the Chi of contact improvisation—the place of incredible fluidity and intuitive meshing of energies. Of course, at any point in the dancing one partner can break the point of contact to separate (either permanently or temporarily) or claim a certain "authorship," leading their partner in a very specific direction. Part of the improvisation is learning how to deal with these situations openly; with curiosity, not determination. Contact improvisation trains one to react without ever being reactionary.

At first, the risks are minimal. Finger to finger, head to head, back to back, beginning contact improvisation exercises build an awareness of how different bodies respond to the simplest movement tasks. Eventually, as the students become more skilled physically, they are introduced to exercises emphasizing falling without tensing up, giving one's weight to another person, as well as visual and spatial dis/orientation. This last discipline is crucial in setting up the exchange of identities that Williams refers to in his essay. Even exercises seemingly as simple as rolling across the floor with another person can be extremely disorienting. These exercises require a very different use of the eyes. In contact improvisation, one learns to see not by fixing one's gaze on people or surrounding objects, but rather by allowing the eyes to rest back in the eye sockets in order to engage a more relaxed, peripheral vision. This small shift in visual attention can radically change one's experience of being in the space. Rolling, spinning, and being upside down in a room with other people moving around every which way forces me to physically negotiate a chaotic field of comings and goings in which I must give up any stable sense of my "position" in the space. What is left, then, is a sense of locating oneself vis-à-vis the other people who are, of course, also moving in the space. While all this dancing around and in between one another can make for a great deal of fun and some rather humorous situations, it also suggests another way of being with others in the world—a kind of existential dance in which this shifting of positions allows for a certain reorganization of social relationships.

Contact improvisation requires a desire to dance in a state of disorientation. Unlike many dance genres, contact improvisation is about being off-balance; about enjoying the loss of control over one's own movements, both physically and psychically. I think that this willingness to experience the vertigo based on a constant exchange of weight, and the inevitable moments of falling and intimacy of catching and being caught, can profoundly affect our intellectual assumptions concerning the stability of categories of "self" and "other." While many of my examples here may strike academics as merely eccentric dance skills (after all, most academics are not interested in rolling around on the floor), the effects of this somatic work are striking and profound. In a university environment where there is a great deal of intellectual activity and talk about mutual respect, acceptance of differences, and building community, the students in contact improvisation classes are building it—from the ground up.

Contact improvisation encourages not only an engagement with another body, but also an understanding of the "other" within one's self. If Elizabeth Grosz is right when she declares that, "alterity is the very possibility and process of embodiment,"[6] then the individual somatic work which is part and parcel of so much contact improvisation training shows us how intertwined that internal alterity is with its external partner. For instance, at the beginning of my contact improvisation class, I often use an exercise known as "the stand." This is a moment where, after moving through the space, the students come to a point of stillness while standing. It gives the students an opportunity to experience the sensations of sweat and air on their arms, their heart beating, the rhythms of their pulses in different places in their body—a way to experience the subtle shifts of weight and muscular action, a chance to feel one's body at once grounded through the feet and extending through the head—a moment to reflect on the position of being suspended between earth and sky.

Later in the exercise, I ask them to imagine opening the pores of their skin so that the world can enter the space of their bodies. This image of one's body as part of the whole landscape, rather than the vehicle which moves through and arranges that landscape, has clear physical results in the released muscular tone of the body. But there is also a profound psychic reorganization here as well. If the world is already inside one's body, then the separation between self and other is much less distinct. The skin is less the impenetrable boundary of the body's integrity (à la the 1950s metaphors of disinfection that dominated both the domestic sector [take care of those germs in the kitchen and bathroom], and the international political climate [be careful of the infectious spread of communism]), as the sensing organ that brings the world closer. By shifting our somatic imagination, we can reorder our cultural notions of selfhood. Rather than the colonialist paradigm of the individual, propelled by his/her will and determination to go out into the world and stake a claim (stand on one's own two feet, make a mark, etc.), the self becomes an interdependent part that flows through and with the world.

Opening one's body up to the world is a profoundly generous gesture. It is the "give" that Williams describes as the "play within the obdurate fixity of corporeal identities." For as bodies begin to become more mobile, exploring the space and exchanging movements between them, this fluidity of boundaries becomes the dance. This generosity dislodges traditional separations of power by refusing to believe in the impermeability of the self as bounded by the body. The dancer says: "Here, take my body, come into me, use me, roll on me, let me support you, let me lean on you." In very physical ways, contact dancers offer their bodies to their partners. But this is an invitation, not humiliation. For even though boundaries are fluid, this is not an existential free fall. In the midst of all these exchanges, we can be attuned to our own physical sensations; the reassuring sense of gravity in the middle of being lifted—a steady groundedness that keeps us safe even while we launch across space and time.

This "give" in stable identities is also at "play" in capoeira. When two people enter the circle (the *roda*) to spar, they are said to be "playing" a "game." Within the protective circle of music and witnesses, the "game" begins with a double handshake—a crossing and touching which indicates a tacit agreement to play by the rules ("look, there are no blades concealed in these hands"). It also sets up a context of mutual agreement—a sign that I will attempt to play well so that you, too, can play your fullest. This gift of a dance (or game) is an opportunity to become, not to prove who you already are. It is a risk, but the payoffs are enormously satisfying. Browning sees it this way: "In a tight, 'inside game' (jogo de denteo) when the players are interweaving spinning kicks, the agility and precision of one opens a precise space for the elegant partnering of the other."[7] This commitment to playing together is also part of the "give" in identity. It is a willingness to move in and out of positions, to mix up who leads and who follows, who attacks and who dodges. As in contact improvisation, sweeping circular motions are critical to this flexibility in the game. They provide the shifting pathways in which an attack can evolve into a defense and a dodge can turn into an offensive strike. Thus, a *compaso* spirals into a *negativa* as the world of the *roda* spins between fighting and dancing.

This blend of partnering and war is part of capoeira's history. It is also, Browning argues, part of its essential character:

> But the strategic blending of fight and dance occurred in Brazil, under specific pressures. And while this strategy appears to have been directed against forces outside the roda de Capoeira, it became the fundamental strategy *within* the game. Dance—as seduction, illusion, deception—became dangerous, and kicks became elements of choreography.[8]

Browning's essay on capoeira is aptly titled "Capoeira's Ironic Inversions," and she sees all the cartwheels, handstands, head spins and other inverted movements as emblematic of capoeira's ability to see the world upside down. I see this as part of the form's double vision—a sign of its willingness to survive its own historical moment and continue to evolve. It is also a strategy of alterity, of being on the outside of the system. What Browning is pointing to in the figure of the inverted capoeirista is a willingness to be disoriented. For me, one of the most interesting correspondences between contact improvisation and capoeira is that both forms train for disorientation—that is, feeling comfortable being upside down, off balance, dizzy, or just plain awkward. These forms train practitioners to circumvent the usual panic at finding oneself in odd positions, retraining one's immediate physical responses (to grip one's muscles, hold one's breath, or shut one's eyes) by substituting a willingness to experience the sensation of being upside down or inside out. This willingness to be caught off guard, at risk, to enter unusual situations, is connected to the improvisational impulse in capoeira and contact improvisation.

Improvisation is a highly misunderstood phenomenon, especially within the dance world. Figured as the opposite of choreography, improvisation is often seen as free, spontaneous, nontechnical, wild, or childlike, as if once improvising, we simply lose all our physical and aesthetic training, becoming this blank slate on which our imagination can "go wild." Of course, as seasoned improvisers know (whether they work in dance, music, or capoeira), improvisation requires rigorous and precise training, which opens the imagination to new narrative possibilities, releases the body from habitual responses, and whets the dancer's curiosity. This is also where training in *dis*/orientation is crucial. Often we think of the "dis" in disorientation as a negative: a non-orientation. But we could reconceive of the word as meaning another sort of orientation, like seeing the world upside down. Sometimes in our linear, visual, cerebral manner we forget that there are many organizing strategies that do not necessarily look like the forms we are used to. The improvisation in capoeira and contact improvisation releases one from a certain way of ordering so that an "other" kind of ordering (often a much less visible one) becomes available. Thus, a structure as simple as moving backwards can force one to use other reflexes and other positions (looking between one's legs, for instance) to orient one's self. Although there are many different kinds of exercises to work on improvisational skills, the true test comes when one enters the circle to join one's partner. This is the moment when everyone—from beginner to the most advanced practitioner—must take a leap of faith and launch themselves across the unknown.

The first few seconds are the hardest, for they create the space of meeting, of understanding, of perceiving his or her rhythms, weight, hesitation, or force. It can be a scary moment, but it does not take place in a void. In capoeira, the *roda* creates a protective ring that insulates the players from outside interference, and keeps them focused. Similarly, in contact improvisation, the round-robin provides an unbroken circle of witnesses whose concentration on the events in the center preserves the almost sacred atmosphere. There is a sense of group responsibility. It is important to keep the circles evenly spaced so that there are no black holes, no breaks in energy. This is a question of safety, of course, but the cohesive energy of the circle also creates an uncanny attentiveness that draws out the magic within these interactions and encourages the participants to realize their fullest potential.

This circle of attentiveness begins as a wild space—a space of improvisation, a space that celebrates the act of becoming (together) something unforeseen. It is a ring of continuity that provides the possibility of transformation and exchange between people. It is, I suggest, an intersubjective space. Not because it magically remakes difference into something that makes no difference (either by erasing the fact of difference or by multiplying it exponentially). No, it is an intersubjective space because upon entering it with another person (the contact improvisation duet, the capoeira game) I meet the "other" in myself. But I do not stop there, arrested by that image of alterity facing me. I move on through the looking glass, passing from the two-dimensional images into three-dimensional movement. Joining another in motion releases me from a position of subjecthood that requires an object as its predicate. It allows me to move beyond my own knowledge of myself to experience my identity in the midst of someone else's energies. This willingness to merge with someone else's energies, movements, rhythms, ideas, is, I believe, one of the most valuable lessons to be had from either contact improvisation or capoeira, and it is something that I am working on engaging in workshops for academics. Negotiating the intimacy of combat or physical contact has made me realize the value of my embodied knowledge and has helped me see how we need to relax into another kind of communication, call on other kinds of corporeal intelligences, in order to open our bodies, expand our imaginations and deal successfully with issues of cultural difference.

In this sense, then, contact improvisation and capoeira are hybrid forms: culturally hybrid because over the years of their existence they have incorporated movement information from modern and postmodern dance, hip-hop, Asian martial arts, and other influences too numerous to list; "internally" hybrid in the sense that they insist on the meeting of two people, energies, and movement preferences every time their respective circles are enacted. This ability to adapt has not only kept these forms alive in many different situations; it has also confounded traditional notions of cultural authenticity and historical lineage, nation, and community. Both forms provide us with important models for living in the twenty-first century, for they orchestrate a confrontation with an "other" person as well as the "other" in one's self. But that meeting takes place within a space receptive to the possibility of movement and change. In this space, the various bodies, energies, and (subject) positions shift back and forth (like the *ginga* or the revolving point of contact) so fast that we can only see the movements in between. The poles of self and other lose their oppositional orientation and meaning as the vibration between them becomes the electrical force powering another kind of exchange.

NOTES

1. In the late 1970s and early 1980s, veteran practitioners of the form for ten years had pretty much crystalized a virtuosic style of dancing that had an easeful, flowing quality, as well as a highly acrobatic edge that frequently looked titillatingly dangerous, as one dancer would spiral up another's body to spin in the air on their shoulder. Highly skilled in falling, rolling, and jumping at high speeds, these dancers focused on the more abstract physical dynamics of the movements rather than the social implications of the dancing. In the latter part of the 1980s and into the 1990s, many contact dancers have expanded this form by drawing out the emotional, theatrical, and political implications of this dancing. A key factor in this development has been the introduction of contact to young children, senior citizens, and differently abled communities. See Novack's, *Sharing The Dance,* and "Dancing With Different Populations," *Contact Quarterly* 1, no. 1 (Winter 1992).

2. Barbard Browning, "Headspin: Capoeira's Ironic Inversions," in *Samba: Resistance in Motion* (Bloomington: Indiana University Press, 1995), 108.

3. David Williams, "(In) the In-Between," *Writings on Dance* (Winter 1996): 26.

4. Ibid.

5. Ibid., 25 (emphasis added).

6. Elizabeth Grosz, *Volatile Bodies* (Bloomington: Indiana University Press, 1994), 209.

7. Browning, 90.

8. Browning, 91.

21

Present Tense

Contact Improvisation at Twenty-Five

From *Taken by Surprise: Improvisation in Dance and Mind,* ed. Ann Cooper Albright and David Gere (2003).

When people ask me how CI25 went, there is one moment I love to describe. It is when I walked back into the main dance studio in Oberlin College at 2:30 a.m. Sunday morning and, much to my delight, saw over sixty sweaty people dancing in the space, with another fifty-some bodies scattered around the periphery of the dance floor chatting, singing, playing music, doing bodywork, sleeping, or just lying back and observing the scene. That this many people were still dancing after twelve days of classes, jams, and various conversations about contact improvisation struck me as wonderful. It was a demonstration of the enduring physical and ethical values and just plain good fun of this particular dance form.

CI25 was a two-week celebration of contact improvisation's twenty-five years of existence, which took place at Oberlin College during the summer of 1997. While a few cynics expressed a belief that this jubilee might actually be more of a wake for a form that had lost its relevancy to our fin de siècle culture, the sheer enthusiasm of the participants and their extraordinary dancing gave ample testimony to the continuing appeal of contact improvisation. Indeed, over the course of the three central events: a three-day intensive contact improvisation training workshop, a mixed-ability weekend, and a weeklong jam and jubilee celebration, I had the very great pleasure of witnessing the finely tuned craft of experienced contact dancing. In addition, there was the excitement of seeing this improvisational form expand beyond the cultivation of virtuosic dancing techniques to explore what kinds of dancing can engage a wide diversity of bodies and cultural experiences.

Giving a coherent description of contact improvisation is a tricky business, for the form has grown exponentially over time and has traveled through many countries and dance communities. Although it was developed in the 1970s, contact improvisation has recognizable roots in the social and aesthetic revolutions of the 1960s. Contact at once embraces the casual, individualistic, improvisatory ethos of social dancing and the experimentation with pedestrian and task-like movement favored by early postmodern dance groups such as the Judson Church Dance Theater. Resisting both the idealized body of ballet as well as the dramatically expressive body of modern dance, contact improvisation seeks to create what Cynthia Novack, in her book on the early development of contact improvisation, *Sharing the Dance,* calls a "responsive" body, one based in the physical exchange of weight.[1] The physical training of contact improvisation emphasizes the release of the body's weight onto the floor or into a partner's body. In contact, the experience of internal sensations and the flow of the movement between two bodies is more important than specific shapes or formal positions. Dancers learn to move with a consciousness of the physical communication implicit within the dancing. Curt Siddall, an early exponent of contact improvisation, describes the form as a combination of kinesthetic forces: "Contact Improvisation is a movement form, improvisational in nature, involving two bodies in contact. Impulses, weight, and momentum are communicated through a point of physical contact that continually rolls across and around the bodies of the dancers."[2]

Two hundred and thirty-nine dancers from nineteen different countries and five continents attended contact improvisation's silver-anniversary celebration.[3] (The Sunday before the event, I answered phone calls from Germany, Japan, Canada, and Brazil—all within the space of an hour!) Some of the participants stayed for all three events, while some just passed through for a couple of days. That so many people would find their way to a small town in Ohio to honor this dance form's coming-of-age was truly extraordinary. Contact improvisation has a strong history at Oberlin College, for it was Steve Paxton's residency and workshop there during January-term 1972 that provided the physical platform for some of the experiments that later took place under the new rubric of contact improvisation at the John Weber Gallery in New York City in June 1972. It was while he was teaching at Oberlin that Paxton met Nancy Stark Smith, who was then majoring in dance and creative writing. Smith joined Paxton in New York City later that year, embarking on a career that would make her one of the most influential figures in the development of contact improvisation. Smith is a widely respected teacher, dancer, as well as the coeditor of *Contact Quarterly*—a journal committed to documenting the various aspects of this contemporary dance form. Inspired by the idea of creating an anniversary celebration at Oberlin, Smith became the central coordinator of an event where the behind-the-scenes organization was as reflective of contact's communal ethos as is the late-night dancing described earlier.

After several preliminary discussions with the board of Contact Collaborations and other calls to check out the feasibility of hosting a dance conference at Oberlin, Smith sent out a letter to over 150 people who taught and/or organized contact improvisation events around the country, inviting them to participate in organizing a celebration of contact improvisation's twenty-fifth anniversary. By November, she had over thirty cocurators, who then took responsibility for different aspects of the celebration, including organizing the teaching-intensive, mixed-ability weekend, the archive and art gallery, documentation, hospitality, and local newsletter. In her editor note in the anniversary issue of *Contact Quarterly*, Smith describes this process: "What a pleasure to work with devoted, intelligent, responsible, creative, playful, funny, dancing organizer-artists, all operating from a love and respect for the work we were there to celebrate, and who never let this fact get too far out of reach. People whose organizing was informed by their dancing: skilled at both initiating and following, listening, offering and asking for support where needed, generating creative ideas, willing to set limits on what they could and wanted to handle."[4] Because one of the most significant tenets of contact improvisation is the marked absence of any hierarchy—be it school, committee, or accrediting association—many contact improvisation dancers quickly become skilled at organizing classes, jams, and retreats simply in order to keep dancing themselves. This grass-roots involvement (Need a dance partner? Teach it to your roommate!) and community facilitating of dance events has allowed contact improvisation to grow in many different communities that otherwise would not have the funds to support a licensed dance school. One of the most interesting pages of Nancy Stark Smith's personal documentation of the early days of contact improvisation was a letter, mostly unsigned, that was meant to trademark the name contact improvisation and certify only certain teachers of the form. Instead of becoming responsible for this kind of technical policing of the form, however, Smith, Paxton, and other early practitioners decided to create "a vehicle for communication in which to report activity and current thinking within the work, to keep the work open by inviting ourselves and others further into the dialogue."[5] The result was *Contact Newsletter*, which later evolved into *Contact Quarterly*—a journal of contemporary dance and improvisation that encouraged dancers to write about their experiences with the form. Each issue of *Contact Quarterly* contains a "contacts" list of teachers and facilitators in the United States and abroad. Indeed, it is not uncommon to hear of people dancing their way across the country, stopping in on jams here and there as they pass through.

The amazing diversity of regional affiliation and nationalities was marked at CI25 by a series of photographs taken on the final day of the jubilee (fondly called Pinnacle Day). Dancers were grouped according to home continents and regional connections, as well as by the number of years dancing, age, facilitator-teachers, original members of the Weber Gallery collective, Oberlin alumni, and whatever other celebratory connections people chose to name. Because this dance form can trace its existence through living bodies, it was amazing to see the interconnections and to trace the various generations of teachers and students present. Many of those present had studied with Nancy Stark Smith, Steve Paxton, or their students. Yet everyone brings their interests and desires to the dancing. This interweaving of physical sources of contact improvisation with one's own focus created one of the most interesting aspects of CI25. People would spontaneously create small discussion/study groups surrounding issues of spirituality, sexuality, race, disability, age, body therapies, and elitism, to mention only a few. But despite this incredible diversity, CI25 often celebrated a specific type of contact improvisation—one that exemplified virtuosic dancing and improvisational ease.

CI25 began with a three-day contact training intensive, with classes taught by Steve Paxton, Nancy Stark Smith, Danny Lepkoff, K. J. Holmes, and Martin Keogh. These experienced contactors gave a demonstration/performance one evening. It was tremendously satisfying to see the depth that a real history of dancing together can give to an improvisational duet, and nowhere was this more evident than in the extended duet that Nancy Stark Smith and Steve Paxton did that evening. CI25 marked not only the twenty-fifth anniversary of contact improvisation, but also twenty-five years of Smith and Paxton dancing together. This recognition of their interconnected movement history provided a highly charged frame for their dancing—a fact recognized by the audience, as well as the other performers. Once Smith joined Paxton in the space, the other performers quickly pulled back to the edges, allowing them an uninterrupted space and energy. The fluidity with which these two dancers' body weight poured into and out of one another's bodies, the sensate, three-dimensionality of their physical awareness, the graceful suspensions and backwards falls, the way that their contact flowed from the center of their torsos through a limb and out into space, not to mention the requisite shoulder lofts, all marked this duet as the classical form of contact improvisation. Grounded by twenty-five years of kinesthetic communication, their dancing was exceptional—paced in a manner slow and sensitive enough to allow the audience a window into their dancing experience. A wonderful moment occurred about halfway through this duet when a spinning movement brought Smith standing about two feet in front of Paxton. As he reached his hand toward her back, his spine began to lean just as she arched her head and pitched sideways. Paxton caught her, and they both dropped towards the floor with an empathetic responsiveness.

Although their duet was improvisational and therefore unscripted in a traditional choreographic sense, Smith's and Paxton's dancing is based on a vocabulary of specific contact improvisation skills. Some of these are the physical skills of falling and rolling, learning to use the head as an extension of the limbs, spatial disorientation, finding strength through spatial extension, and lofting the pelvis. Underneath these physical skills is a whole complex of psychic skills that set up the real foundation for their improvisational dancing. At its best, contact improvisation reorders our traditional Western conceptions of the body and identity. The sense of self as an ego that goes forth to make its mark on the world (the frontier mentality) is subtly reshaped into a sense of one's own body as it exists in space and with others. While this radical reorganization of the psyche can be emotionally complicated for specific individuals, the contact improvisation exercises that train for these kinds of awarenesses are often deceptively simple.

There is, for instance, the stand, developed by Paxton as the final section of *Magnesium,* a piece he made while at Oberlin in January 1972. The stand is just that—a stand with feet placed about hip-width apart, knees and ankles relaxed. Although each teacher will use slightly different images (my favorite is to imagine that your body is a fountain with water pushing up through your feet, legs, and spine, shooting out through the top of your head into the air five feet, then washing back down over your skin and draining down into the core of the earth), the point is to feel the small internal shifts one's body necessarily makes to stand "still." It is an awareness of one's body in a space with other bodies; a relaxation of the pores of one's skin so that the world can flow through you. It is a mutual moment of interpenetration and interdependency—one that always strikes me as a potentially transformative (and ecological) moment. Of course, I realize that not all contact improvisers appreciate, internalize, or even understand the psychic implications of this work. Yet I have taught enough contact improvisation classes to realize that something very extraordinary can happen to a group of thirty individuals working within this form over the course of a semester.

It is this kind of psychic (re)training of self and other that lies at the core of the work showcased in CI25's mixed-ability weekend. Bruce Curtis, Karen Daly, Sue Stuart, Riccardo Morrison, and Teri Carter all contributed to curating and facilitating the weekend workshop, but it was Alito Alessi, one of the most influential figures in this area, who led the opening workshop and introduced the parameters of the experience to those who were new to this work. Alessi teaches a form of contact improvisation that focuses on movement as a form of physical communication rather than a form of physical virtuosity. Touch becomes a window into one's partner's physical experience. In this way, Alessi replaces the *dis* of disability with dance, calling his work DanceAbility. Although this mixed-ability work makes a special effort to accommodate dancers with disabilities, Alessi is quick to assert that these dancing experiences do not just inspire or enable the disabled participants; they create a mutual physical dialogue that can empower and inspire the nondisabled participants as well.

Saturday night featured a mixed ability performance followed by a jam. One of the most exciting pieces on the program was a dance on wheels—Rollerblades, skateboard and wheelchair—in which the signifier of disability (the wheelchair) blended in with the various technologies of mobility. The participants—Bruce Curtis, Karen Nelson, Caroline Waters, Riccardo Morrison, Ray Chung, and Tom Giebink—used the fluid mobility of the wheels to play with momentum and speed. Also featured was an improvisatory piece by the Brazilian Compannia 100 Habilidades. While many of these pieces were interesting, the truly extraordinary dancing came in the jam after the performance.

Unlike a structured workshop or a performance, the contact improvisation jam setting allows for an open-ended type of dancing—a mode particularly conducive to dancers with different abilities. For one thing, it is a lot easier to rest or stop and talk with your partner. This space to dance, talk, and experiment was very helpful in getting the temporarily able-bodied participants who had little previous experience dancing with disabled folks to give it a try. And vice versa. A student who was struggling physically with an enormous cast on her broken leg went to the jam expecting to watch, but by the end of the evening, she had joined the forty people rolling, crawling, and spinning around the room. Even though it is a major ideological shift for many people to see disabled movers as dancers, the elements of much contemporary dance—breath, rhythm, extension, release, various effort qualities, partnering, humor, etc.—were all abundantly present within the dancing that evening.

More than any other genre of dance, contact improvisation has nurtured and embraced dancing that can integrate multiple abilities and limitations. In fact, many of the most renowned nondisabled contact improvisation practitioners (including Steve Paxton), spend a lot of time teaching, facilitating, and dancing with disabled communities. Then, too, there are the contact improvisation teachers and performers that are disabled themselves. (As Steve Paxton once remarked, "Have we previously heard of a paraplegic dance teacher? No, we have not.") This is because the contact improvisation aesthetic does not try to create a static, "classical" representation of the ideal body, but rather focuses on the process of the dancing communication between two bodies.[6]

Still, it would be disingenuous to pretend that all contact improvisation situations embrace such a democratic aesthetic. It seems to me that there is, in fact, a very real tension within the larger contact improvisation community between two kinds of dancing: one that emphasizes virtuosic movement skills and one that emphasizes movement communication that is accessible to anybody. (The two are not mutually exclusive, of course.) This tension was clearly embedded in the very structure of CI25. The first three-day contact training intensive was generally focused on skills only the most able bodies could do. There were no disabled teachers, nor were there classes that specifically addressed mixed-ability work. Most people who attended this workshop were hungry to improve their dancing skills, and a lot of the jam dancing during these days was acrobatic and fast-paced. This beginning of the celebration set up a dancing energy and an aesthetic mindset that had to shift gears radically for the mixed ability weekend to be successful. Fortunately, one of the most telling principles in contact improvisation (originally articulated by Nancy Stark Smith) is "replace ambition with curiosity." This openness to new experiences, combined with a willingness to be disoriented and feel awkward (two of the best lessons that contact improvisation has to offer) helped the dancers move from one dancing situation and aesthetic into another space—one open to a new definition of contact improvisation.

In the time since CI25, I have been wondering what it would have been like to begin this event with a mixed-ability training—whether that would have immediately deflected any prioritizing of different modes of dancing; whether it would have shaken up everyone's expectations. It is hard to say. It might actually have further marginalized the work, inadvertently positioning it as a "preconference" event. For although participants had to shift gears from the intensive training to the mixed-ability workshop, this shift helped to create an inclusive atmosphere for the following week of open jubilee dancing, talking, and celebrating the continuing presence of contact improvisation.

NOTES

1. Cynthia Novack, *Sharing the Dance: Contact Improvisation and American Culture* (Madison: University of Wisconsin Press, 1990), 186. For references to Judson Dance Theater see Sally Banes's work on the era, especially *Terpsichore in Sneakers* and *Democracy's Body: Judson Dance Theater 1962–1964*.

2. Curt Siddall, "Contact Improvisation," *East Bay Review,* September 1976. Cited in John Gamble, "On Contact Improvisation," *Painted Bride Quarterly* 4, no.1 (Spring 1977): 36.

3. For a more complete discussion of CI25 see *Contact Quarterly* 1, no. 1 (Winter/Spring 1998).

4. Nancy Stark Smith, "Editor Note," *Contact Quaterly* 23, no. 1 (Winter/Spring 1998): 11.

5. Ibid., 35.

6. See "Strategic Abilities" in the Occasional Pieces section of this book.

22

Feeling In and Out

Contact Improvisation and the Politics of Empathy

Talk for the Kinesthesia and Empathy in Dance conference, part of the Languages of
Emotion symposia at Freie University of Berlin, July 2011.

In his poetic short essay on Rembrandt's paintings, art critic John Berger
traces the differences between the artist's drawings and his paintings, particularly the late portraits. Whereas in his drawings Rembrandt is a master
of proportion, in his paintings this realistic perspective is radically altered.
Berger asks: "Why in his paintings did he forget—or ignore—what he could
do with such mastery in his drawings?" Alluding to the historical context of
Rembrandt's time, Berger suggests: "He grew old in a climate of economic
fanaticism and indifference—not dissimilar to the climate of the period we
are living through. The human could no longer simply be copied . . . the
human was no longer self-evident; it had to be found in the darkness."[1]
Berger searches for language to address what is not directly visible in Rembrandt's painting, and postulates that "Something else—something antithet-
ical to 'real' space must have interested him more."[2] Vital yet elusive, palpable yet not immediately visible, this "something else" present in Rembrandt's
work is defined by Berger as a "corporeal space." By distorting a part or
parts of the bodies he was painting, Rembrandt was able to give them what
Berger calls a "special power of narration." Tellingly, this corporeal space is
incompatible with architectural, measured space. It is connected to energy,
not geometric lines. Berger writes: "Corporeal space is continually changing
its measures and focal centers, according to circumstances. It measures by
waves, not meters. Hence its necessary dislocations of 'real' space."[3]

In order to give his readers a sense of the different orientations of this
corporeal space, Berger charges us to "leave the museum" and go the emergency room. It is there, Berger insists, that we will find:

> each sentient body's awareness of itself. It is not boundless like subjective
> space: it is always finally bound by the laws of the body, but its landmarks, its
> emphasis, its inner proportions are continually changing. Pain sharpens our
> awareness of such space. It is the space of our first vulnerability and solitude.
> Also of disease. But is also, potentially, the space of pleasure, well-being and the
> sensation of being loved.[4]

For Berger, this corporeal space can be felt by touch more clearly than it can be seen by sight, which is why it is the space that nurses occupy more often than doctors. "On each mattress, within each patient, it takes a different form."[5]

I am intrigued by Berger's notion of a corporeal space—one that requires another "way of seeing" to register its potency. In this essay, I want to explore how this space prioritizes touch and "feeling" rather than seeing, shifting the traditional subject/object dynamic of these exchanges. Of course, I am talking not only about the social and political relationship between painter and model, or even that of an art critic and the work of art, but also of the relationship between one's self and an "other." Over the course of this essay, I argue that by attending to the practice of feeling rather than its affects, contact improvisation can help us revise Western notions of empathy that are based on a psychological conception of the individual subject and an object of sympathy.

But first, let's talk about the word *feeling*. Anybody who knows me or has read my work will recognize my fondness for gerunds and for words that carry multiple meanings at one time. In English, feeling is both a noun and a verb form. Its many definitions span the gamut from the strictly material—such as to finger, palpitate, or touch something—to the highly cerebral. It can be used to describe a physical sensation (I feel something sticky), an intellectual perception (I have a feeling that), or an emotive state (feeling blue). Feeling can refer to both the surface of the body and the interior self. Feelings, of course, are closely linked to empathy. Nowhere is this more obvious than in the German term *einfuhlung,* which can be translated as "feeling in" or "feeling into." As Susan Foster outlines in her recent genealogy of empathy, this term was originally coined in 1873 by German aesthetician Robert Vischer and subsequently translated into English as empathy.[6] In its late nineteenth-century German context, feeling into (or empathy) was primarily used to describe the experience of contemplating, moving into, and merging with a work of art—something that John Berger does very well in his writing. In an early twenty-first-century context, however, empathy usually refers to the experience of relating to someone else's circumstances, and constitutes the stuff of daytime talk shows à la Oprah Winfrey. As feeling moves from a verb to a noun, from the physical sensing of touch to a projected image of another's experience, it can take on the colonial baggage of sympathy and the psychic mantle of emotion.

But what if we were to refuse this stabilizing of a verb into a noun—of an active experience into a passive object? What if we kept feeling at the surface of the body, rather than letting it sink into what Foster describes as the late nineteenth century's "newly constructed interiority whose proclivities for repression, identification, transference, and sublimation were just beginning to be explored and whose defining consciousness could be fathomed only through intensive introspection."[7] What if we approached *einfuhlung*, or feeling into, as a kinesthetic practice rather than a psychological state? By holding our attention to the physical I am not trying to suggest that this realm is any more authentic, natural, "real," or less culturally grounded than the psychological. On the contrary, I am quite interested in foregrounding the sociopolitical moorings of corporeal training. But it is crucial for us to recognize just how quickly and easily we tend to elide feeling with emotions, setting up a subject position based on possession (I have emotions) rather than one based in sensation (I am feeling).

Contact improvisation has been around for almost four decades and I have been involved with the form for three of those decades. I have participated in and taught workshops in many different communities all over the world. Although the form has changed and moved as it adapts to different historical circumstances and geographic locations, there are some fundamental elements that comprise the core of the physical training, no matter whether it is conducted in German, English, Mandarin, or Tamil. One of these is a focused attention to sensation at the level of the skin.

As we know, skin is the largest and one of the most sensitive of our organs. It covers our entire body and it is impossible to exist in the world without one's skin. However, many people go through their everyday lives with little awareness of their skin as a perceptual faculty. This is because our current postindustrial culture reifies the visual almost to the exclusion of our other senses, including those of sound and smell. Most of us use sight to navigate the world—off-line as well as online. Generally speaking, in the West, seeing is believing and feeling is suspect. We tend to become aware of our skin only in extreme situations such as fear (the skin crawling up the back of my neck), awe (it gave me goose bumps), or pleasure (the tingling sensation of a lover's caress). Much of the foundational training in contact improvisation attempts to reverse this cultural hierarchy by reducing our dependency on the visual and bringing awareness to the nuances of the tactile. In contact improvisation, one's skin becomes a primary site of communication.

The first step in this process of retraining our corporeal habitus is to release the tension that is a direct result of what I call a territorial approach to the body's integrity. We can conceive of our skin as either a boundary or a conduit, and this shift in perception leads to a radically different understanding of the relationship between myself and the world. If my skin is seen as a barrier to disease, infection, or any kind of "otherness," I might well approach life with a certain Cold War mentality—shoring up any breeches in my defense system and using my skin as a wall or a container meant to keep me safe from the outside world. If, on the other hand, I experience my skin as the porous interface between my self and the world, then I will be more apt to engage my skin as a permeable, sensitive layer that facilitates that exchange. As Corey Spiro, one of my students in a recent contact improvisation class, suggests:

> I feel as though we live in a world where the boundary between self and 'other' is constantly being defined, labeled, and monitored. This is especially apparent in our perceptions of the ownership of space. MY PROPERTY, MY ROOM, etc. Nowhere is this line more clearly drawn than at our skin . . . It's all too easy to convince oneself that the skin represents the ultimate energetic boundary between self and other. Of course, this barrier works both ways, just as it stops the world from coming into us, it similarly prevents our conception of self from expanding beyond the limits of our physical bodies.
>
> I would expect then, that opening the pores of my skin wide enough to let the world in would be a frightening experience. Rather than an upsetting intrusion, however, I was surprised to find out that it was actually extremely refreshing. My energy in class was perhaps lagging a little bit today, but I felt that by opening myself up I was able to simultaneously expand outward into the energy of Wild Main Space and also feel more acutely the electro-magnetic fields of everyone else standing around me. In short, opening my pores did more than just "let the world in," it also let me out. The feeling was one of freedom and relief, as I was no longer alone within the prison-like confines of my injured and fatigued frame.[8]

In this dialogue between the self and the world, one becomes aware of the intriguing possibilities of interdependence, including a deeper sense of responsibility. I think of responsibility not as an oppressive duty towards others, but rather as an ability to respond, an ability to be present with the world, and as a way of being present with oneself. If the world is already inside one's body, then the separation between internal and external—self and other—is much less distinct. The skin is no longer the boundary between the world and myself, but rather the sensing organ that brings the world into my awareness. However, given the anxiety swirling around boundaries and bodies in contemporary society, this latter sensibility requires a bit of practice.

One of the earliest exercises that I give in my improvisation classes is referred to as "the small dance" or "the stand." First developed by Steve Paxton in the early 1970s as he explored the physical skills that would lead towards defining the form of contact improvisation, the stand allows one to focus on the internal movements created by the shifts of bones, muscles, and breath required to stand "still." After they have been warming up, moving through the space for awhile with big, vigorous movements, I ask the students to choose a spot and stand in a relaxed, but active manner. Engaging one's peripheral vision is crucial to this process, and I tell the dancers to try and release the fronts of their eyes, allowing images and colors to come into their head instead of straining their eyes in order to go out and grab the visual image. Often, I will call their attention to the sensation of the moisture on their skin, asking them to feel the difference between air and clothing. Next, I ask them to concentrate on opening their pores so that their skin becomes like a screen window, allowing air, smells and sounds to come in from the outside. I ask them to try to breathe through their pores. Only once they sense the responsiveness of their own skin, are my students ready to work with a partner and feel their weight shifting back and forth between two people. I emphasize the homonymic connections between pore (of the skin) and pour (as in pouring water from a pitcher), asking the students to reflect in writing on what it feels like to open their pores wide enough to let the world pour in. Here is how Isabel Roth, another of my recent contact students, responds to this physical practice:

> I think the idea of opening pores as being similar to the idea of opening your mind. It's not as if you can actively think to open pores and actually feel the individual pores opening. But it is a palpable feeling of release, of spreading and opening your skin to the physical space and people around you . . . Just like opening the pores of the skin allows you to be ready to receive, it also makes you ready to give. Skin is such a pliable and ever-flexible organ, constantly shifting and regenerating, depending on movement and contact. By opening the pores you prepare the skin for contact and for the willingness to open up to another's touch. Now ready to accept that touch, it is easier to reciprocate pouring weight from open pores to a partner.[9]

As you may have noticed, each of my students' responses uses feeling as both noun and verb—an active state of sensing and also a reflection of that experience. These two meanings of the word resonate with one another, vibrating in an ambiguous space between a subject (who feels) and an object (of feeling). Reading the students' descriptions of their experience, I am reminded of Berger's sense that corporeal space is measured in "waves, not meters," and is predicated on touch, not sight. The somatic state of responsiveness that these students articulate is crucial in preparing the body to enter safely into a contact duet. But before I move into an analysis of the physical dimensions of touch and sharing weight, I want to look at two different ways of thinking about empathy by making a distinction between introspection and interoception.

Etymologically, introspection means to look into one's self, which is usually specified as one's own mind or feelings. This interior space is the site of empathy—envisioned as contained within one's self until it is drawn out by the object of one's gaze, sympathy, or even pity. As Foster demonstrates in her earlier-cited study, introspection is implicated in the scopic economy of the nineteenth-century self. Interoception, on the other hand, replaces the visual emphasis (*spect*) with the more tactile sensibility of *cept*. Used mostly in neuropsychology, the term interoception references one's ability to feel sensations arising from within the body—specifically, one's visceral organs—giving us the term "gut feelings." Advances in brain imaging have helped scientists locate interoception in the right frontal insula—a part of the brain also identified with emotional intelligence. It could be easy to collapse these two terms into an overall feeling of empathy. But as any Zen master will tell you, feeling does not necessarily have to evolve into emotion. In fact, I want to suggest that the physical mind of interoception can produce an entirely different kind of empathetic exchange—one that stays with feeling without getting stuck in the emotional baggage of feelings.

Once my students are comfortable with opening their pores, we begin the infinitely interesting process of learning to pour our weight, like water, into one another's bodies. Starting with two hands, one partner will firmly, yet openly, touch another person on the back or shoulder, kinesthetically "asking" their partner to pour their weight into the receptacle of their hands. The asking partner can regulate how much weight is given by resisting and pouring back even as they accept the responsibility for the other person's weight. This mutual pouring creates an energetic dialogue that continuously loops between the partners. Eventually, the partners begin to pour their weight back and forth, using different body parts as their physical contact revolves around the space and across their bodies. As the dancers gain fluidity in the giving and receiving of weight, the dancing tends to speed up. This is the moment when the responsiveness of one's body is critical. There is no time for the lengthy processing of emotions here; one has to focus entirely on keeping up with the point of contact.

This point of connection is sometimes referred to in contact improvisation parlance as the "third mind." Allowing their dancing to be led by this "third mind," the two partners endeavor to follow its spatial and rhythmic journey throughout the studio space. At first it may seem clear which partner is leading and which one is following, but eventually those roles evolve into such a fluid and subtle exchange that the categories of leader and follower lose their oppositional moorings. This does not mean, however, that all difference is collapsed. For me, this third mind marks an intersubjective space in which one is aware of sensations both internal and external without necessarily categorizing those feelings into socially recognizable roles. The notion of a third mind directs attention away from the oppositional poles of self and other, stretching a single line into a more open field of play. Contact trains for a physical interconnectedness that is akin to what Deidre Sklar calls "empathic kinesthetic perception."

> Emphatic kinesthetic perception suggests a combination of mimesis and
> empathy . . . Whereas visual perception implies an "object" to be perceived
> from a distance with the eyes alone, empathic kinesthetic perception implies a

bridging between subjectivities. This kind of "connected knowing" produces a very intimate kind of knowledge, a taste of those ineffable movement experiences that can't be easily put into words. Paradoxically, as feminist psychologist Judith Jordan points out, the kind of temporary joining that occurs in empathy produces not a blurry merger but an *articulated perception of differences* (emphasis added).[10]

It is this "articulated perception of differences" that I want to focus on here. When I am teaching contact improvisation and I use terms such as "interconnected, "feeling one's partner's experience," or "moving together," I emphasize that this going with the flow does not mean one becomes a neutral container; nor does it suggest a blurry merger of energies such that the dancing homogenizes into one long fluid chain of rolls and lifts—quite the contrary. The sensitivity to another's experience also creates an awareness of subtle differences—differences that can be celebrated within the improvisation. While I do not have time to fully engage with Merleau-Ponty's ideas about intersubjectivity and touch in this context, I do think it is important to point out that in French the verbs for touch and feel are both transitive and reflexive verb forms. That is to say that one feels an "other" at the same time that one feels oneself feeling. Similarly, one can touch something and feel oneself being touched at the same time. (This is Merleau-Ponty's famous example of one hand holding the other.) This looping across to another and then back to oneself intrigues me, for it loosens up the psychological patterns of relating to an "other" as an object (of empathy, scrutiny, or desire). This play of difference can be accentuated in another dance score that I give to my students. Here are my instructions:

> *This is a duet, not an exercise. A dance, not an activity. To begin, one person lies down, completely passive, allowing their weight to sink fully into the floor. Their partner begins to move their body with attention to giving the passive person an experience of the weight of their bones and the mobility of their joints. As anyone who has ever done any kind of body work or physical therapy knows, a passive body allows one to feel sensations unavailable to a body that is self-engaged, even the most released one. Focusing on their breaths, the partners establish a vibration of energetic exchange. Bit by bit, percentage point by percentage point, the passive partner becomes increasingly active, engaging first the core of the body's structure and working outwards to mobilize the limbs—arms, legs, head and tailbone. Both partners dance together in a fully active state. Eventually, the originally active partner becomes progressively passive until they are lying on the floor, enjoying the sensations of their own body through the manipulations of their partner's.*

The implications of this score are pretty obvious. Over the course of this duet one experiences the entire continuum of possibilities of being active or passive. Normally in our culture, these various positions of active and passive are pathologized into power dynamics, where the passive figure is seen as not having control, as being either infantile or lazy, rendering them an object of pity. But my experience and that of many of my students is that the experience of being totally passive, rather than feeling powerless, actually opens up a great deal of feeling that can create its own pleasures and sense of agency. Experiencing both extreme ends of these positions can be truly revelatory. For instance, Heather Sedlacek writes:

> I also found novelty and enjoyment in being able to dance at a different level than my partner . . . It was clearly stated that we were at different levels, that this was okay, and that the high intensity partner would take care and responsibility for the low intensity partner. Thus, for the first time I didn't have to resist when my partner resisted or attempt to match her intensity. I didn't have to be fire when she was fire, or wind when she was wind. I could simply revel in the percentage that our teacher called out every few minutes . . . Reaching 100% intensity and then helping my partner down to 0% provided another new and powerful experience . . . I felt a sense of responsibility that I have not felt before in Contact. Instead of moving with my partner and following the point of contact, as my partner decreased in intensity, I began to control her movements and direction. I had a unique sense of agency in the dance that for me is usually left up to the Third Mind, not to an individual partner.[11]

Throughout this discussion, I have tried to articulate how contact improvisation creates a corporeal space in which feeling allows for an interconnectedness with another person without solidifying that relationship into the subject/object dyad implicit in classic conceptions of empathy. I have highlighted how attention to skin as porous and open to the world can facilitate a dancing based on an interchange and multiplicity of subject positions. Moving with the point of contact requires a willingness to stay engaged with feeling (verb) in the present moment, refusing to allow any one kinesthetic exchange to get stuck in a particular feeling (noun). This is not to suggest that relationships in contact improvisation are so fluid as to be meaningless—quite the contrary. But we need to enter something like Berger's corporeal space with the dancers in order to read the meaning of their connection differently. Watching two people explore the continuum of energies available in contact improvisation, we become aware of the basic generosity at the core of the form. To dance with you, I need to first feel you, recognizing that this feeling can change. The improvisational possibilities of this dancing can teach us that *einfuhlung* does not have to be only an introspective process, but rather can open us up to feeling both in and out.

1. John Berger, "Rembrandt and the Body," in *The Shape of a Pocket* (New York: Pantheon Books, 2001), 105.

2. Ibid., 106–7.

3. Ibid., 109.

4. Ibid., 107.

5. Ibid., 107.

6. Susan Foster, *Choreographing Empathy* (London and New York: Routledge, 2011), 127.

7. Ibid., 154.

8. Corey Spiro, in *Encounters with Contact: Dancing Contact Improvisation in College* (Oberlin, OH: Oberlin Theater and Dance Program, [distributed by *Contact Quarterly*], 2010), 40.

9. Isabel Roth in *Encounters with Contact*, 38.

10. Deidre Sklar, "Five Premises for a Culturally Sensitive Approach to Dance," in *Moving History/Dancing Cultures*, ed. Dils and Albright (Middletown, CT: Wesleyan University Press, 2001), 31–32.

11. Heather Sedlacek in *Encounters with Contact*, 17.

V

PEDAGOGY

I have always tried to be thoughtful about my teaching, which spans a wide range of theoretical and practical classes both in and out of the academy. As reflected in most of the writings collected here, I have spent much of my life intentionally drawing connections between our physical experiences and (meta)physical responses, recognizing that how we move through the world affects how we think about it, and vice versa. Sometimes ideas can help us stretch our notions of what is important in dancing or choreography; at other times our bodies can learn a new physical practice much faster than our minds can comprehend it. In the last few years, I have delighted in teaching courses outside the dance program (such as my first-year seminar Bridging the Body/Mind Divide) that ask liberalarts students to bring their embodied knowledge into the process of learning intellectual debate and critical writing skills. These classes combine philosophy, feminist and queer theory with somatic exercises intended to engage those ideas directly in the body. This section traces different modes of engaging bodies and minds across a variety of teaching situations, from contact improvisation to a cross-cultural dance history course to *Girls in Motion*—the after-school program that I run in the local middle school.

Generally, I think about teaching in terms that reflect my physical engagement with my students. For instance, one of the realizations I had early on in my teaching career is that resistance is support. Indeed, it is much easier to feel my own weight and position if someone pushes their weight into me. This physical truth comes from my training in contact improvisation and guides many of my pedagogical strategies, although I hasten to add that the resistance of which I speak is a firm but open resistance, not a rigid, inflexible reactionary resistance. I like the feeling of mutual engagement when one body leans into another. In the classroom, this engagement allows the students to feel their own reaction and access their own point of view as the teacher "leans" on their body or thinking. The physical work clarifies very quickly what it means to commit one's self to a point of view; to feel one's weight is an intriguing way to think about agency and voice in academic discourse.

The first essay, "Dancing Across Difference," was written early in my academic career for a special issue of *Women and Performance* focused on pedagogy. Here I extrapolate the lessons about positionality and proximity that I learned from teaching contact improvisation in order to think about the negotiation of bodies and power in other classroom settings as well. On the one hand, contact improvisation fits uneasily into an institutional framework. Learning how to deal with the risk, uncertainty, and complexities of teaching thirty young people how improvise in close contact—how to roll together and jump on each other—stretches me every time I teach the class. On the other hand, being able to engage students in the learning of this dance form for two-hour classes, three times a week for fourteen weeks, means that we move beyond the initial euphoria of tactile connection into a more layered experience of this deeply interpersonal dancing. Then too, I have found that teaching within the context of a liberalarts college setting has enriched my sense of the political, sociological, environmental, and feminist potential of contact improvisation immeasurably, as students bring the knowledge of their other courses to lean on this form.

The second essay, "Channeling the Other: An Embodied Approach to Teaching across Cultures," was originally given as a talk for an International Federation of Theater Researchers (FIRT) conference in Jaipur, India, and was subsequently published in *Research in Dance Education*. In this, I confront the complex power dynamic involved with teaching dance history across cultures. An animating question for me in this investigation was: how can I engage my students' bodies in learning about a dance culture with which I may have no physical history and certainly little cultural background? While I want to be attentive to the differences between cultural appropriation and cross-cultural inspiration, I find myself urging teachers to take some risks and encourage students to use their bodies to kinesthetically imagine other forms and contexts for dance. Using my experience with teaching a section of my cross-cultural dance history course on classical Indian dance, I propose several strategies for consciously including students' bodily learning even when dealing with forms of dance that are embedded in completely different cultural experiences.

The final essay, "Training Bodies to Matter," traces three different teaching contexts (from adolescent girls to college students) in which I consciously intervene in what I consider to be the negative corporeal effects of a twenty-first-century Internet lifestyle. This essay presents a number of my favorite physical exercises that encourage young bodies to experience the support of gravity and the sense of being grounded to the earth at a moment when so many young people feel dislocated. I also explore the ways that certain somatic skills engage internal, proprioceptive states—the same ones that recent studies in neuroscience have linked to the areas of the brain involved in empathy. This essay's title hinges on the double meaning of matter—as both making a difference in the world and the physical stuff that is being reshaped in the process.

All three essays in this section make extensive use of my students' journals and published writings. As someone who truly engages with my students' reflections about their embodied experience, I find myself thinking about and being influenced by (and sometimes even deeply inspired by) words written two or three years earlier. From time to time, when I mention to a student that I am still thinking about their response to a classroom exercise or the metaphors they used to describe an experience, they are amazed and most likely have forgotten what they said back then. But teaching and learning are life processes that have their own time frames, and oftentimes the most powerful lessons crystalize many years later, making teaching a sometimes frustrating and yet inherently joyful pursuit.

23

Dancing across Difference

Experience and Identity in the Classroom

Women and Performance 1, no. 2, 1993.

The lights fade up slowly, creating a diagonal pathway and gradually illuminating two figures leaning—shoulder to shoulder—on one another. As they advance into the light, that physical connectedness shifts across their backs and over the other shoulder until they are standing chest to chest, their heads leaning on one another's shoulders. This image of a human bridge changes abruptly as one dancer jerks away from her partner's support, but is caught again before she hits the floor. Hands intertwined, the women lean away from each other, tenuously balanced. This moment of suspension is interrupted by a playful game of pushing and pulling that becomes progressively more violent until they are forcefully launching their bodies at one another. At one point, they slam into one another and drop, exhausted, to the floor. Spread-eagled across each other, they rest for a moment, as their breathing eventually becomes synchronized—their chests rising and falling together in a single motion. Slowly they begin to move, rolling across the floor in a series of intertwined spirals in which their bodies alternately surface and dive back under, like two sea lions in slow motion.

This is a description of a dance performance that took place as part of a senior dance concert at Oberlin College in May 1992. The duet grew out of a contact improvisation class taught in the dance department during the spring semester. The dancers were a student and a professor. This essay is committed to understanding what that particular confluence of identities and bodies might mean in an academic setting. How, in other words, did Naomi and I move across the traditionally separate and static positions of our institutional identities as a "teacher" and a "student" to engage in a dance form in which physical movements and their social implications are open to negotiation at the very moment of dancing? How had we learned to trust one another well enough to risk dancing across a continuum of physical intimacy and physical struggle? And how was I, a professor at Oberlin College, willing and able to suspend the authority of that role in order to dance in close physical contact with a student who was ten years younger than I?

In the following pages, I want to explore how the movement training of contact improvisation—specifically, its focus on disorientation and physical contact—can shape a radically new perspective on and approach to the dynamics of classroom interaction, whether that class is a dance class or a philosophy class. It is my contention that in order to deal effectively with the issues of identity and the politics of institutional locations that are currently at the forefront of many feminist discussions of pedagogy, we have to be willing to look at the ways that these identities get negotiated through our physical bodies. Paying attention to this body politic can help educators understand the practical as well as the theoretical significance of actually locating ourselves—both intellectually and physically—in each and every class we teach.

Teaching—whatever one's discipline or pedagogical focus—is an intellectual, social, and a physical activity. Often the very architectural conditions of the room help to determine the social dynamic of the bodies that inhabit that space. (For instance, are the desks arranged in rows or in a semicircle? Is there a seminar table for everyone to sit around, or does the professor have a larger desk at the front of the room?) As someone who teaches a variety of courses in both the theater and dance and the women's studies programs (ranging from advanced classes in feminist theories of representation to beginning studio courses in modern dance) at a small liberalarts college, I have frequently occupied radically different teaching environments within the same afternoon—occasionally with a few of the same students. Although I never stand behind a lectern (partly because I do not lecture), I have taught classes from various vantage points including: from the back of a darkened auditorium next to a slide projector; in front of forty-five students packed into a room that was meant to hold twenty-five people comfortably; in a circle with twelve students and another professor; in my office; in front of a mirror in a traditional dance studio; from the floor of a big gymnasium; as well as in the woods. As I move from one class to the next, I am aware of the ways in which these physical conditions affect my relationship to the students, their relationship with me, and their relationship to one another.

When I teach an advanced theory seminar, for instance, I try to get to class early in order to rearrange the rows of chairs into a circle. Generally, however, the large table in front of the chalkboard forces me to be satisfied with a semicircle. After I announce readings, upcoming events, lectures, etc., and the class discussion has been launched, I find that I need to avert or lower my gaze momentarily so that the students can begin to address their comments to one another and not just to me. I try to demonstrate my attentiveness by visually taking in the whole class's participation (not just assuming that to talk is to participate; active listening is important as well) or asking questions. I realize that this can be unsettling to a student who expects the teacher to constantly nod approval. I find, however, that if

I do not shift my gaze—if I continue to look directly at each student while they are talking—the class discussion tends to become a series of individual conversations between myself and each student in turn. In my contact improvisation class, I can use the openness of the large studio space to send the class moving through space right away. Walking in and among the students, I direct their focus verbally. Soon, the students learn that they do not have to stop what they are doing and look at me in order to hear the next directions or images for their movements. I feel as if this shift releases me from the students' gaze (and them from mine) and allows me to participate in the class as well as direct it.

On one hand, it may seem that these different locations are minor and mundane details that divert attention away from the fact that they are all located in some way or another within a much larger institutional framework that is undeniably grounded in sexist, racist, classist, and ablest assumptions about the world. It is true, of course, that the physical structure of a classroom does not necessarily guarantee a specific class dynamic. Certainly, the overall atmosphere of a class can be oppressively authoritative in the midst of a very open physical space. I have experienced dance classes in which the teacher was positioned as a master, one who is giving the students the pearls of wisdom from his or her dancing experience. Even without tables and chairs, these teachers position themselves at the head of the room and the students are aligned in rows and expected to maintain these spatial forms as they dance across the floor. I do not want to argue for a deterministic one-to-one correspondence between architectural dimensions and pedagogical styles. I do want to suggest, however, that an increased awareness of the physical contours of a learning environment can help us recognize these psychophysical patterns so that we can use the physical space we occupy more consciously. I am always struck when reading articles that address issues of identity and location in an academic classroom, to find that very few people ever discuss the physical ramifications of the spatial arrangements in which these interactions take place. Although concerns of institutional power and individuals' stakes in that power are often at the core of these writings, they are frequently completely dis-embodied. Simply listing the identificatory labels such as I am a ——, ——, —— professor, and my students are ——, ——, ——, does not help me understand the physical politics present in any classroom.

I believe that this focus is particularly important in the midst of current debates concerning diversity in academia. At Oberlin, especially in the women's studies department, we have had ongoing discussions about pedagogy and diversity, and many of the tenured women faculty members have expressed their ideological commitments to diversifying not only the women's studies curriculum, but also their own syllabi. Adding books written by people of color, people of different age groups, abilities, and sexual orientations, however, does not automatically make students with parallel commitments feel "at home" in one's class. For me, it is in the physical dynamics of these interpersonal interactions that issues of class, race, gender, sexuality, and body image emerge in all their complex intersections. Although many of the faculty have learned to adopt a very middle-class "politeness," which can include keeping an "appropriate" distance from one another (frequently euphemized as "academic freedom"), the students do not always demonstrate the same temper, patience, or worn-down mellowness. I have seen situations in which faculty have winced or shuddered when a Latino male student throws a ball of verbal energy in their direction, or smiled and patted an African-American female student who was similarly exploding with frustration in class. Even in less extreme circumstances, there is frequently an implicit assumption that the faculty member will not change energies to meet the student even halfway, and will instead wait (either patiently or impatiently) until the student calms down enough to "make sense." But I keep wondering why, when we are dealing with very personal issues of oppression, we think that we can somehow contain these discussions in a "rational," or a disembodied (i.e., nonemotional) frame. Most academics shy away from the vitally important (albeit extremely difficult) project of trying to incorporate ambiguity—intellectual or emotional—into their own teaching. For me, this means accepting a certain unease—the result of realizing that there are no easy answers or politically correct methodologies with which to shield one's own vulnerable position as a teacher.

As a dancer, I try to think of these sticky pedagogical situations as places to move through and learn from. I neither want to ignore, nor to become mired in them. Theoretically this means that if we, as teachers, could reconceive of who we are and what we teach in terms of movement rather than a single static position, then we might just be able to imagine opening up to different kinds of intellectual performances in our students and other colleagues.[1] Often when I speak about this physical side of diversity, I am accused by other faculty members of asking them to participate in and understand cultures that are not a part of their history or experience. I do not want to suggest that teachers should all become penultimate cultural chameleons, or that there are not significant connections to be made with a student or fellow faculty members who share one's own cultural commitments. But it seems to me that while issues of diversity are never confined to the physical body—they are always implicated in social contexts and representational structures—they are made present through our bodies. Therefore, if we are going to learn to teach across cultural differences, we have to understand how to move (theoretically as well as physically) in different, potentially uncomfortable, directions.

I believe that nonverbal behavior plays a significant role in negotiating identity politics in the classroom, despite my trepidation at invoking the dangerously simplistic approach that pop psychology brings to discussions of the body. How we approach, walk, talk, and dance with one another means a lot. I am not suggesting that if we all hold hands in a circle, some kind of precolonial unity will rest, like a halo, above our heads. As a feminist, I realize that bodies are deeply constructed by cultural attitudes and economic conditions. As a dancer, I am aware that bodies can also be physically retrained and consciously re-theorized. It is in the conscious use of this possibility that I find a very intriguing potential for a pedagogy that strains at the seams of its own institutional context.

Contact improvisation—a dance form developed in the early 1970s—involves a willingness to experience a state of disorientation.[2] Unlike many genres of dance including classical ballet, classical Indian dance, and traditional forms of American modern dance, contact improvisation is about being off-balance; about enjoying a certain loss of control over one's own movements, both physically and psychically. I think that this willingness to experience the vertigo based on a constant exchange of weight, and the inevitable moments of falling and intimacy of catching and being caught, can profoundly affect our intellectual assumptions concerning the stability of categories of "self" and "other." Even exercises seemingly as simple as rolling across the floor or writing bold graffiti on the space around you with an imaginary marker attached to the top of your head, can be extremely disorienting. These exercises require a very different use of the eyes. In contact improvisation, one learns to see not by fixing one's gaze on people or surrounding objects, but rather by allowing the eyes to rest back in the eye sockets and relying on a more relaxed, peripheral vision. This small shift in visual focus radically changes one's experience of being in the space. Rolling, spinning, and being upside down in a room with other people moving around every which way forces me to physically negotiate a chaotic field of comings and goings in which I must give up any stable sense of my "position" in the space. What is left, then, is a sense of locating oneself vis-à-vis the other people who are, of course, also moving in the space. While all this dancing around and in between one another can make for a great deal of fun and some rather humorous situations (as well as warming up the dancers by getting their blood flowing), it also suggests another way of being with others in the world—a kind of existential dance in which this shifting of positions allows for a certain reorganization of social relationships.

The contact improvisation course that I teach at Oberlin College meets for two hours, three times a week, with an optional Sunday jam that is open to anyone who wants to join in. I insist on carving out this amount of time from a university scheduling system that balks at any course that does not fit tidily into the official one hour-and-twenty-minute class slots. Yet I have found that I need the two hours in order to work in and out of a high group energy, sustained personal concentration, and partnering skills. After a group warm-up and before we work in pairs, I usually lead the students through a visualization exercise that first asks them to attend to their own movement style, sensation of weight, and postural alignment. As they progress from a simple head nodding exercise to more complex coordinations, as their movements become larger and begin to travel through space, I ask the students to become increasingly aware of the other people in the space around them without losing the attentiveness to their own internal sensations with which we began. This kind of dual focus training helps the students become more conscious of how they can locate themselves in movement and with other people—not just when they are still and alone.

Although I am currently fascinated by the way that contact improvisation helps me think through the body in ways that problematize contemporary debates about identity and poststructuralist theory, I choose to start the semester without directly addressing this material. Instead, I begin with physical skills, for the movement training in contact improvisation works to build a sense of trust within the class within which we can take individual risks. One of the most disorienting aspects of contact improvisation, especially for people who are new to the dance form, is the whole issue of bodily contact—of physical touch. Like most contact improvisation teachers, I introduce touch through a series of exercises based on following a specific point of contact. For example, two people stand facing one another. Pressing their right forefingers together, they wait until they feel that joined point of contact begin to move in space. Following that point as it takes on a life of its own, the dancers concentrate on the qualities of that touch; letting their bodies move with little thought to the specific shapes they are making. In another introductory exercise that focuses on feeling and giving weight, partners lean back to back on one another; sinking down to and rising up from the ground. This is usually a comfortable and fun exercise, as most people remember doing something similar in elementary-school gym class. The back is a good spot to initiate contact, as it is a fairly neutral physical place, with no sex organs or facial features to cause an initial embarrassment. Yet within this exercise, I start to call attention to the physical sensuality and connection of their bodies, to their mutual breathing, and the warmth, texture, and support of their joined backs. After a few minutes or so, I ask them to separate and take notice of the physical traces of the other person's body on their own. These sensations then become the impetus for a solo improvisation. Later, as they become more sophisticated with sharing weight and taking responsibility for one another's weight, the students begin to dance while maintaining the point of contact, allowing that physical connection to inspire their duet.

Physical contact, of course, is societally determined. One of my most difficult tasks, therefore, is to create a dancing environment in which everyone feels safe enough to push their focus beyond the mere fact of touching and being touched to the how of that interaction. In order to build this trust, I begin with simple mirroring exercises, choosing the more neutral points of bodily contact like the forefingers, wrists, and forearms, and the back. Often, I will have the class work on the same exercise with different partners so that everyone gets a sense of how different bodies hold weight and everyone experiences how the various combinations of bodies negotiate the physical tasks I set them. Even within the most elementary rolling or stretching exercises, we focus on the fluid exchange of movement, weight, spatial direction, and power from one partner to the other, and back and forth. Talking about our various experiences, the class acknowledges the physical communication that is operating between two bodies, exploring the muscular indications that might suggest a resistance to, or willingness for, a particular physical adventure. This very specific focus on the nuances of movement coordinations helps the students begin to process the profound experience of touching, smelling, and dancing with one another before we work into a fully weighted body-to-body contact—a moment in which the issues of power, trust, body image, sexuality, and fear suddenly explode in class.

Besides the more informal communication networks that are frequently set up outside of class, I give the students time to talk with their partners in between exercises. These short conversations often spark comments in the final discussion circle with which we end each class. In addition, I ask students to keep a regular journal documenting their dancing experiences and their sense of participation in the course. It is important for me that the issues of the body that become so urgently foregrounded in dance forms such as contact improvisation begin to be addressed in verbal, as well as physical, terms. I have found that students often first think about an issue in their journals, and then later bring up these concerns in class. This effort to articulate what may feel like a vague sense of dis-ease forces the students to recognize the critical intersection of cultural and physical discourses in contact improvisation.

> There are many issues involved in giving my weight and taking someone
> else's. What does my weight feel like to another I wonder. Do I feel heavy, do I
> constrict her breathing or am I just heavy enough so the pressure on her back
> feels like a massage? When I take weight, I often question my ability to secure
> the person. I want to take weight and be trusted by my partner, but am I strong
> enough? I know I am but I question myself anyway. The part of me that ques-
> tions is the same part that sometimes feels fragile. (Jenny Pommiss, student)

While we take time in the class to acknowledge and discuss the social and emotional baggage we all experience in giving over our weight and taking on someone else's, I also try to structure specific physical exercises that will give students like Jenny the opportunity to experiment with giving and receiving weight in ways that they feel comfortable with. For a woman like Jenny, this kind of physical training can help overcome both her sense of fragility and her fear of imposing too heavily on someone else.

Another exercise that extends one's awareness to the shifting nuances of self and other through an exchange of weight and energy is an improvisational duet score in which one partner is completely passive while the active partner manipulates her limbs, head, or torso for her. Bit by bit, that passive partner becomes more and more active. Later, after a period of equal "activeness," the originally active partner gradually becomes less and less active until her passive body is being manipulated by her partner in an inverse of the original relationship. As the following entry in a student's journal make clear, one of the most extraordinary experiences that contact improvisation offers is this opportunity to become vibrantly aware of one's own body, even in the midst of a duet that is stretching and challenging that body.

> The active-passive partner work really did a lot for me . . . when we were both equally active, with no set passive, I noticed that that connection remained surprisingly strong between us. We had relatively low amounts of contact, but the responsiveness was there without further effort. And it was more than responsiveness. There was, for example, one place where we were doing a flowing, repetitive movement in synch with each other. And we both stopped at the same moment and turned away. It wasn't a case of one person stopping and the other reacting and stopping a split second later. It just happened so smoothly—I didn't even realize how amazing what had happened was until several seconds later.
>
> That's why it worked today—I had relaxed myself into a new kind of concentration—not even concentration—more like awareness and focus. My movement felt like it was really me—not what I should do. And I didn't not think—my mind was working very clearly, thinking things like this feels good, I'm off balance, here's the floor. I did it with my eyes open and I didn't "clunk" once. It was wonderful, but I didn't want to talk about it right away. I wanted Selinda to find it for herself. And as I watched her I thought that. It was, I think, an experience for her like mine. When I watched her—she looked like a four year old dancing in the sun barefoot—it wasn't about how she looked but how she felt. And it looked great. (Catherine O'Keefe, student)

Catherine's euphoric description of her dancing experience is telling in a number of ways, not the least of which is her enthusiasm for the moments of "connection" and "responsiveness" in her duet with Selinda. It is important to note, however, that the movement synchrony that these two women experienced is not a Zen-like goal of becoming "one" with each other or the world. (Besides being politically dangerous, that kind of cloning makes for rather boring dancing.) Rather, what Catherine is describing is a sense of what I call intersubjective dancing—a physical connectedness based on both partners being equally present (but in different ways) in the duet. What is particularly interesting for me in Catherine's comments is the way her phys-ical concentration within the duet gave her a sense of fully participating in her own movement; engaging her body in a way that "felt like it was really me—not what I should do." The personal sense of power and interpersonal connection that Catherine describes here is not an end goal for me, but it is a crucial step in creating a basis of safety and community within the class from which we can then move onto riskier territory.

In the first half of the semester, issues of power, trust, desire, sexuality, as well as cultural norms and biases about what constitutes an able body surface intermittently through discussions of our physical experience in con-tact improvisation. Later, the class begins to address these issues explicitly, bringing them into our dancing on a much more conscious level. For ex-ample, we explore the dramatic possibilities of social hierarchy in contact improvisation duets, as well as the various ways to "make contact" that do not require touch, such as kinesthetic synchronicity and visual, vocal, and rhythmic connections with one another. Similarly, we might question the assumption of "following" the point of contact, and look instead for the possibilities which lie in willful resistance. It is at this point in the class that I introduce a series of tasks that consciously explore the emotional content implicit in certain physical states. For example, we might set up the gym mats and do a wrestling exercise that compels the students to confront their potential for physical strength, rage, and even destruction. The act of trying to pin your partner (now positioned more like an opponent) down to the floor with all the weight and strength you can muster can be especially dif-ficult for women, for instance, who have had little experience with this kind of rough physicality. Some students may initially resist the competitive over-tones of the wrestling match, but, interestingly enough, they often change their minds once they have experienced it. Occasionally, there is a student who refuses to participate, but usually the flushed and excited faces of their classmates as they come off the mat after a two-minute bout convinces even the most reluctant to give it a try.

During the second half of the semester, we also work with contact impro-visation as a performance form, dancing in a structure called a round-robin, which is based on a revolving series of solos, duets, or trios. The idea is that the dancing is continuous and evolves as a new person enters the duet while another (usually the one who has been in the longest) eventually leaves that dance. The audience and those class members who are not dancing sit in a circle around the dancers, creating a heightened energy with their focus. This format tends to create a more external, performative style of dancing, which often comments on the social relationships, gender roles, and physical hierarchies that are rolling, shifting, and sliding in and out of view. Later, we talk about how we all feel watching and being watched, about what we are seeing and what we feel others see. Informed by the critical readings on contact improvisation and by watching videotapes that present a historical overview of the form's evolution, the students become increasingly aware of and interested in the cultural implications of these kinds of physical experiences.

> I've been thinking all semester about Contact and sexuality. When I first entered class, I was apprehensive about dancing with men because I was scared to be attracted to them. I was apprehensive about dancing with women because I was scared I would be attracted to them as well. I was thinking about issues of homosexuality and I was wondering if I was dancing with any.
>
> I don't think there is anything wrong with these thoughts. And the fears are still there. But, I've learned to enjoy the sensuality a lot more now. It's perhaps more gratifying than raw sex. The level of sensualness in class is very high, and sometimes I wonder why they give credit for this stuff. It doesn't seem very . . . academic.
>
> I must admit that while the class has helped me to overcome many social assumptions about sexuality, it hasn't helped to overcome them all. I feel myself consistently challenged to maintain a level of acceptance of the other bodies in the class, and the personalities that go with them . . . Maintaining this high level of sensual intimacy along with an acceptance of the egalitarian standards of contact is a tough thing to do. (Michael Sherman, student)

Sometimes students will resist talking about differences—sexual, physical, and emotional—insisting that contact improvisation brings out the "human" qualities of each individual. Usually, however, most students (like Michael, whom I quoted earlier) are willing to confront the various experiences of dis-ease present in even the most connected duets. For me, these disjunctions within the larger frame of a mutual commitment to improvising together are what make this dance form so continuously challenging even after one masters the physical skills needed. Although Naomi and I had worked together many times before we performed in her concert, we never knew exactly what might emerge from our dancing. We originally met as a teacher and a student in a classroom, but over the course of our performance we danced in and out of various relationships. Improvising across these differences, we were willing to experience and work with whatever material arose from our physical interaction.

Perhaps the most radical part of teaching contact improvisation within an academic institution is the physical contact between the professor and the student. This is absolutely clear to me each time the class is outside on a nice spring day and the deans, provost, and assorted suited administrators walk by as I am rolling on the grass with a student. As an improvisatory form in which relationships, movements, and social situations are all open to negotiation and invention, contact improvisation refuses the traditional student-teacher paradigm. I cannot teach contact improvisation from behind a desk and I can't keep an "appropriate" distance from my students. Even the most liberal-minded colleagues are shocked when they see me dance—body to body—with a student. Of course, I am aware that physical contact between a professor and a college student can be (and has frequently been) used to manipulate that student. However, besides making sure that I dance with each one of my students within the public setting of the classroom, I also feel that I present my body to the students within a very different physical dynamic. Lying down on the floor so that a student can roll over me, or meeting a student in a contact improvisation duet helps me to engage with that person in a way that neither erases nor insists upon my position as the teacher. By allowing myself to physically support and be supported by students, I feel as if I am negotiating a relationship with them in which they, at that moment, are equally responsible for the direction of our duet.

My experience with the form of contact improvisation helps me to set up inventive physical exercises that will facilitate the students' dancing within a safe environment. But because the form is improvisatory, it is always redefining its own priorities depending on who is dancing, when, where, and how. As the person "in charge" of this open situation, I rely on my dancing experiences to guide me through a class in which I do not directly control the outcome of the day's dancing. The importance of the physical training in disorientation is still relevant when we come together to air any thoughts or issues that arose during the dancing. This is often the moment when the students articulate the emotional and social implications of their physical experiences.

Confronting the uncomfortable moments that are inevitable when thirty people begin to deal with issues of self and other, identity and the body, feels very different to me when it is done in a class that already has a history of dancing and improvising together. I feel that our dancing exchanges allow us to take the intellectual risks necessary in order to talk about sex, gender, weight, body image, race, physical strength, smell, and touch in ways that are often not accommodated within most institutional contexts. These are difficult, often divisive discussions. Yet, within the frame of a contact improvisation class, these discussions are accommodated by a generous willingness to plunge into unknown situations and experience awkward moments. One thing that helps at this stage of the game is that, in addition to dealing with this kind of heat, we are also experiencing (both in our watching and our dancing) some amazing improvisations together. That physical connectedness gives us both the ambition and the safety net to attempt to risk jumping into situations we can't always control.

Contact improvisation is only one of ten different courses that I teach on a rotating basis. Many of the other classes are taught in a more conventional academic setting. I like the critical focus that those situations afford me, but I am aware that in the interest of academic rigor, I tend to be less open about what constitutes "appropriate" critical commentary from my students. I enjoy working with students on their writing and it is deeply satisfying to see them really refine their rhetorical skills over the course of a semester. But I often wonder what gets left out of this pedagogical focus, particularly for students who are not interested in writing academic essays for the rest of their lives. At the same time, I react strongly against any simplistic notion of "empowering" the students, because too often I sense that this is a pedagogical excuse for certain laziness on the part of the teacher—a desire not to ruffle any feathers by confronting a difficult issue or critically rubbing up against a student's entrenched position.

Because it locates its practice in the moving body, contact improvisation can deconstruct the notion of a singular, stable identity without destroying the presence of that material reality, the physical body, which insistently foregrounds the importance of gender, race, class, and body image—issues which are currently so critical to feminist thought. By incorporating experiences of self and other, marginality and centrality, dependence and autonomy, difference and sameness, in a way that actually complicates those very categories, contact improvisation provides a space of improvisation—a space for experimentation—in which individuals can physically negotiate the minefield of identity politics, without losing contact with one another. Bringing this kind of embodied experience into the classroom is, I find, a very potent pedagogical tool.

As I think about how to transfer some of the more successful teaching strategies from a contact improvisation class into my other, more academic, courses (without making every course I teach into a dance class), I realize that I would like to create the same willingness to improvise that I find in contact improvisation, within the framework of an intellectual discourse. So far, I have come up with two strategies to help me facilitate this translation: (a) try to find a way in the beginning of the semester to radically break up the physical and psychic arrangements of the learning environment while still maintaining intellectual contact. In other words, see what happens if the activity of learning can set up its own classroom dynamic and then find a corresponding spatial structure best suited to the particular priorities of that course; (b) translate the physical movement of contact into metaphors for a certain intellectual flexibility. For me, this means learning how to locate ourselves in the classroom not in order to dig in our heels and nervously guard those positions, but in order to chart the spaces we must travel—intellectually and physically—to meet one another with the sort of open generosity necessary to begin a dance.

1. I believe that the same logic holds for students as well, but I am assuming that my audience here is academic faculty.

2. For a discussion of the development of contact improvisation see "Open Bodies" and "Present Tense" in the Contact Improvisation section of this book.

24

Channeling the Other

An Embodied Approach to Teaching across Cultures

Research in Dance Education 4, no. 2, 2003.

The potent intersection of dance theory and cultural studies has contributed to a much needed theorization of embodiment (the processes by which cultural values are internalized and represented by social bodies), and has led to an increasingly sophisticated elucidation of cultural difference within the dance field. This discourse of difference has helped dance scholars and dance teachers in both the United States and the United Kingdom to reevaluate dance traditions and experiences that have been long overlooked by mainstream histories of theatrical dancing. Thus, for many dance educators, a history course focused on twentieth-century dance in America now begins with discussions of minstrelsy and the influence of African-America dance, rather than a romanticized narrative of Isadora Duncan as the "mother" or "originator" of modern dance in the West. This revisionist cultural framing does not necessarily diminish Duncan's contributions to dance history, but it does help students to recognize the class-based and racist rhetoric in her writing, as well as the wonderfully feminist dynamics in her dance practice. An awareness of cultural difference has shattered any easy assumptions about modern dance as "natural," "authentic," or the undisputed origin of most twentieth-century and contemporary dance forms. The resulting deconstruction of historical canons and aesthetic assumptions has created a certain amount of unease for dancers and teachers alike. Unfortunately, as the specificity of our bodies (white, female, middle-aged) becomes radically highlighted, the complexity of these issues tends to lead us away from our own physical experience. In this essay, I argue for a pedagogical space in which we can at once honor cultural difference while at the same time affirming a willingness to engage our bodies in historical and cross-cultural analysis. In other words, how can we learn to use our own bodies to think about culturally different bodies?

I teach dance history at Oberlin College—a small, progressive, liberalarts college in the Midwest. When I teach twentieth-century dance history, I endeavor to find ways for the students to understand that sense of evangelistic mission and revolutionary fervor so endemic to modern dance in the early part of the twentieth century. For example, when I teach a section on Isadora Duncan, I move back and forth between guiding the students through Duncan-based exercises that might approximate an experience of that earlier physicality, and challenging them to understand some of her writings through their own bodies and histories, asking them to imagine what movements might give them a similar sense of committed kinetic energy and power. I also ask my students to do an in-class movement and writing exercise in which their bodily experience becomes a primary source for their historical reflection. This studio class takes place after several weeks of introductory readings. I give the students Abraham Walkowitz's famous sketches of Duncan's movement and Gertrude Stein's prose poem on Duncan, "Orta, or one dancing."[1] I then ask them to improvise movement based on the kinesthetic information they derive from these images and words by artists who were contemporaries of Duncan. Once I have given them about forty minutes to "think through their bodies," so to speak, I ask them to write an essay that incorporates the information from the readings, as well as the embodied knowledge gleaned from their physical improvisations. These writings are often quite wonderful, with a marvelous interweaving of movement description and cultural context. Indeed, I often find a seamless blending of kinesthetic and historical discussions held together with an unusually strong sense of the writer's voice and bodily experience.

Generally, the students I teach enjoy this kind of adventure in the physical as well as the intellectual realm; they are happy to be challenged to move beyond the studio/classroom dualism still maintained by most dance curricula in this country. Oberlin students are delighted to be improvising, and seem to feel quite comfortable exploring this slightly nebulous area of historical research. One of the reasons for this may be that I, their professor, get right in there with them, allowing them to see my own critical and creative process as I try to articulate my relationship with this movement style, and discuss how I have dealt with the tensions that arise in negotiating the more racist and class-based aspects of Duncan's rhetoric with an appreciation of her visionary zeal. Of course, my students are often somewhat familiar with Duncan's name if not the details of her dance career, and I am lucky enough to have found an old Oberlin dance club scrapbook from the early part of the twentieth century, which has programs from annual dance events, including Ted Shawn's visit (with his all-male company) in the thirties. These early programs feature pictures of women in Grecian tunics dancing outside in a pastoral setting, thus bringing Duncan's legacy of "natural" dancing into the college's history as well.

At Oberlin, I teach three different dance history classes: twentieth-century American dance; contemporary dance; and cross-cultural dance history (a course that focuses on a comparative analysis of classical Indian dance, European court dance, and the development of ballet; West African dance forms; and Native American dance traditions). For a long time in my cross-cultural dance history class, I contented myself with the occasional studio master class. Usually this class was taught by someone steeped in the particular dance tradition we were studying. In one special class session, these teachers would attempt to give my students a small taste of the dance training and physical dynamic of the form that we were studying. I soon found this token class in "ethnic" dance to be unsatisfactory. For one thing, I became tired of always having to ask the same local dancers to come in and teach the same sort of broad introductory class. I also felt that, despite my protestations to the contrary, I was reinforcing a racist dynamic implicit in this situation of white professor on a tenure-track line teaching the history end of a class, while the African, East Indian, or Native American guest artists came in to add the physical spice, so to speak.

The question that confronted me in this course was how to keep some aspect of the learning physical without tokenizing that experience? How could I introduce embodied thinking in a cross-cultural situation in which I had much less kinesthetic grounding in the forms we were studying? How could I engage my students' physical experiences, when those experiences (for the most part) arose out of a completely different cultural framework? I decided to try to develop an exercise similar to the one on Duncan (which I described earlier), that would ask the students to use their bodies not simply to follow or imitate—but as vehicles for analytic thinking.

I begin my cross-cultural course with a section on classical Indian dance. We start with a number of classes devoted to tracing the evolution of classical forms such as bharata natyam and Odissi dance from the early Vedic times through to contemporary revisionist performances in India, as well as in the United States. Looking at the issues of religion, the position of women within the culture, structures of artistic patronage, the status of dance as an art form as well as a devotional act, and the effects of feudal and colonial occupations (including the internalization of a Christian morality), the class traces the historical changes within these classical traditions. We document how these spheres of influence merge and separate according to the shifts in the political and economic landscape. In addition to secondary-source readings, the class looks at historical surveys, aesthetic texts, personal memoirs, and official government documents.[2] The readings are interesting and I feel that this introduction to a world dance form gives the students a solid intellectual grounding. Nonetheless, it disturbed me to only study world dance as an intellectual adventure in cultural theory. One semester a few years ago, I decided to take the risk and launch into a somatic exploration of this cross-cultural material—not in an attempt to approximate the dance form, but rather to see if we could experience something of the changing performative context and shifts in representational frames through our respective bodies. In other words, how did the history of classical Indian dance affect the relationship between the dancers and their audiences, and what might that have felt like from the inside?

Deciding to work improvisationally in this context meant that I asked my students to confront a myriad of disturbing questions about cross-cultural interaction, authenticity and appropriation of ritual experience, colonial voyeurism and the representation of women's bodies, as well as the romanticization of community within non-Western cultures. As if this was not hard enough, I wanted them to both be critically aware of their privileged position, and to be open and humble enough to enter an improvisation in which I was asking them to channel an "other" bodily experience. I wanted them to be conscious, but not overly self-conscious, so that they could use their body to cross over into some kind of physical understanding. After the end of two weeks study on classical Indian dance, I asked the students to enter the dance studio and experience these different historical moments through a guided physical exploration.

The space is arranged so that there is only natural light, and there is an altar set up at one end with flowers, rice, a statue of Nataraja, and incense burning. I ask the students to lie down and focus on their breathing; emptying their minds and releasing their weight into the floor. I proceed to give them a sense-based visualization of different historical contexts as I understand them. Then I am quiet while they stand up and begin a ten-minute movement improvisation, trying to feel how dancing as worship at that time felt, and how that physical context affected the movement qualities of the dancing. After they finish, the students free-write for another ten minutes.

We begin with the Vedic period in which dance was used in the temples as part of a spiritual offering. Here, there is no mortal audience, no stage, only an omnipresent and yet deeply internal gaze—for the gods are found both within the self and everywhere outside. Next, we proceed to feudal time in India to experience what it would be like for a dancer to be asked to dance in a court setting. What does the shift from Hindu temple to royal court do to the relationship of the dancer to her audience? Finally, we explore how this dance form (which has been outlawed in the early twentieth century by another colonial power, Britain) was reconstructed to serve a new nationalist agenda—albeit one with very different take on issues of gender, performance and eroticism. Having experienced these moments in their physical improvisations, the students are then asked to write on the different aesthetic and cultural relationships between the dancer and their audience. In this writing they incorporate their embodied knowledge with their academic study of the dance form to talk about how the changing contexts effected the movement and agency of the dancer.

The students' writings and our class discussions afterward have convinced me that it is an important and ultimately valuable exercise. For instance, a number of students had experiences similar to the following student, who captures in her free-writing a sense of the difference between dancing internally and dancing for an external audience that did not share her religious convictions.

> Feeling ME as a devadasi was a sensual, personal experience. I began moving very internally, slowly, almost subconsciously, with thought of a whole, larger energy . . . The dance felt really good. I was beautiful, loved by the universe and my idea of God, nurtured by my own devotion. The movement began stretching, ribs and torso, arms reaching into space with soft energy, feeling the earth and the sky; it moved downward into my pelvis and legs, swaying and turning. I could feel not only an appreciation and love through what I was doing, but also an honor in return—a comfort because I belonged here in this temple space, I was dancing with the gratitude of the people in my community behind me . . . Moving into a space where I was being watched, I became modest, even defensive. I would not show these strangers the beauty of what I could really express for what I believed and worshipped . . . I danced sideways, hiding my face. The dance was no longer for me, but them. My movements became more detached and angular. (Katie Hopkins)

Other students had much less comfortable experiences in this movement exploration. Sometimes that discomfort arose from a fear of imitating someone else's religious devotion, or from a sense of violation of an other's religious space. One student described it as a feeling of trespassing, and wondered if she would be angry if someone came into her temple without knowing much about Judaism. Another student began to recognize how her experience of dance has always been strongly secular and technically based. She also realized (when improvising to the Mughal court entertainer section) how much being judged by outside, critical eyes was part of her dance background. Issues of control over one's dancing (as in was I moving or being moved by an outside force), and the pervasive separation of mind, spirit, and body came up for many students. We spent a long time talking about questions of spirituality in dance, and how that same energy manifested itself differently across cultures.

Pedagogically speaking, I think this kind of exercise can be extremely valuable because the physical engagement forces students to evaluate their own preconceptions and assumptions with a depth rarely present in purely intellectual classroom discussions. It is the kind of exercise that stays with the student throughout the semester and comes up again in the end of the course evaluations. As much as I think that it is useful, it also rubs a lot of students the wrong way. Like many small liberalarts colleges, Oberlin fosters a climate of extreme self-consciousness about issues of oppression—including the litany of race, gender, class, sexuality, and ability. Most often, my teaching contributes to this kind of critical awareness of social positions and cultural privilege. But I must say that frequently, in terms of cross-cultural dance studies, I find this hyperawareness of difference to be somewhat limiting. It would be much easier for both me and my students to approach a cross-cultural dance class from a safely academic, physically detached, position. Reading essays, watching videos, maybe even taking a West African dance class—these are all ways of learning well within our comfort zones. What is the usefulness of pushing ourselves further? In order to explore this question, I would like to relate how I became intrigued with the study of classical Indian dance, and to share with you one of my most enduring experiences of cultural exchange—the exchange of an embodied idea.

I first became interested in classical Indian dance when I was fortunate enough to witness a performance by the late Sanjukta Panagrahi, a great Odissi dancer. Later, I took a short workshop with her. Although her performance was my first exposure to live classical Indian dance, I have to say that I felt as if I immediately understood the form in some deeply intuitive way. Now I certainly do not want this last statement to sound like some kind of cultural hubris—I am not pretending that I saw Sanjukta's dancing as an "expert"—but rather that I was brought into her dancing, her experience of the movement in such a way, that seemed to bridge over the cultural differences that informed our separate dance styles, to give us a mutual experience of the dance. When I took the workshop, these cultural differences erupted again as I tried to mimic the facial gestures of the various moods or emotional states that we were trying to learn.

As I continued to study the history of classical Indian dance, I began to think of that moment of mutual energy that I experienced in Sanjukta's dancing in terms of the Indian aesthetic theory of Rasa—a theory that binds much Indian art and performance to a larger sense of the cosmic universe. For me, Rasa suggests a very potent way of reframing how dance performances are constructed in Western culture. I think that Rasa provides us with a theory of watching dance that is closer to witnessing in the interactive sense of that word. Rasa is based on the notion of a mutual responsibility between the performer and the audience. I mean that in the sense of a real "responsiveness"—an ability to "respond" to the energy of that moment. This kind of "responsiveness" assumes a willingness to refuse static definitions of beauty or grace, a willingness to give up expectations of what this dance should look like, and an ability to commit to a joint process of building an aesthetic experience together, no matter what culture one comes from.

The exchange of energy in Rasa is not unique to Indian dancing, of course. Many cultures believe in the same kind of interaction, but describe it differently. Yet my experiences with classical Indian dance have inspired a sense of affinity with that form that eludes words and spills away from critical analysis. When I reflect on my own evolution—both physical and intellectual—through the dance form over the past decade, I realize how profoundly this form has influenced how I think, see, and move in my own life. This influence is not necessarily visible or directly referenced in my work. It does not translate into the "look" of classical Indian dance at all. Nonetheless, it is through my exposure to this form that I am able to imagine an "other" reality—one based in a belief that dance could be a transformative practice. When I ask my students to improvise different moments in the history of classical Indian dancing, I am asking them to understand this kind of exchange corporeally. This does not mean that I am asking them to forget or refuse the historical facts that separate the dancers we read about from their own cultural situation. But it does mean that I believe we can engage in a conscious crossing-over to learn through our bodies what can never be taught through our books. Sure, I want to be conscious and articulate about the processes of power and representation, identity and appropriation. But I also want to allow the reverberations of other dancing to register in my body. That channeling is never simply an academic gesture.

NOTES

1. See Abraham Walkowitz, *Isadora Duncan in Her Dances* (Girard, KS: Haldeman-Julius Publications, 1945), and Gerturde Stein, *Two* (Freeport, NY: Books for Libraries Press, 1969).

2. See the work of Kapila Vatsyayan, particularly her *Classical Indian Dance in Literature and the Arts* (New Delhi: Sangeet Natak Akademi, 1968), and Avanthi Meduri, "Bharatha Natyam—What Are You?," in *Moving History/Dancing Cultures,* ed. Albright and Dils (Middletown, CT: Wesleyan University Press, 2001).

25

Training Bodies to Matter

Journal of Dance and Somatic Practices 1, no. 1, 2009.

This essay traces three different pedagogical situations in which I try to shift what I see as the negative corporeal dynamics of our contemporary moment, one body at a time. Drawing examples from my experiences with the body-to-body interactions of contact improvisation—the dance form that first brought me into dance thirty years ago—Bridging the Body/Mind Divide, a first-year seminar taught to a general range of students at Oberlin College, as well as *Girls in Motion,* the after-school program I run for adolescent girls at a local school, I present a series of physical skills that I believe create an important somatic foundation for a more mindful being in the world. Over the past decade, I have become increasingly interested in drawing out the cultural implications of many somatic exercises. I want to push these practices beyond the sphere of personal experience to think about how to engage different populations of people in this type of bodily awareness. In these examples of what Deidre Sklar would call "corporeal rhetorics," I consciously harness the persuasive force of movement experiences to convince my students there is a better way to dwell in their bodies and in this twenty-first-century world.[1]

When I first began teaching dance technique and contact improvisation in the mid-1980s, my students were hungry for the physical experience of disorientation and the intellectual sensibilities of deconstruction. They loved to spin and fall, and they clearly connected these wild displacements of the body with a sense of possibility in the world. Nowadays, as I enter my third decade of university teaching, I am struck by the shifting needs of young peoples' bodies. Generally, they do not want to be pushed too hard, or thrown off-balance. Indeed, I believe that the experience of growing up in a time where some part of life—for many of my students a significant part—is lived out on a two-dimensional screen, has created a real fear of falling; a fear of losing stability in a world that is already so chaotic. As a result, I have become aware of the pedagogical need to address this existential state, and I am increasingly interested in the connections between the physical sensation of gravity and the spiritual sense of being grounded in the world.

It is rare that I am committed to my current place. It seems that location has become less important now that we are all connected, and I find myself living in a chronic state of dislocation . . . I am at a desk in Shakespeare class, but my head is in the clouds. My roommate is on her bed looking up what the weather is like in Australia. I call home in Tennessee and forget that I am living in Ohio. (Katherine Dohan, student)

These comments written by Oberlin College student Katherine Dohan are (unfortunately) common sentiments on my university campus these days, where it is common practice to spend many of our waking hours in front of a computer screen. Most of my students are conscious when pressed of the very real danger of addiction to the Internet's easy information and to their ever-evolving social networks. In addition, the oddly disembodied mobility of much contemporary communication has severed many of my students' connections with grounding aspects of location—the experience of feeling one's feet planted in the earth, so to speak. This is reflected not only in the most obvious postural dysfunctions, but also in the way students use their eyes (myopically, from the front of the lenses, looking at small screens, short distances, with no awareness of their peripheral vision), as well as the resulting overuse of one aspect of cognition (the visual, symbolic synapses of the frontal lobe). The more people focus only on the screen in front of them, the less they are aware of the three-dimensionality of their bodies, including their backspace.

Because I recognize the reality of our globally interconnected world, I am not suggesting that we all go off-line or retreat into a more traditional model of physical placement or identity location. As a teacher, I need to accept (albeit not uncritically) the twenty-first-century framework of my students' lives. Throughout this essay, I chart some of the shifts in my teaching as I work to balance grounding with training in re (as opposed to dis)location. Here, I try to articulate the theoretical implications of paying attention to gravity and weight while simultaneously training for disorientation and shifting global perspectives (including survival in an economic crisis). Using students' writings as well as descriptions of exercises and improvisational scores I have developed over the last ten years, I argue for the vital importance of introducing gravity to a generation of students whose bodies are rarely in the same place as their minds.

I taught a dance class the day after 9/11. After leading a vigorous warm-up, I introduced an improvisational score that I find myself using repeatedly these days. It is a very simple score—the implications of which have shifted over time. It begins as people spread out across a space, each facing a different direction. Slowly, each person on his or her own time sinks to the ground, rolls over across their back, and then slowly uncurls through their spine to rise up into a standing position. Staying there for a moment, we acknowledge the space around us, playing with the soft balance of muscles and bones that makes maintaining an upright posture into an intricate dance. Sink, rise, and stand; sink, rise, and stand. Each time we roll in toward the center such that we move closer and closer to one another until we are in a tight clump. Nine years ago, the class went outside to the town square to perform this score, and I interpreted the folding and unfolding as a metaphor of the crumbling and rising of the twin towers. These days, I use this practice as a warm-up, where the images are much less explicit. Instead, I ask students to attend to the different relationship to gravity as they sink down into and grow out of the earth.

Not surprisingly, given how much time we spend in front of computers these days, the visual and verbal synapses in our forebrains are deeply rutted—both quick to fire and worn down with repeated use. The sensation of gravity, on the other hand, can activate the mid- and lower brains—the more bodily and less symbolic areas of the brain that connect to the parasympathetic systems of our being. Keeping those systems active in our modern, industrialized culture requires placing the body in situations where physical reactions must operate faster than the verbal mind. Thus, once I have given students an opportunity to digest individual sensations of gravity, I begin to introduce the experiences of momentum and falling. For those of us involved in contact improvisation, of course, falling is a crucial skill.

As we know, one of the essential aspects to teaching falling is retraining the instinctual impulse to grip or hold our breath when we feel our bodies lose their grounding. (Think of the classic comic routine triggered by the act of leaning against something that suddenly gives way.) One way to train students to fall without fear, to enjoy that suspension of the upright orientation and the loss of control in that moment of release, is to learn to fall with light support. At first this requires becoming used to the experience of falling within a tight circle and always with a sensation of physical touch that registers possible support. Later in my classes, we haul out the gymnastics mats and practice falling and catching. Then I introduce a score in which there is one catcher and up to four people falling. The trick is to create a rhythm of suspension and fall that allows the catcher to coordinate catching one person after the other in very quick succession. Often, the timing is such that the catcher can only offer a quick counter balance to ease the descent. Sometimes, a person who is suspending for too long needs a little push. Eventually, all the participants, but especially the catcher, learn to trust their instincts, and a kind of magic transpires where people can turn and catch someone behind them as if they had eyes in the back of their head.

At its core, movement is a series of falls (some small, some more spectacular) that propel the body through time and space. Using gravity, we can attune our sensibilities to the more subtle of those displacements. This is the practice of what contact improvisers call the "small dance," where one stands with one's eyes closed, feeling the smallest shifts of muscle and bone as the body aligns itself between sky and earth. The proprioceptive tuning that is acquired with this practice gives us an awareness of the physical location in which the body is both grounded and open to moving in any direction. Reflecting on the students who have passed through my classes over these past years, I realize the sad irony of some of their lives—that they are stuck in one place, all the while floating aimlessly in cyberspace. Dancing with an attention to falling and gravity can help keep them both moving through space and connected to the world. As Katherine Dohan recognizes:

> Within my tragically fractured existence, dancing is one of the few times when I can be in one place. It is rather ironic that the time when I can best become a part of a specific location is while I am moving. Yet in this world that is becoming more and more disconnected through constant connection, in which the need to move is declining every day, moving might be more important than ever.

In an essay in *The Body Eclectic: Evolving Practices in Dance Training,* Melanie Bales describes an underlying feature of many contemporary release techniques that resonates with this particular training in contact improvisation: "In many somatic practices, the body's relationship to gravity is examined on and off the vertical axis, through exercises or experiences that require lying, sitting, or getting up and down from the floor. Alignment is not about standing straight or upright but rather about the changing relationships within the body, sensing balance, and avoiding unnecessary muscular holding so the body is open to possibility."[2] The shift here is to a pedagogy based in experiencing the sensate dimensions of one's physical state of being. Most dance training today, at least in universities in the United States, carries this emphasis on what I would call "physical mindfulness," the awareness of sensations inside one's body. But I believe that we could move this potent practice beyond the studio and into more general classrooms or work places. Recent studies in neurology reveal that this facility of internal perception, which is called *interoception,* is fundamental to reading another human being's emotional state. That is to say, the more aware we are of our own internal sensations, the more empathetic we are.

There is a similar corporeal logic at work in my first-year seminar, Bridging the Body/Mind Divide. Bridging the usual spatial divide between academic and practice courses, this class is taught in a large studio, with a seminar table in one corner such that we can easily shift from reading texts and intellectual discussions to physical exercises that ground those ideas (or stretch them) through our bodies. Throughout the classes, I match somatic awareness training with key texts from Western philosophy and Eastern Buddhist traditions, along with contemporary feminist discussions of embodiment. These eighteen-year-old students read Maurice Merleau-Ponty's *The Phenomenology of Perception* in its entirety. Over the course of the semester the students learn to reflect on how their bodily approach to the world has clear implications on their thinking.

Let me give an example. Often, I begin with the class moving through the space, shifting directions to walk with different facings. There is a moment where, after moving vigorously through the space, the students come to a point of stillness while standing. This gives them an opportunity to experience the subtle shifts of weight and muscular action—a chance to feel one's body at once grounded through the feet and extending through the head—a moment to reflect on the position of being suspended between earth and sky. Sometimes, I ask them to imagine opening their pores so that the world can enter the space of their bodies. This image of one's body as part of the whole space has clear physical results in the released muscular tone of the body. Even the eyes work differently if we imagine the world entering the space of the head, rather than the eyes having to strain to capture the world visually. As the front of the face relaxes, the eyes can release into their sockets, thus opening up our peripheral vision, increasing our awareness of the space around us, allowing us to see ourselves in the world, not just the world from our point of view (which, as we know, can be quite narrow).

There is also, I believe, a profound psychic reorganization here as well. By shifting our somatic imagination, we can reorder our cultural notions of selfhood. Rather than the colonialist paradigm of the individual, propelled by his will and determination to go out into the world and stake a claim (stand on one's own two feet, make a mark, etc.), the self becomes an interdependent part that flows through and with the world. Similar exercises with breath can cultivate a mindfulness of the constant exchange between inhalation and exhalation, teaching us that air is not a void, the absence of solid objects, but a manifestation of the interchangeability of self and the world. In addition, I draw their attention to both their skeletal structures and the different body systems such as fluids, endocrine system, etc., to provide a physical referent for developing new connections between our bodies and the environments we inhabit.

I am often surprised at how receptive these nondance students are to working on Merleau-Ponty's notion of intersubjectivity through their bodies. In my Bridging the Body/Mind Divide seminar, I introduce the point of contact, but expand its meaning to think about how we are with others in the world. Facing a partner, one presses a forefinger against that of their partner. Attending to how the energy of his or her whole body can move through their spine out their arm and into their finger, the partners wait. The point created by the joining of two energies is sometimes referred to as a *third mind* in contact improvisation, and it is that which becomes the focus of their mutual attention. Allowing their motion to be led by the point of contact, the two partners endeavor to follow its spatial and rhythmic journey throughout the room. At first, it may seem clear who is leading and who is following, but eventually, with time and practice, the shifting back and forth evolves into such a rapid and subtle exchange that the categories of leader and follower begin to lose their oppositional meaning. That binary is subverted as the attention shifts onto the play of space and touch between the two movers. Embedded in this exercise is a fluidity of experience that can change our perceptions of the boundaries between self and other.

In my seminar, this exercise is paired with our discussion of Merleau-Ponty's own description of touching and being touched and his concept of intersubjectivity in *The Phenomenology of Perception*. In class, we confront this question of the differences between self and other by asking: can one really know another's experience? Asking this existential question without a physical basis would lead to a very abstract exegesis. But in the context of our physical exercises, it becomes a mode of engaged inquiry that is grounded in their bodily experience. It is exciting to me as a teacher to see these young students become both critically articulate and thoughtful about their lives.

I run an after-school program for girls at the local public school, which is like a mini-urban environment, with many of the same problems of poverty and behavioral issues. The mission statement for *Girls in Motion* reads: "The *Girls in Motion* program seeks to introduce girls at risk for academic failure and low self-esteem to a series of fun and integrative movement experiences that will allow them to develop more holistic relationships with their bodies. The program's motto *Move Smart—Talk Smart—Be Smart* reveals the philosophy behind it. *Girls in Motion* provides a safe place for girls to discuss and explore issues of body image and peer pressure through movement forms—including dance, yoga, and sports—aligned with creative activities and writing projects, with the aim of developing physical fitness, mind-body awareness, and increased self-esteem." I think we would all agree that these are admirable goals. The question is how to achieve them? How, exactly, does one teach integration to sassy twelve-year-olds, especially when much of one's energy is spent on getting them to show up regularly?

Needless to say, I have no easy answer; no fabulous combination of skills that can shore up self-esteem the way Pilates can tighten one's abs. The college-student mentors who work in the program and I have introduced a variety of activities—from step-dancing, to hip-hop, to climbing walls, to yoga, to ultimate Frisbee. Here is one example of a modified sun salutation, which we do to focus and warm up at the beginning of the program. While it is a simple physical exercise (so that everyone can do it, and it is easy to remember), the crucial part is the verbal litany that accompanies the movement. Half Girl Scout pledge, half yoga mantra, these words provide a framework in which to realize the larger implications of that physical exercise. We begin standing, stretching the hands to the sky ("I reach to the sky"), then bend over and touch the ground ("I press into the earth"), and spiral the body around ("I gather all the energy around me"). Next, we take our right legs back into lunge and trace a semicircle with the right arm ("I open to one side"), and coming back to facing front with the palms together in front of the chest ("and I center myself"), repeat to the other side ("I open to the other side, and then center myself"). Next, we jump back into plank pose ("I create a bridge from my school to my community"), and then come into child's pose ("I gather into myself") and walk back to the front of the mat to stand in mountain pose ("and walk forward to become present in the world.")

To become present in the world. Just standing, aware of the sensation of that line of energy running from the earth, through one's spine, to the sky. Many of us take this moment for granted. We do it every day rising from our chairs, or in technique or yoga classes. And yet, in the context of a middle-school environment with its chatty, attitude-filled street energy, this can be an amazingly profound experience. Much to my surprise, the adolescent girls in this program enjoy this sequence so much that they often insist on ending most sessions with it as well. In fact, one of the most pleasurable moments for me was when a mentor told me one of her students had gone up to her room and done the sun salutation instead of yelling and arguing with her mom. But what exactly are they being taught? I believe that on some level, they are learning to find the connections between breathing and inspiration, to feel the stability of gravity, to mobilize their pelvis, to find resistance through internal strength rather than external tension, to rely on lines of energy to support their bodies, to realize the three-dimensionality of their bodies, and finally, to recognize the importance of what is inside (their organs), as well as on the surface of their skin.

In her work from the early 1990s on the physical attributes of gender conditioning, Iris Marion Young articulates the phenomenological basis for feminine bodily comportment by distinguishing three modalities of women's movement: ambiguous transcendence, inhibited intentionality, and discontinuous unity. Basically, this is fancy philosophical language for throwing like a girl—which is to say using a body part in a manner that is totally disconnected from the rest of one's weight and strength. By analyzing the ways that young girls and women are trained not to take up the space around them, not to use the capacity of their whole body when engaging in physical activity, and not to fully project their physical intentions onto the world around them, Young describes the tensions between experiencing one's body as both a thing and as capacity for action—as both a passive object and an active subject. This dichotomy is rarely stronger than in middle school, when most girls become acutely aware of the social dynamics of attractiveness and social success. Working to resist and unpack the sexist, racist, and class-based foundations of these cultural discourses, *Girls in Motion* tries to teach these kids to take up space, to activate their weight, and thus to learn to commit themselves to engaging fully in the tasks (both physical and academic) at hand.

The title of this essay is "Training Bodies to Matter," and much of what I have articulated here hinges on the double meaning of *matter*—as both making a difference in the world and the realization that that difference has a material basis. This focus on the process of embodiment, rather than on the product of a particular style or technique, gives me the opportunity to explore the ways in which bodies and cultures are mutually informative. At the same time, it helps me avoid the depressingly deterministic effects of so many academic discussions of the regulated or submissive body. I realize, of course, this work represents a utopian vision—one that can easily be swept away by several hours spent in front of a computer, in a faculty meeting, or in line at the Visa office. My sense, however, is that many of my students are searching for physical hope and a community in the flesh. Used to spending hours floating in cyberspace, they are immensely relieved when someone helps them to reconnect with the earth's gravity and the sensation of their own weight. In addition, having an opportunity to share those somatic experiences with adolescents allows the college students to intervene in a critical moment in many girls' lives. My experiences in the studio and in the classroom affirm my belief that for a person who has come of age surrounded by screens, it is truly powerful to feel—concretely, through a connection with gravity and community—that bodies really do matter.

NOTES

1. Deidre Sklar, "Introduction to On Corporeal Rhetoric Panel," presentation at the Society of Dance History Scholar's annual conference, Paris, 2007.

2. Melanie Bales, *The Body Eclectic: Evolving Practices in Dance Training* (Urbana: University of Illinois Press, 2008), 157.

VI

OCCASIONAL PIECES

This section's title comes from that of a folder on my computer where I store presentations, papers, articles, book reviews, and essays that I have produced for very specific occasions. These could be an invitation to write something for an anthology, or a request that I speak at a conference, or contribute to a thematic issue of a journal. These pieces are inspired by the particular themes of those occasions and are written with that audience in mind. Unique opportunities to think about subjects I may not have previously considered, these short studies do not necessarily evolve into longer projects or books. Often, they exist only as a response to that occasion. Nonetheless, I am quite fond of some of these writings. Like patches in a crazy quilt, their relationship to one another can be unscripted and elusive, but stitching them together in this section made me realize that they represent important pieces from the fabric of my writing life.

I find it supremely interesting to be called upon to address a topic or area that I might never have considered on my own. For instance, in the fall of 2012, I was asked to address the Abrace conference in Porto Alegre, Brazil. The theme of that gathering was memory. At once filled with trepidation (I had never thought about memory in dance) and intrigued (memories are often disorienting, a metaphysical concept that I have been spending a lot of time thinking about), I embraced the possibilities and wrote a presentation called "Falling into Memory," which focused on a 2002 dance entitled *Fallen* by Jess Curtis and various oral histories of 9/11. Book reviews can also be opportunities to read and think about someone else's work that I might not have previously been aware of, especially if the author is not an American scholar. At times these intriguing opportunities seriously stretch my comfort zone—witness my involvement with the Screendance network and the *International Journal of Screendance,* on whose editorial board I sit with curiosity as well as skepticism, for at times I am not even sure I like screen images very much. And yet there is something compelling about working with ideas from the place of a slight resistance, especially if one's coparticipants are engaging and persuasive. I have left many of these conferences or meetings inspired and grateful that I had had the opportunity to participate. I derive a great deal of pleasure thinking about dance with others.

Because originally many of these pieces were written for an interactive situation—a conference, network meeting, symposium, roundtable, even Skype events—I am hopeful that their informal tone helps to evoke the proximity of the audience I was addressing and reveals the kind of rich exchange of ideas and passions that these public occasions cultivate. Echoing the wide range of intellectual curiosities that animate the rest of this collection, these writings run the gamut of my interests from an early essay on the structures of improvisation and play to a semiautobiographical essay on disability, to a discussion of the politics of teaching and presenting African dance in North America, to a talk on the global economies of artistic exchange, as well as a longer discussion of shifting cultural contexts of late twentieth-century dance. I have also included three short editorials that I wrote for *Movement Research Journal*—a publication connected to the dynamic downtown arts organization of the same name, as well as a series of discussions of dance on screens, a very short piece about graduate programs in dance, several book reviews, and a final essay, "Falling," which points towards my current book project, *Gravity Matters: Finding Ground in an Unstable World*.

Although they address many different kinds of dance, these eclectic writings share a personal tone with which I reflect on my embodied experience, all the while focusing on an issue of critical importance in contemporary dance. Whether I am discussing the time when I was temporarily disabled and refused surgery, choosing instead to make a dance; or my time spent learning West African dance with Chuck Davis at the American Dance Festival; or describing the palpable, yet invisible presence evoked by the loss of a loved one, I try bring a corporeal thoughtfulness to the topic I am addressing. At times fiercely political, at other times elegiac, these short pieces weave my dancing through my writing, revealing another aspect of my engagement with the bodies and ideas that animate the field of dance studies today.

26

The Mesh in the Mess

Contact Quarterly, Winter 1987.

Out of the silence, her small, lithe body shotputs into a mass of shiny build-ing blocks. Still, but alert and ready to move, she crouches with her head cocked, listening to sounds from a distant world, a jungle world. Always close to the ground, this tiny figure in white stands out against the huge, still, black emptiness of the space all around her. Moving tentatively at first, she crawls with an ease and grace unknown to most human adults. Suddenly, something or some energy seizes her. Her body hums with urgency as light tremors dart through her limbs. She strains her upper body, twists, and pulls back to catapult through the air. Her voice cries out, "I want to know I'm alive," as she lands with the sure-footed sheerness of a cat.

Two women vault spread-eagled through the air and land onstage as if the floor were a trampoline propelling them upwards and forwards. Transfer-ring the crash momentum into a forward roll, they emerge from their tumult long enough to glance over and smile at each other before another spurt of energy sends them reeling backwards into an arch that peels off the floor and spins them headlong into three other dancers.

Three girls are building castles on the sand table. They are utterly absorbed in the task of placing plastic forms filled with sand on the table, and the suspense as they wait to see if the sand will hold its shape after the form is removed. All the while they keep shifting their positions and muttering to themselves. One girl looks up and places a foot on the table. Steadying herself by stretching her arm forward, she climbs up onto the table. Without any hesitation and with barely a glance up, the other two girls also step up onto the table. For a moment they seem dazed—then they look at one an-other and giggle. Just as quickly as they all jumped up, they begin flinging sand and containers off the table. A torrent of sand and plastic forms flies every-which-way. Enthusiastic—with the job well done—they grab hands and start skipping around in a circle on the table. The faster they go, the more they lean out and let their heads drop back, laughing with the joy of the momentum. After a few circles, one girl begins to sing "Ring around the rosy," and soon the initial burst of chaotic energy settles into a regular rhythmic game.

These paragraphs describe three movement events. The first traces the opening few minutes of Kei Takei's solo in the latest section of her ongoing dance saga, *Light Part 20 and 21*. The second describes a brief duet sequence in Pooh Kaye's dance, *Wildfields* (1984), and the third recounts an episode from an afternoon of watching the sand box in Washington Square Park. Although the contexts and the specific movements of these three events are different, they share a noteworthy feature: they all communicate a sense of play or playfulness. The last two situations, however, contain another level of complexity. Two dancers in one, and three girls in the other, are playing together. It is not only their individual movements that evoke playfulness, there is a dynamic structuring in their movement interaction that also seems characteristic of play.

The whole concept of play elicits an enormous amount of speculation concerning its meaning, purpose, function, and place in society. The literature on primate behavior abounds with parallels between the play activities of primates and humans. Developmental psychology places emphasis on the connections between children's play and their growing sense of themselves. Anthropologists, sociologists, and performance scholars often view play, including ritual and contests, as a socially sanctioned way for people to release tensions. Even aestheticians attribute artistic creativity and poetic imagination to a mysterious drive that they label as the "play impulse."

But first, what is play? What is playful movement? What are the interactions of play? And what are the underlying structures that guide play? Webster's *Seventh New Collegiate Dictionary* defines the noun *play* as "an activity of children, free or unimpeded motion, brisk, fitful or light movement and frolic." The verb is described by the same source as "to move or operate in a lively, irregular or intermittent manner; to discharge, fire or set off with continuous effect; to move or function freely within prescribed limits." It is the verb's definition that most intrigues me: it suggests a dynamic organization within the activity of play.

In a chapter entitled "The Play—Concept as Expressed in Language" in his study of the play element in culture, *Homo Ludens,* Johan Huizinga traces the sources and etymologies of play throughout the ancient and modern languages of the world. While most languages center their play-related words on rapid movement or physical activity, there are several interesting tangents from this generalized meaning. In Sanskrit, for instance, the word for play can designate a certain radiance, or shininess. The roots of play in German, Latin, and Sanskrit all serve to identify the movement of the wind or waves. The oldest definition of the Dutch word *plegan* (play) is "to take a risk, to expose oneself to danger." Huizinga's linguistic history of the word also uncovers various other attributes of play, among which are "lightness, tension, uncertainty as to the outcome, and free choice."[1]

Any arena of movement or activity whose definition can slide from "the movement of the waves," to "taking a risk," to a certain "radiance," to "uncertain as to the outcome," must either encompass a wide range of behavior or allow for a certain elasticity in its perimeters. Play does both, and almost defies definition by its own flexibility. Definition means the action or the power of making definite and clear. Yet play is a fluid state and is thus never completely definite and clear. To make it so may well change the very essence that we are trying to identify.

Enter any playground and watch for an hour, or four hours, and then try to define what play is. Is play a girl running furiously after a ball? Yes, but . . . Is play four children sliding "as a train" down the slope? Yes, well, but . . . Is play one girl spinning with her head thrown back, eyes closed, and another girl watching her intently and then starting to spin too? Yes, well, but, there is . . . Is play a boy who thinks he is a bear, chasing another boy, who, laughing and running around the jungle gym, is trying to decide whether he is a tiger or a dog? Yes, well, but . . . there is also . . .

Play is a mess. But there is a mesh in that mess, which holds, but does not bind, that mess together. It is this mesh, or what I refer to as the *dynamic structuring* of play, that I explore throughout the remainder of this essay.

My raw observation material is culled from four weeks of watching children move and interact in playgrounds throughout the city, and repeated viewings of a videotaped performance of Pooh Kaye's *Wildfields,* which I have also seen live on two occasions. I chose this dance because of its striking use of play-like movements. The prevalence of words like *play, playful,* and *playfulness* in the reviews of the piece confirm my sense of the dance.

After a week or so of watching children in playgrounds, especially in the large sandboxes, I realized how sporadic their attention and their play activities are. Unlike the dancers in Pooh Kaye's constructed rompings, children rarely bound and scamper nonstop for twenty minutes. While the dance, *Wildfields,* has clear boundaries in its clear beginning and ending, children's play activities merge with various distractions—a detour to the water fountain, a foray beyond the fence for an errant ball, a shoe-tying session with a parent or caregiver.

Two girlfriends, one with a ball, approach a third girl and ask her if she wants to play a game. The rules are negotiated and one girl, the "it," goes over to the side fence to count to fifty. The other two run off with the ball. All the while darting glances back to the "it" to see if she's still counting, they confer and decide to go over to the sliding board. They eagerly climb the stairs, stamping their feet on each step. At the top they settle down to wait for the "it" to finish counting. At first tense and poised for action, the girls soon relax and later become impatient. The "it" was taking too long. The girl without the ball on the slide soon loses interest, slides down, and walks over to the drinking fountain. Finally "it" is finished counting and runs over to the slide. As the "it" gets closer, the girl with the ball slides down while throwing the ball to her other teammate at the drinking fountain. The intended catcher misses, and the ball ricochets off the fountain and bounces away on the loose. Attentions snap to action as the three girls scramble for the ball. Pursuing it back and forth across the playground, the girls shriek with excitement and pull at each other's arms in an effort to grab the ball.

The movements of these three girls feature elements commonly seen in children sliding, running, swinging, maneuvering around the jungle gym, and playing tigers and bears. These children are completely unself-conscious while moving. They exhibit no sense of "performing" for others; there is no "presentational" focus, nor is there the formal attention to space that one might expect from an actor or a dancer. While excited, the girls seem to be mostly aware of their bodies and the physical sensations of running or dodging the ball. Their attention is largely action oriented, with the engaged physical alertness disappearing after each action (sliding, running, or catching the ball and throwing it) is completed. The personal rhythms of each child are fluid, and they respond with great spontaneity to each other and to outside attractions.

This quality and type of movement seems completely normal in the frame of the playground. Its eccentricity is highlighted, however, when the steel fence is replaced by a stage setting. Pooh Kaye's *Wildfields* incorporates much of the spontaneity, physical aliveness, idiosyncratic phrasing and fun of playground activities. Although the specific movement lexicon is more complex technically in *Wildfields,* the general performance attitude remains charmingly close to that of children. None of the dancers actively "present" themselves to the audience. They smile—even laugh outright—at one another. The movement is not danced in a way to show shapes or specific forms. Rather, it is danced with a real sense of the dancers experiencing the momentum in their own bodies. Although many of the movements are large, they are not particularly focused spatially. Their phrasings do not draw out the movements unnecessarily, and there is little attempt to smooth over the breaks of action.

All these movement and qualitative similarities between *Wildfields* and playground activity set the stage on which to see a more revealing affinity. I have already described somewhat the mess of play. Because play is usually linked in our culture to children and to a certain freedom from convention ("to move in a lively, irregular manner; to move freely," etc.), we rarely look to playground activity for any sense of structure. We are accustomed to looking for structure in dances, however, and it was by looking again and again for a structure in *Wildfields* that I began to understand certain basic dynamics in play. Like play, *Wildfields* is a mess. But also like play, it has its own kind of mesh.

One by one, three dancers enter the stage with a lazy, looping, elephant walk. Just as the group stretches across the stage in a diagonal line, another dancer walks behind a scrim and the three dancers explode into separate movements. Thrashing their limbs and hurling their bodies through space in a curiously frenetic, yet nonchalant manner, they first orbit individually and then cluster to the side. Separate movements connect in a single suspension and they all shoot to the floor, each one finding a different path downward. Two more dancers vault onto the stage, just in time to pick up the speed and energy of the others, who now rest subdued on the floor. They dance in unison for a while and then split off into two unrelated tangents. This action spawns another reaction that sends all five dancers reeling and tumbling through the space in individual explosions of wild vigor. Everyone is doing everything, every which way. And then almost magically, like a blurry picture brought into focus, this chaotic field etches itself out across the stage in a single, long diagonal line. The dancers squat and pause, crystalizing a moment of stillness and visual simplicity.

The structure of *Wildfields* is similar to the spontaneous organization of many play activities. As in the example of the three girls playing on the sand table, where a common rhythmic circle blossomed spontaneously out of individual pursuits, *Wildfields* is colored by the juxtaposition between a chaotic texture of many individual movements and distilled moments which center around one movement theme.

This carefully crafted alternation between independent activities and group cohesion in *Wildfields* seems to present a dichotomy between non-structured and structured phrases. The structured elements include moments of clear spatial design, such as when the dancers make a line or specific shape on stage. There are also periods of unison dancing, as well as clearly recognizable patterns, such as a series of canons, a dance game of follow-the-leader, or a transposed version of "London Bridge is falling down," where the bridge is made with joining feet and the dancers hop on all fours under it. The nonstructured sections are collections of arbitrary spatial designs, separate movement, and disparate rhythms. There is a problem, however, in this conventional distinction between structured and nonstructured elements in that it limits the concept of structure to the most basic and obvious coordinations of space and time.

Structure is most often defined as a static form, a skeleton, a scaffolding, or a floor plan. But it can also be approached dynamically, as a patterning of forces, or a mesh. Mesh is a good word for the type of structuring that pervades *Wildfields* and much playground activity. A mesh is something mobile and flexible, a loosely woven or knit fabric, with a more or less open texture. There are two threads in the mesh fabrics of *Wildfields* and playground activity that guide independent actions into clear moments of connectedness. These are the structuring forces of synchrony and dynamic interchange.

Synchrony is the extraordinary phenomenon where two or more beings coordinate their movements or their conversation or their lives. Nonverbal communication studies teem with examples of gestural or postural synching. To be in sync with someone does not mean to mirror the other's movements, but it does suggest a sort of unconscious coordination and reaction to another person or thing. In any group of four people conversing, it is likely that certain gestures—head nods, chin strokes, and even nose wipes—will occur simultaneously or in a sequence. Likewise, shifts in body position by one person may precipitate shifts in posture by the others. We often sync, as well, to music, sports events, and dance concerts.

E. T. Hall recounts a fascinating example of synching among children in a chapter on rhythm and body movement in his book *Beyond Culture*.[2] Commenting on a film made by one of his students in which children are seen romping in a school playground, Hall notes:

> At first, they looked like so many kids each doing his own thing. After a while, we noticed that one little girl was moving more than the rest. Careful study revealed that she covered the entire playground. Following procedures laid down for my students, this young man viewed the film over and over at different speeds. Gradually, he perceived that the whole group was moving in synchrony to a definite rhythm. The most active child, the one who moved about most, was the director, the orchestrator of the playground rhythm![3]

What is particularly interesting here is that all the kids seemed, at first, to simply be doing their own thing. As in sections of *Wildfields*, there was little visual structure. One saw children laughing, screaming, yelling, and running all through the playground. Later in this study, when the synchrony was fully documented, the film was shown to schoolteachers at the regular speed. Even though they were told that "an unconscious current of synchronized movement tied the group together," these new observers had trouble seeing or understanding this connectedness.

Synchrony, as a thread in the mesh, is a structuring force that can organize children, animals, communication, dancers, and even adults in ways we often fail to see. Take for instance the example of the three girls who were building on the sand table and suddenly jumped up and started dancing together. They seemed at first to be doing independent things. And they were. But there was probably a kind of synching in their playing that facilitated that final impulse to dance together.

There are a number of places in *Wildfields* where movement synchrony is a cohesive thread that wanders among a chaotic splattering of independent actions. Within these literal wild fields, dancers have separate steps, foci, body attitudes, and rhythms. Nonetheless, large changes of level (usually from high to low) or major variations in the dynamic range will occur simultaneously. Dramatic sparks of movement such as plopping or diving to the floor, explosive surges, suspensions, and rapid streams of flicks, dabs, and wiggles blanket the stage momentarily and then dissolve as each dancer reenters her own particular style and pathway.

The second cohesive thread in the mess of play and *Wildfields* is that of dynamic interchange. Something as simple as a child with a ball running up to a standing child, giving him or her the ball and watching while the new ball carrier runs off, is an exchange of both the ball and the running. So often in play activities, balls become symbols of action and their exchange, an exchange of dynamics. While there are no balls in *Wildfields*, the dance sometimes looks like a special soccer game, where the ball has been replaced by movement energies. One dancer has it, then passes it down the line to another, who dribbles and maybe transforms the energy, then passes it along.

Because there is usually so much going on in *Wildfields*, this dynamic interchange is not always as clear as a silent soccer game. Moments of energy-passing surface here and there, diving back down into the dance and resurfacing somewhere else, like a dolphin that is playing hide-and-seek. Playground activity has a similar flux between clear flashes of dynamic interchange and the muddle of uncoordinated passes. These threads of synchrony and dynamic interchange ignite some of the most exciting bursts of movement in play and in *Wildfields*. Not only does an awareness of these structuring forces help make clear the processes embedded in the flow of play; they also help reveal what is going on compositionally in the wild field of the dance. And while illuminating as an analytic device, they do not interfere with the fun and invention of play. Luckily, they do not clean up the mess.

NOTES

1. Johan Huizinga, *Homo Ludens: A Study of the Play Elements in Culture* (Boston: Beacon Press, 1950), 28–45.
2. Edward T. Hall, *Beyond Culture* (Garden City, NY: Anchor Press, 1976).
3. Ibid., 66.

27

Through Yours to Mine and Back Again

Reflections on Bodies in Motion

Movement Research Journal, Fall 1993.

Pre/face

My face

reflecting back from the blank sheet of paper in front of me.

How do I begin?
writing from my body to other bodies
about the place of bodies
and states of being.

It comes from my flesh, from my heart.

I THINK BECAUSE I CARE . . .

about dancing bodies and the stories they tell.

Twenty years ago, most dancers, when asked what the medium of dance is, would probably have replied "movement" or perhaps "movements of the human body." In those heady days of abstraction and anarchy, the body was recognized as a wonderful source of movement possibilities. The 1970s reification of abstract movement and the notions of choreography as formal arrangements of bodies in space and time has largely given way to a focus on the content of the body itself. Today, the dancing body is more often seen as a source of identity—a physical presence that moves with and through its cultural meanings. With a renewed emphasis on personal narrative and social issues, combined with an increasing involvement with movement trainings inspired by an awareness of Asian, African, and Afro-Caribbean performance practices and new body therapies, contemporary experimental dance focuses on the dancer's physical and emotion experience within the moment of dancing.

As a dancer and feminist scholar, I am interested in this interweaving of physical experience and cultural representation in contemporary dance. I believe that dance offers a uniquely relevant context in which to look at the interconnectedness of identities and bodies that are currently at stake in contemporary cultural politics. From issues concerning freedom of choice and antifeminist backlashes, to social diversity and the politics of multiculturalism, to regulating representations of the body through arts censorship, to managing the AIDS crisis, to the debates surrounding the acknowledged presence of homosexuals in the military, it is clear that representations of identity and experiences of the body are completely intertwined with representations of the body and experiences of identity. What fascinates me about the work I have seen over the past seven years is the way in which the dancing body can both fully embody its own cultural markers such as gender, physical ability, race, sexuality, and class (to mention only the most obvious), and, at the same time, explode these very categories by moving beyond them in performance.

It's hard to articulate what these bodies know and yet I feel compelled again and again to try.

Constantly moving through time and space, the dancing body is physically present and yet always in the midst of becoming absent. Learning how to really see that body is a complex task that requires an awareness of the kinesthetic and aural, as well as the visual and intellectual implications of dance. While we may know whether the dancer is a he or a she, Anglo or Latino, able-bodied, etc., the action or theatricality of the performance can place that knowledge in jeopardy. In performance, the dancing body can work over, play with, and exceed its own socially marked identity to disrupt those categories and disconcert the audience's reception of that bodily image. By moving through instead of locating her (him) self in such narrative positions, the dancer is thus able to slip in and out of meaning before it becomes stabilized.

Watching: first I unlock the tension in my neck, allowing my skull to rest easefully and loosely on the top vertebrae of my spine. Then I imagine all the pores of my skin opening and expanding so that the movement can enter and affect my body.

When I watch dance, I try to approach the experience with all of my intellectual, physical, and emotional capacities. That means that I bring my history as a dancer and a feminist scholar with me as well. The meaning that the dance holds for me shifts as I digest it through journal writings, physical associations, and conversations with the dancers and friends. Dances have a way of taking up residence in my body. They often start out whispering to me, but eventually their voices become clearer and clearer and then I begin to know which words will follow that motion. I never pretend to know the whole dance, and yet I never assume that I've lost the immediacy of that physical experience as I begin to articulate the cultural implications of those dances. This process of unraveling the meanings of these images, movement, bodies, and identities, can take a long time, and I frequently find myself in the position of thinking deeply about certain dances when the choreographer and dancers have long since moved onto other projects.

Writing: I begin with descriptions of the most compelling moments. If a remembered image does not take me close enough, I repeat the movement or gesture, letting my body help me to verbally articulate what was going on in the dancing.

I have spent the last twenty-five years of my life watching, writing about, and dancing with many different bodies. In addition to training in Hawkins, Cunningham, contact improvisation, and release techniques during that time, I have also spent those years thinking about the ideological functions of the body (particularly the feminized body) in American culture. This work has placed me at the center of cultural debates concerning the primacy of biological nature versus cultural conditioning as constituting the "essence" of one's identity. Ultimately, however, the specific intersections of my interests have led me to refuse the limited terms of this discussion. Clearly cultural values resonate throughout the bodies that constitute them, and often these structures are physically internalized and thus rendered as "essential" elements of human nature. Yet the body is at once social and personal, internal and external. Indeed, bodies, particularly dancing bodies, are always simultaneously registering, creating, and subverting cultural conventions. By becoming conscious of the cultural consequences of their physical techniques and dancing styles, dancers can effectively challenge oppressive cultural ideologies concerning the body.

I want to write about dancing
and I want to dance in writing
to move my body and my pen together in a virtual space that is at once real and imaginary.

What would it be like to enter my mind with my body and slide in and among my ideas?
to work out the language in a dance,
to touch bodies and words with one gesture,
one breath.

I think of my writing as tracing the dances that I have seen. They are translations into another medium. But translation is not a linear, but rather a cyclical, dynamic process. The dancing I see inspires my writing as much as my writing affects (hopefully) how people think about the dancing. Ultimately, I am trying to contribute to building respect (both financial and aesthetic) in our culture for dance and dancing bodies. Bodies, words, and motion. My life is dedicated to that ongoing dialogue.

28

Physical Mindfulness

Movement Research Journal, Spring 1998.

The first year I realized I would be dancing for the rest of my life was when I was a junior in college. I was living in Paris for the year and searching for a dance studio where dance was more than a form of body-toning exercise. Although I was not very fluent in French yet, I knew I was interested in what the French called *danse expressive*. It seemed like a pretty old-fashioned term to me at the time, but I came to realize it signified exactly what I wanted—dance that had meaning; that expressed social as well as aesthetic visions. As fate would have it, I noticed an advertisement for an atelier (I love the resonance of tradesmanship in that French term for studio) whose poster of two children rolling over one another on the floor was framed by the words: *Epanouir vos corps sans violence.* The language, the notion of spreading one's body without violence, fit perfectly with my own movement experiences with release work and contact improvisation. After searching through back alleys for over an hour, I finally found the studio in a small, concrete bulding, five floors up. A small, silver-haired woman was just finishing her practice when I entered. I spoke my desires in halting French. She turned to me and smiled and said, "Here, dance is a way of life." Those words began a relationship of movement and minds that has lasted through time and into memory.

Language is important to me, it helps me understand what I'm doing.

Names have meaning. How one names one's organization or studio is significant. By the time I finished college and an MFA in choreography, I knew I wanted to move, to make dances, to think and write about bodies in motion, and to live a life grounded in the physical and psychic work of contact improvisation. **Movement Research.** A name that intrigued me with its suggestions of an ongoing inquiry, a commitment to exploration, to work that was grounded in process. The name also held that tantalizing combination of dancing (movement) and writing (research), which, although I did not realize it at the time, would mark the exact intersection of my own work in this field. To me, Movement Research became a code for physical mindfulness.

I am a second-generation Movement Researcher. I moved to New York in 1985 and immediately began taking workshops and classes. This was back when Movement Research was housed on Varick Street in the Ethnic Folk Arts building. In 1987–88, I was the studies project coordinator for Movement Research. The artists who founded it were my teachers, dancers a generation older than me—people whose work and life decisions I followed and learned from. I was inspired by their patience with developing forms, their commitment to improvisation, their enthusiasm for working in a loosely organized, barely paid, wildly creative moment of artistic and institutional collaboration. Very few of them had children. This fact seems oddly significant, if only as a distinction between the first and second generation of dancers involved with the organization.

One of the things I've always appreciated about Movement Research was its strong self-consciousness of its role in history—a living dance history. This clarity and awareness came out of a mission—a utopian one at that—to encourage, present, document, and sustain a certain kind of dance and performance exploration that was increasingly threatened by the cultural and economic practices of the Reagan years. Striving to keep up with the realities of shrinking arts support, increasing poverty, depleted physical resources, and AIDS, Movement Research pulled together a group of activist/ artists willing to change the way they worked in order to work with more people.

Movement Research had always been dedicated to having dance artists— those people most fully defined in our culture as bodily and therefore nonverbal (a weird logic that I have spent most of my life trying to debunk)— talk about their work. Indeed, the forum of the studies project and, more recently the journal, is a perfect place to investigate the consequences of what we are doing; to use language to articulate our experience as cultural workers. One of the first studies projects I was involved in was on improvisation. I still remember what it was like to witness dancers try and articulate their process of working, and what the implications of that process were, are, can be. I also organized a panel on autobiography and dance, as well as one on writing and dancing. This was all back in my mid-twenties, before I had any idea where my own journey in dancing and writing and improvisation and autobiography would take me. **Physical mindfulness**. In many ways, Movement Research was my model for this.

Memory is a funny thing. Usually we remember an experience in light of our present realities. Sometimes I wonder, how do memories influence what histories get written, and which ones get written out? How are histories remembered in living bodies?

I no longer live in New York City. Each time I visit, however, I go back to Movement Research to study, to teach, to talk, to watch, to get a sense of where the organization is these days. I also send my students there as interns—to study and to work. This journal also helps me feel connected, and for that I am grateful.

29

Researching Bodies

The Politics and Poetics of Corporeality

Movement Research Journal, Spring 2004.

Movement Research was founded on a tension. A tension that has remained embedded in this organization for most of its twenty-five-year history. At times, this tension has been incredibly productive; but it also has been frequently ignored, like an irksome old injury one hopes will go away on its own. Thinking about what I might contribute to this issue of the journal honoring Movement Research's legacy, I decided to out the tension. Why not? Any reckoning of an arts organization's contributions at the end of a quarter-century of service to experimental dance and dancers should include airing a little dirty laundry, don't you think?

Before I continue, allow me a moment of personal reflection. I moved to New York City in the fall of 1984 with about $500 in cash. As I went looking for work and dance classes that first week, I happened upon an ad in The Village Voice for a workshop with Simone Forti, and one for an ongoing series of classes in contact improvisation. I glanced up to see what organization was hosting these classes, and there it was, at the top of the advertisement, "Movement Research, Inc." Eureka! Suddenly, I felt like I was home! Because that's exactly what I wanted to do at the ripe old age of twenty-three, Research Movement—in all its manifestations. Twenty years later, I am still involved in researching movement in ways that were fundamentally informed by my time studying under the auspices of this organization.

Nonetheless, (note the rhetorical shift—here comes the tough love part) I feel that it is important for Movement Research to come to terms with its internal contradictions, not in order to erase them, but rather as a point of departure for a dialogue about them. As a multifaceted arts organization, Movement Research sponsors workshops in experimental dance (including a wonderful focus on improvisation), presents the work of emerging artists, hosts Open Movement, and produces the studies project, as well as *Movement Research Journal.* I was thinking about Movement Research while at a conference entitled "Perceiving Gender and Performance" at Denison University. Intriguingly enough, most of the performers who were a part of the conference were Movement Research alumni: dancers such as K. J. Holmes,

Chris Aiken, David Beadle, Peter Bingham, and Angie Hauser. Even though they were performing under the auspices of this focused inquiry, most of the dancers were not really all that interested in thinking about gender in their performances. In fact, a few thought that their training in forms such as contact improvisation had neutralized any internalized gender training they may have grown up with. While the program order was consciously organized in terms of a range of gender dynamics—a male-male duet, a female-female duet, and a male-female duet—there was a significant refusal among the dancers to engage with gender as a conscious element within the improvisation. That is when I realized how much the tension between movement exploration as a product of a natural body, and dance as a form of cultural representation (and therefore necessarily a discourse about social identity and political power) lay underneath the workings of Movement Research.

Tension is an interesting concept, especially in light of the emphasis in American contemporary dance on release techniques. In the midst of our efforts to yield (into the floor, into our partners), tension gets a bad rap—somehow, it smacks of corporate ambition. And yet the word itself does not just imply hardness, or blocked energy—it can also mean a stretch, or a state of balance, something along the lines of what it takes to engage a half-moon pose in yoga. In other words, it can connote a "productive tension."

There have been moments in the history of Movement Research where experiences of the body's physicality and how those experiences operate in representation—be it visual, written, or performed—polarized the organization. One such moment was the December 1983 studies project with Bill T. Jones and Steve Paxton. Another was the brouhaha surrounding the 1991 gender performance issue of *Movement Research Journal*. Instead of sweeping those uncomfortable moments under the proverbial carpet, I think there is something to be gained by considering those lines of tension more fully.

In both these situations, the issues at stake revolved around the tension between cultural meaning and personal experience; between politics and art. For instance, the studies project was designed as an opportunity to see artists' work and hear them discuss their conceptual and physical processes. But when Steve Paxton and Bill T. Jones got together, the dialogue got a bit dicey as Bill started pressing Steve on the question of audience reception. Bill was asking Steve to shift perspectives from one of process and investigation to one of representation. At the time, Bill was highly focused on how his own body—black and gay—was read by an audience. (Remember all those early solos with texts that confronted the audience with their own racialized gaze?) Paxton, whose identity had never been at stake in his dancing (a result of both privilege and choice), resisted and things got a bit personal. A lot was learned during that afternoon, but it did heat up. In an editor's note describing her experience that afternoon in the Fall 1984 issue of *Contact*

Quarterly, Nancy Stark Smith articulated the moment of tension: "What I saw light up in the heat of that friction was each man as an individual; his unique perspective came into focus as it was forced to narrow from a more general *field* of vision to a distinct *point* of view, teased and poked and pushed into the light. And though I squirmed in the heat of that confrontation, I was at the same time struck by the commitment behind the stand."

Both Bill T. and Steve warm to resistance; they like a feisty interaction. But after their afternoon session, each went back to his own corner. This was unfortunate, because that afternoon held a challenge for Movement Research to understand its own point of view. Like whiteness, the primary focus on experimental dance within Movement Research has been unexamined ideologically. Being a liberal organization, Movement Research supports the artistic focus of individual artists on their specific identity (i.e., if you are black or queer), but that kind of work is seen as separate from much of the physical investigations done in workshops and classes.

I think a lot about this dichotomy these days, because my artistic and critical work straddles both the realms of internal investigations of movement possibilities informed by contact improvisation, release work, body-mind centering, authentic movement, as well as questions of identity and cultural representation fomented by studies in feminist and queer theory. Each area carries a certain truth for me, and I like the tension between them. Interestingly enough, my willingness to submit to that pull in both directions at once, comes directly from my improvisational training and practice that was formed and informed by Movement Research. Yet, I believe the potency of improvisational practices today lies less in the opening up of more movement options, but rather in understanding how to encourage a willingness to cross over into uncomfortable territories—to move in the face of what is unknown. Improvisation can lead us out of our habitual responses by opening up alternative experiences, encouraging dancers to explore new possibilities and desires—not only physically, but critically too. Why not let our improvisational practice, as well as the physicalities that experimental dance cultivates, lead us into an engagement with the world instead of away from it? On the eve of its silver anniversary, I challenge Movement Research to start teaching attention to the political, as well as the personal, meanings that bodies carry. Only then will Movement Research really be able to realize their mission in the twenty-first century.

30

Strategic Abilities

Negotiating the Disabled Body in Dance

Michigan Quarterly Review 1, no. 3, Summer 1998.

The dance's opening image of a naked back in a backless wheelchair haunted me long before I ever choreographed the piece. Indeed, it was the power of this image—its visual and physical effect on me—that gave me the courage both to create a performance about the undoing of my life as I knew it and to stage it in the middle of a dance concert. Through this process of performing the unperformable, of telling the untold story, of staging the antithesis of my identity as a dance professional, I began to reclaim the expressive power of my body.

What do you see? A back? A backless wheelchair? A woman? A nude? Do you see pain or pleasure? Are you in pain or pleasure? How do you see me?

Most likely you do not see a dancer, for the combined discourses of idealized femininity and aesthetic virtuosity which serve to regulate theatrical dancing throughout much of the Western world refuse the very possibility of this opening moment. As a dancer, I am a body on display. As a body on display, I am expected to reside within a certain continuum of fitness and bodily control, not to mention sexuality and beauty. But as a woman in a wheelchair, I am neither expected to be a dancer nor to position myself in front of an audience's gaze. In doing this performance, I confronted a whole host of contradictions both within myself and within the audience. The work was a conscious attempt to both deconstruct the representational codes of dance production and communicate an "other" bodily reality. It was also one of the hardest pieces I have ever performed.

I take my place in total darkness, carefully situating myself in the back-less wheelchair set center stage. Gradually, a square frame of light comes up around me to reveal the glint of metal and the softness of my naked flesh. I am still for a long time, allowing the audience time to absorb this image, and giving myself time to experience the physical and emotional vulnerability that is central to this performance. I focus on my breathing, allowing it to expand through my back. Soon, I can feel the audience beginning to notice the small motions of the constant expansion and contraction of my breathing. This moment is interrupted by a recorded voice that tells the mythic story of another woman many centuries ago, whose parents carved the names of their enemies into her back. The first image fades into blackness as my voice continues:

> Two years ago, when I was severely, albeit temporarily, disabled, this scene from Maxine Hong Kingston's *The Woman Warrior* kept reappearing in my dreams. I see now that disability is like those knives that cut and marked her skin. Sometimes it leaves physical scars, but mostly it marks one's psyche, preying upon one's sense of wellbeing with a deep recognition of the frailty of life.

What followed when the lights came up again was a performance about disability—both the cultural constructions of disability and the textures of my own experiences with disability. The spoken text was structured around stories—stories about my son's frantic first days of life in intensive care, about my grandfather's life with multiple sclerosis and the recent diagnosis of MS in one of my students, as well as the story of my own spinal degeneration and episodes of partial paralysis. These bodily histories interlaced with my dancing to provide a genealogy of gestures, emotional states, and physical experiences surrounding many of our personal and social reactions to disability. I introduce my experience in creating and performing this autobiographical work as a point of departure for my discussion of the intriguing intersection of physicality and ideology when disability meets dance. By comparing the representation of disability in three integrated dance groups, Cleveland Ballet Dancing Wheels, CandoCo, and the duets of Alito Alessi and Emery Blackwell, I argue that we must look past the mere presentation of disabled bodies onstage and engage in a thorough analysis of the cultural implications of different aesthetic frames within dance.

Because my performance was staged on a body at once marked by the physical and psychic scars of disability and yet unmarked by any specifically visible physical limitation, I was consciously challenging the usual representational codes of theatrical dance. Indeed, I wanted the audience to be put off-balance, not knowing whether this was an enactment of disability or the real thing. Was this artistic expression or autobiographical confession? Did I choose not to do more technical dancing (artistic interpretation), or was this all that I could accomplish (aesthetic limitation)? And why would I, a dance professor, want to expose myself (including my ample buttocks and disfigured spine) like that anyway? Given that Western theatrical dance has traditionally been structured by an exclusionary mindset that projects a very narrow vision of a dancer as white, female, thin, long-limbed, flexible, heterosexual, and able-bodied, my desire to stage the cultural antithesis of the fit, healthy body disrupted the conventional voyeuristic pleasures inherent in watching most dancers. Traditionally, when dancers take their place in front of the spotlight, they are displayed in ways that accentuate the double role of technical prowess and sexual desireability (the latter being implicit in the very fact of a body's visual availability). In contrast, the disabled body is supposed to be covered up or hidden from view—to be compensated for or overcome in an attempt to live as normal a life as possible. When a disabled dancer takes the stage, he or she stakes claim to a radical space—an unruly location where disparate assumptions about representation, subjectivity, and visual pleasure collide with one another.

I originally performed this piece at the Spring Back Dance Concert at Oberlin College (April 10–12, 1997). On that occasion, it was placed between more conventional dances that displayed the grace of line, technical virtuosity, and the beauty of the female body. Within this context, my piece was disorienting for the audience as well as myself. Yet it also proved to be a catalyst for many people who saw the work, including a woman with MS whose daughter (a young dancer in the department) refused, at first, to talk about her mother's condition. My performance helped them begin a conversation about their bodies and loss, and love. Throughout the weeks following my performances, I found out about a myriad of small ways in which this piece had helped various people come to terms with their own bodies. Although I certainly believe that performances can change lives, that is not why I did this work. I did it to change my life. For even though I had successfully rehabilitated my body from two spinal injuries, regaining much of my strength, if not all of my range of motion, I found myself resisting dancing before an audience. I even resisted publically identifying myself as a dancer rather than simply a dance scholar. Even though intellectually I had deconstructed societal conventions of feminine beauty and able-bodiness, I was not truly at ease with my own changed corporeality. Creating a piece that so directly brought attention to the body I have instead of the body I am supposed to have, helped me recognize the performative power of my own flesh.

This is an essay about dance and disability. It is an essay which, on the one hand, will detail how American culture constructs these realms of experience oppositionally in terms of either fit or frail, beautiful or ugly, and, on the other hand, will discuss the growing desire among various dance communities and professional companies to challenge this binary paradigm by reenvisioning just what kind of movements can constitute a dance and, by extension, what kind of body can constitute a dancer. It is an essay about a cultural movement (in both the political and physical senses of the word) that radically revises the aesthetic structures of dance performances and just as radically extends the theoretical space of disability studies into the realm of live performing bodies. This intersection of dance and disability is an extraordinarily rich site at which to explore the overlapping constructions of the body's physical ability, subjectivity, and cultural visibility that are implicated within many of our dominant cultural paradigms of health and self-determination. Excavating the social meanings of these constructions is like an archeological dig into the deep psychic fears that disability creates within the field of professional dance. In order to examine ableist preconceptions in the dance world, one must confront both the ideological and symbolic meanings that the disabled body holds in our culture, as well as the practical conditions of disability. Watching disabled bodies dancing forces us to see with a double vision, and helps us to recognize that while a dance performance is grounded in the physical capacities of a dancer, it is not limited by them.

Over the last twenty years, I have followed the evolution of various dance groups that are working to integrate visibly disabled and visibly nondisabled dancers. I use the term "visibly" to shift the currency of the term disability from an either/or paradigm to a continuum which might include not only the most easily identifiable disabilities such as some mobility impairments, but also less visible disabilities, including ones such as eating disorders, and histories of severe abuse. It seems to me that all of these disabilities profoundly affect one's physical position in the world, although they certainly don't all affect the accessibility of the world in the same way. Each year, the list grows longer as groups such as Mobility Junction (NYC), DanceAbility (Eugene), Diverse Dance (Vachon Island), Cleveland Ballet Dancing Wheels (Cleveland), Light Motion (Seattle), and Candoco (England) inspire other dance communities to engage with this work. In addition, there are several dance companies such as Liz Lerman's Dancers of the Third Age, which works with older performers, as well as various contemporary choreographers who consistently work with nontraditional performers from diverse backgrounds and experiences. These include dance artists Johanna Boyce, Ann Carlson, David Dorfman, and Jennifer Monson, to mention only a few. Unfortunately, the radical work of these groups is often tokenized in the dance press in terms of "special" human-interest profiles rather than choreographic rigor. Of course this critical marginalization implicitly suggests that this new work, while important, will not really disrupt the existing aesthetic structures of cultural institutions. For instance, when Dancing Wheels, a group dedicated to promoting "the diversity of dance and the abilities of artists with physical challenges," joined up with the Cleveland Ballet in 1990 (to become Cleveland Ballet Dancing Wheels), it was as an educational and outreach extension of the mainstream arts organization. The Dancing Wheels dancers rarely perform in the company's regular repertoire, and certainly never in classical works such as Balanchine's *Serenade*. Even in the less mainstream examples of integrated dancing, the financial reality of grassroots arts organizations often means that nondisabled dancers receive much more touring and teaching work than even the most highly reknowned disabled dancers. It is still prohibitively expensive to travel as a disabled person, especially if one needs to bring an aide along.

Issues of disability eventually affect everybody's life. Yet even though many of us are familiar with the work of disabled writers, artists, and musicians, physically disabled dancers are still seen as a contradiction in terms. This is because dance, unlike other forms of cultural production such as books or painting, makes the body visible within the representation itself. Thus when we look at dance with disabled dancers, we are looking at both the choreography and the disability. Cracking the porcelain image of the dancer as graceful sylph, disabled dancers force the viewer to confront the cultural opposite of the classical body—the grotesque body. I am using the term "grotesque" as Bakhtin invokes it in his analysis of representation within Rabelais. In her discussion of carnival, spectacle, and Bakhtinian theory, Mary Russo identifies these two bodily tropes in the following manner:

> The grotesque body is the open, protruding, extended, secreting body, the body of becoming, process, and change. The grotesque body is opposed to the classical body, which is monumental, static, closed and sleek, corresponding to the aspirations of bourgeois individualism; the grotesque body is connected to the rest of the world.[1]

I realize, of course, that by using the term "grotesque" within a discussion of disability and dance, I risk invoking old stereotypes of disabled bodies as grotesque bodies. Clearly, this is not my intention. I employ these terms not to describe specific bodies, but rather to call upon cultural constructs that deeply influence our attitudes towards bodies, particularly dancing bodies. Over the past few years, I have felt this opposition of classical and grotesque bodies profoundly as I have fought my way back to the stage. Look again at the opening image of my performance and then at any other image of a dancer in *Dancemagazine,* or another popular dance magazine. The difference is striking, and I believe that it has much to do with the cultural separation between these bodies.[2]

In the rest of this essay, I would like to explore the transgressive nature of the "grotesque" body in order to see if and how the disabled body could deconstruct and radically reform the representational structures of dance performances. But, just as all disabilities are not created equal, dances made with disabled dancers are not completely alike. Many of these dances recreate the representational frames of traditional proscenium performances, emphasizing the elements of virtuosity and technical expertise to reaffirm a classical body in spite of its limitations. In contrast, some dances, particularly those influenced by the dance practice of contact improvisation, work to break down the very distinctions between the classical and the grotesque body, radically restructuring traditional ways of seeing dancers. While all dance created on disabled bodies must negotiate the palpable contradictions between the discourses of ideal bodies and those of deviant ones, each piece meets this challenge in a different way.

> At the start of *Gypsy*, tall and elegant Todd Goodman enters pulling the ends of a long scarf wrapped around the shoulders of his partner, Mary Verdi-Fletcher, gliding behind him. To the Gypsy Kings, he winds her in and out with the scarf. Her bare shoulders tingle with the ecstasy of performing. She flings back her head with trusting abandon as he dips her deeply backward. Holding the fabric she glides like a skater, alternately releasing and regaining control. At the climax he swoops her up in her chair and whirls her around. Did I mention that Verdi-Fletcher dances in her wheelchair?[3]

Gus Solomons's account of a romantic duet describes one of the first choreographic ventures of Cleveland Ballet Dancing Wheels—a professional dance company comprised of dancers on legs and dancers in wheelchairs. Essentially a pas de deux for legs and wheels, *Gypsy* extends the aesthetic heritage of nineteenth-century Romantic ballet into several intriguing new directions. Like a traditional balletic duet, *Gypsy* is built on an illusion of grace provided by the fluid movements and physics of partnering. The use of the fabric in conjunction with the wheels gives the movement a continuous quality that is difficult to achieve on legs. When Solomons describes Verdi-Fletcher's dancing as "gliding," he is describing more than a metaphor; rather, he is transcribing the physical reality of her movement. Whether they are physically touching or connected by their silken umbilical cord, the dancers in this pas de deux partner one another with a combination of the delicacy of ballet and the mystery of tango.

Solomons is an African-American dance critic and independent choreographer who has been involved in the contemporary dance scene since his days dancing for Merce Cunningham in the 1970s. An active member of the Dance Critics Association, he has spoken eloquently about the need to include diverse communities within our definitions of mainstream dance. And yet Solomons, like many other liberal cultural critics and arts reviewers, sets up in the earlier-mentioned passage a peculiar rhetoric that tries to deny difference. His remark, "Did I mention that Verdi-Fletcher dances in her wheelchair?" suggests that the presence of a dancer in a wheelchair is merely an incidental detail that hardly interrupts the seamless flow of the romantic pas de deux. In assuming that disability does not make a (big) difference, this writer is, in fact, limiting the (real) difference that disability can make in radically refiguring how we look at, conceive of, and organize bodies in the twenty-first century. Why, for instance, does Solomons begin with a description of Goodman's able body as "tall and elegant," and then fail to describe Verdi-Fletcher's body at all? Why do most articles on Verdi-Fletcher's seminal dance company spend so much time celebrating how she has "overcome" her disability to "become" a dancer rather than inquiring how her bodily presence might radically refigure the very category of dancer itself?

The answers to these questions lie not only in an examination of the critical reception of *Gypsy* and other choreographic ventures by Cleveland Ballet Dancing Wheels, but also in an analysis of the ways in which this company paradoxically acknowledges and then covers over the difference that disability makes. There are contradictions embedded within this company's differing aesthetic and social priorities. While their outreach work has laid an important groundwork for the structural inclusion of people with disabilities in dance training programs and performance venues, the conservative aesthetic that guides much of Cleveland Ballet Dancing Wheels' performance work paradoxically reinforces, rather than disrupts, the negative connotations of disability.

Dancing Wheels began as a joint adventure between Mary Verdi-Fletcher, who was born with spina bifida and now uses a wheelchair, and David Brewster, the husband of a friend who enjoyed social dancing as much as Mary did. In those heady days of disco fever, they mostly competed in various social dance competitions. Soon, however, the notion of a dance company of dancers with and without disabilities crystalized. In 1980, Verdi-Fletcher founded Dancing Wheels and began concentrating on outreach and audience development, doing lecture-demonstrations at community centers and performances in schools and nursing homes. Although they have now merged with the Cleveland Ballet, the company still produces work independently, collaborating with a number of ballet and modern choreographers to perform their works in various theatrical venues across the country.

The genesis of the company is described by Cleveland Ballet's artistic director Dennis Nahat, who recalls meeting Verdi-Fletcher at a reception when Verdi-Fletcher introduced herself as a dancer and told him that she was interested in dancing with the Cleveland Ballet. In the annotated biography of Verdi-Fletcher's dance career, which was commissioned for Dancing Wheels' fifteenth anniversary gala, Nahat is quoted as saying: "When I first saw Mary perform, I said 'That is a dancer,' . . . There was no mistake about it. She had the spark, the spirit that makes a dancer."[4] I am interested in pursuing this notion of "spirit" a bit, especially as it is used frequently within the company's own press literature. For instance, in the elaborate press packet assembled for a media event to celebrate the collaboration with Invacare Corporation's "Action Technology" (a line of wheelchairs that are designed for extra ease and mobility), there is a picture of the company with the caption "A Victory of Spirit over Body" underneath.

I find this notion of a dancing "spirit" that transcends the limitations of a disabled body rather troubling. Although it seems, at first, to signal liberatory language—one should not be "confined" by social definitions of identity based on bodily attributes (of race, gender, ability, etc.)—this rhetoric is actually based on ablelist notions of overcoming physical handicaps (the "supercrip" theory) in order to become a "real" dancer, one whose "spirit" does not let the limitations of her body get in the way. Given that dancers' bodies are generally on display in a performance, this commitment to "spirit over body" risks covering over or erasing disabled bodies altogether. Just how do we represent spirit? Smiling faces, joyful lifts into the air? The publicity photograph of the company on the same page gives us one example of the visual downplaying of disabled bodies. In this studio shot, the three dancers in wheelchairs are artistically surrounded by the able-bodied dancers such that we can barely see the wheelchairs at all; in fact, Verdi-Fletcher is raised up and closely flanked by four men such that she looks as if she is standing in the third row. But what is most striking about this publicity shot is the way in which the ballerina sitting on the right has her long, slender, legs extended across the bottom of the picture. The effect, oddly enough, is to fetishize these working legs while at the same time making the "other" mobility—the wheels—invisible. I am not suggesting that this photo was deliberately set up to minimize the visual representation of disability. But this example shows us that unless we consciously construct new images and ways of imaging the disabled body, we will inevitably end up reproducing an ablelist aesthetic. Although the text jubilantly claims its identity, "Greetings from Cleveland Ballet Dancing Wheels," the picture normalizes the "difference" in bodies, reassuring prospective presenters and the press that they will not see anything too discomfiting.

In August 1995, Cleveland Ballet Dancing Wheels presented a gala benefit performance at the Cleveland Playhouse's State Theater. The program opened with a reconstruction of a dance choreographed by May O'Donnell in 1959. Originally a member of the Martha Graham dance company, O'Donnell has developed a choreographic style more reminiscent of Doris Humphrey's. In its use of space, fall and recovery, and breath rhythms, *Dance Energies* evoked Humphrey's great modern epic, *New Dance*. The connection between May O'Donnell's work, with its signature early modern dance's expressive, communal style of movement is Sabatino Verlezza, the new co-artistic director of Dancing Wheels and resident choreographer, who was a dancer with O'Donnell for many years. Verlezza's background in modern dance brings a welcome shift of physical vocabulary to Dancing Wheels. Unlike ballet, modern dance was created by working-class, female bodies, and its early democratic spirit was based in a belief that one should create movements specific to one's own body. Ideally, then, this form would seem to lend itself to working with and without wheels.

While he still often choreographs within his group pieces a central theme for dancers with legs, leaving the dancers on wheels to provide an architectural backdrop (a process which works against the democratic principles of the company's stated claims), Verlezza has begun to experiment with creating movements specifically for the wheelchair dancers. Whereas most of Dancing Wheels' previous choreography involved dancers on legs leading or swinging dancers on wheels around the stage, in the present repertory there is, at least, some effort to explore momentum and other movement possibilities unique to the wheelchairs. The premiere of 1420 MHZ on August 19, 1995, presented one of the most physically challenging works, and provided a very good opportunity to see what extraordinary moves were possible on wheels. The fact that the piece was made for three women on wheels allowed the audience to experience a truly enabling representation of difference without the physical comparisons inevitable when women on wheels dance with men on legs.

Another piece by Verlezza entitled *May Ring* completed the evening's program. I was absolutely stunned by the final image of this dance, and I find it hard to believe that neither Verdi-Fletcher nor Verlezza were aware of how this image might read to some of their audience members. *May Ring* ends with a long fade as Verlezza lifts Verdi-Fletcher, arms spread wide and face beaming, out of her wheelchair, and high above his head. This is clearly meant to be a climactically transcendent moment. Yet its unavoidably sexist and ableist implications—reinforced by the fact that Verlezza dances on legs and Verdi-Fletcher dances on wheels—deeply disappointed me. Like Disney narratives and pop songs of my youth that promised salvation through love, this image portrays Verlezza as a Prince Charming, squiring Verdi-Fletcher out of her wheelchair in order to make her into a "real" woman. Now, it is possible to argue that this image is, in fact, a deconstruction of the ballerina's role, a way of winking to the audience to say that yes, a disabled woman can also fulfill that popular image. But the rest of the work does not support this interpretation. Verdi-Fletcher's smiling, childlike presence suggests little personal agency, much less the sense of defiance or chutzpah it would take to pull off this deconstruction.

In a short but potent essay reflecting on the interconnected issues of difference, disability, and identity politics entitled "The Other Body," Ynestra King describes a disabled woman in a wheelchair whom she sees on her way to work each day. "She can barely move. She has a pretty face, and tiny legs she could not possibly walk on. Yet she wears black lace stockings and spike high heels . . . That she could 'flaunt' her sexual being violates the code of acceptable appearance for a disabled woman."[5] What appeals to King about this woman's sartorial display is the way that she at once refuses her cultural position as an asexual being and deconstructs the icons of feminine sexuality (who can really walk in those spike heels anyway?). Watching Verdi-Fletcher in the final moments of *May Ring* brings us face-to-face with the contradictions involved in being positioned as both a classical dancer (at once sexualized and objectified), and a disabled woman (an asexual child who needs help). Yet instead of one position bringing tension to or fracturing the other (as in King's example of the disabled woman with high heels and black lace stockings), Verdi-Fletcher seems here to be embracing a position that is doubly disempowering.

Since this performance, I have been searching for the reasons why, in the midst of an enormous publicity campaign that seeks to present Mary Verdi-Fletcher as an extraordinary woman who has overcome the challenges of spina bifida to realize her dream of becoming a professional dancer, she would accept being presented in such a fashion. In retrospect, I think that this desire has everything to do with the powerfully seductive image of the romantic ballerina. It seems to me that when Verdi-Fletcher closes her eyes and dreams about becoming a dancer, she still envisions a sugarplum fairy. Although she has successfully opened up the field of professional dance to dancers on wheels by creating Dancing Wheels, Verdi-Fletcher has not fully challenged this image of the sylph yet. Despite its recent forays into modern dance, her company still seems very much attached to an ideology of the classical body.

Mary Verdi-Fletcher is a dancer, and like many other dancers, both disabled and nondisabled, she has internalized an aesthetic of beauty, grace, and line which, if not centered on a completely mobile body, is nonetheless beholden to an idealized body image. There are very few professions where the struggle to maintain a "perfect" (or at least near perfect) body has taken up as much psychic and physical energy as in the dance field. With few exceptions, this is true whether one's preferred technique is classical ballet, American modern dance, bharata natyam, or a form of African-American dance. Although the styles and looks of bodies favored by different dance cultures may allow for some degree of variation (for instance, the director of Urban Bush Women Jawole Willa Jo Zollar talks about the freedom to have and move one's butt in African dance as wonderfully liberating after years of being told to tuck it in modern dance classes), most professional dance is still inundated by body image and weight issues, particularly for women. Even companies, such as the Bill T. Jones and Arnie Zane Dance Company, who pride themselves on the physical diversity of their dancers, rarely have much variation among the women dancers (all of whom are quite slim). If a dancer's body is not completely svelte, the press usually mentions it. In fact, the discourse of weight and dieting in dance is so pervasive (especially, but certainly not exclusively for women) that we often do not even register it anymore. I am constantly amazed at dancers who have consciously deconstructed traditional images of female dancers in their choreographic work, and yet still complain of their extra weight, wrinkles, gray hair, or sagging whatevers. As a body on display, the female dancer is subject to the regulating gazes of the choreographer and the public, but neither of these gazes is usually quite as debilitating or oppressive as the gaze that meets its own image in the mirror.

I find it ironic that just as disability is finally beginning to enter the public consciousness and the independent living movement is beginning to gain momentum, American culture is emphasizing with a passion heretofore unfathomed the need for physical and bodily control.[6] As King makes clear in her essay this fetishization of control marks the disabled body as the antithesis of the ideal body:

> It is no longer enough to be thin; one must have ubiquitous muscle definition, nothing loose, flabby, or ill defined, no fuzzy boundaries. And of course, there's the importance of control. Control over aging, bodily processes, weight, fertility, muscle tone, skin quality, and movement. Disabled women, regardless of how thin, are without full bodily control.[7]

This issue of control is, I am convinced, key to understanding not only the specific issues of prejudice against the disabled, but also the larger symbolic place that disability holds in our culture's psychic imagination. In dance, the contrast between the classical and grotesque bodies is often framed in terms of physical control and technical virtuosity. Although the dancing body is moving and, in this sense, is always changing and in flux, the choreography or movement style can emphasize images resonant of the classical body. For instance, the statuesque poses of ballet are clear icons of the classical body. So too, however, are the dancers in some modern and contemporary companies which privilege an abstract body, for example those coolly elegant bodies performing with the Merce Cunningham Dance Company. Based as it is in the live body, dance contains the cultural anxiety that the grotesque body will erupt (unexpectedly) through the image of the classical body, shattering the illusion of ease and grace by the disruptive presence of fleshy experience—heavy breathing, sweat, technical mistakes, physical injury, even evidence of a dancer's age or mortality.

How the disabled body gets positioned in terms of a classical discourse of technique and virtuosity is not unaffected by gender. Gender is inscribed very differently on a disabled body, and there has been a great deal written on the way that disability can emasculate men (whose gendered identities are often contingent on displays of autonomy, independence, and strength), as well as desexualize women. Yet the social power that we accord representations of male bodies seems to give disabled men dancers (with a few exceptions) more freedom to display their bodies in dance. My own observations and research suggest that disabled men dancers can evoke the virtuosic, technically amazing body (even, as we shall see, without legs), while nevertheless deconstructing that classical body, allowing the audience to see their bodies in a different light. In the section that follows, I look at various dance groups (including Candoco and groups working with contact improvisation) whose work has, in different ways, revolutionized notions of ability in contemporary dance. While Candoco has established new images of physical virtuosity and technical excellence—exploding assumptions that virtuosic dancing requires four working limbs, it is within the integrated work based in contact improvisation that we see dancing which actually redefines the dancers' bodies, refusing the classical/grotesque binary and opening up the possibility of looking at the dancing body as a body in process, a body becoming. This attention to the ever-changing flux of bodies and the open-endedness of the improvisation refocuses the audience's gaze, helping us to see the disabled body on its own terms.

Candoco is a professional British dance company that evolved from conversations between Celeste Dandeker, a former dancer with the London Contemporary Dance Theater, who was paralyzed as a result of a spinal injury incurred while performing, and Adam Benjamin, a dancer who was then teaching at the Heaffey Centre in London, a mixed abilities recreation center connected to the Association for Spinal Injury Research, Rehabilitation, and Reintegration (ASPIRE). In 1991, these two dancers began a small dance class for disabled and nondisabled dancers. Since then, Benjamin and Dandeker have established a professional company that includes eight dancers and an extensive repertoire of works by some of the most interesting experimental choreographers in England today. Candoco has received various awards in recognition for its work, and the company was selected for BBC's Dance for Camera series. Introducing the company's philosophy to the press and the general public, artistic director Adam Benjamin has chosen to redefine the term "integration." In his manifesto of sorts about the company's history and goals, "In search of integrity," Benjamin writes:

> Time and again ones sees the use, or misuse of this word "integration" to describe a group or activity that has opened itself up to include people with disabilities. To integrate a group of people in this way of course implies a norm into which they need to be fitted. If however, you're using that word, integrate, from the Latin *integratus,* it forces you to acknowledge that they are already an integral part of the whole, even if you haven't found them a place yet.[8]

Although Benjamin's philosophy is quite radical in many ways and although Candoco has commissioned some very intriguing choreography, which does not just "accommodate" the disabled dancers, but recasts cultural perceptions about an "able" physicality, Benjamin is still committed to classical elements of technical virtuosity. For Benjamin, true integration means insisting on high standards of professional excellence in order to create interesting choreographic works for *all* the dancers in the company. He criticizes companies,

> in which highly trained dancers "dance circles round" those with disabilities who share the stage but little else, in which there has been no real attempt on

the part of the choreographer to enable the performer to communicate . . .
Worse still are dances in which trained, able-bodied dancers drift inconsequen-
tially, as if embarrassed by their own skills, used instead to merely ferry about
the bemused occupants of wheelchairs.[9]

Recognizing the need to create their own style of dancing that will accommodate different physical possibilities, the dancers in Candoco are constantly trying out new ways of using momentum, working in a variety of
levels including the floor, and coordinating legs and wheels. In a review of
the fall 1992 London season, Chris de Marigny registers his own astonishment at Candoco's work.

> Indeed *all* the dancers perform with amazing skill. This is rendered possible by
> the extraordinary choreographic solutions which have been invented to allow
> these people with very different disabilities to create the most startling and
> beautiful images. New concepts of falling, leaning, and supporting have been
> created to make both lyrical and at other times energetic work.[10]

The press discussions of Candoco's first few seasons repeatedly emphasize the extent to which this company has stretched people's notions of what
is possible in mixed ability dance companies. Yet because they rely on one
very exceptional disabled dancer to break down the public's preconceptions
about disability, Candoco sometimes re-creates (unwittingly) new distinctions between the classical (virtuosic) and grotesque (passive) bodies within
the company.

Victoria Marks was one of the first choreographers to work with Candoco (she was a member of their first class at the Heaffey Center, creating
The Edge of the Forest for them in 1991), and it is her choreography that
is showcased in Margaret Williams's dance film for the BBC, *Outside In*.
A lyrical film that interweaves surreal pastoral landscapes with the urbane
suspended rhythms of tango and the beat of world music, *Outside In* begins
with an extended kiss, which is passed from one company member to another. The camera lingers on each face, registering everyone's delight in receiving the kiss and allowing the viewer to see how each kiss is transformed
en route to the next person. A jump cut transports the action to a cavernous
space in which a single empty wheelchair rolls into the camera's focus. The
company then quickly assembles and reassembles, each time leaving a maze
of white patterns on the floor, as if they had just stepped in chalk. This is the
first time that the viewer sees the dancers' full bodies and individual styles
of locomotion. One of the most striking is David Toole's ability to career
across the space with his arms. Toole is one of three disabled dancers, but
he is the only one who moves easily in and out of his wheelchair. Toole has
no legs. Instead, he relies on his strong arms to walk. Ironically, the fact that

Toole has no lower body gives him an incredible freedom of movement. His presence is wonderfully quixotic, and he can practically bounce from his chair to the floor and back up again within the blink of an eye.

Toole's abilities as a dancer are remarkable—and amply remarked upon. Indeed, Toole's dancing is often the subject of extended discussions within reviews and preview articles about Candoco. Adjectives such as amazing, incredible, stupefying, are liberally sprinkled throughout descriptions of his dancing. For instance, in an article in *Ballet International* that reviews the performances of several British dance companies during the spring 1993 season, Toole's dancing is the central focus of the short section on Candoco: "David Toole is a man with no legs who possesses more grace and presence than most dancers can even dream of . . . Toole commands the stage with an athleticism that borders on the miraculous."[11] This language of astonishment reflects both an evangelistic awakening (yes, a disabled man can swagger!) and traces of freak-show voyeurism (see the amazing feats of the man with no legs!). David Toole's virtuosic dancing comes at a price—a physical price. Recently, on the advice of his doctors, Toole had to quit dancing. His extraordinary mobility is predicated on his ability to support and carry his entire body weight on his arms, allowing him to walk, run, or even skip across the stage. These astonishing feats, however, are actually destroying his arms and shoulders. Because of his status as a virtuosic dancer, however, Toole cannot seem to envision the possibility of continuing to perform in a way that would not hurt his body (such as in a wheelchair, or with fewer athletic feats).[12]

Although the medium of film is notorious for its voyeuristic gaze and spectacle-making tendencies, and although Toole is one of the most visible dancers in *Outside In,* the combination of skillful cinematography and inventive choreography in this film actually directs our gaze away from the extraordinary sight of Toole's body to the interactive contexts of his dancing. Even when he is moving by himself, Toole is always in dialogue with another person's movements. For instance, in the second scene, after the group has left the space, one woman remains, stepping among the circular patterns created by the wheelchairs. We see her choosing an interesting pattern and improvising with it—a skip step here, a shimmy there. That she is translating the pattern of the wheels onto her body only becomes fully clear when the camera jumps to Toole, who is approaching a similar task—that of translating cheeky Arthur Murray footprints onto his own body. At first he seems to hesitate, running his fingers across the black outlines of a shoeprint. But then he looks directly at the camera and, squaring his shoulders with a determined look, he launches into a dashing rendition of the tango. This solo leads, after a brief tango sequence with the full company, into an extended duet with Sue Smith. The usual negotiation of desire in a tango is replaced here by the respectful negotiation of level changes. From the moment that

Smith climbs aboard Toole's chair, to the last shot of them rolling away, the choreography refuses the implicit ideology of standing upright by placing most of the movement on the ground. The cinematography follows suit, filming them both at eye (that is to say ground) level. The camera's ability to shift viewpoints so seamlessly provides one of the most ingenious ways of breaking up (by breaking down) an ablelist gaze—the one that is forever overlooking people who are not standing (up) in front of its nose.

While the mobility of the camera itself allows for wonderful new ways of viewing dancers, the medium of film itself tends to reinforce images of the classical body by making the dancers always look pristine and unmussed. In *Outside In* we lose the experiential impact of breathing, the sound of thuds and falls, the sweat and physical evidence (hair out of place, costumes messed up, etc.) of this very kinesthetic dancing. This is particularly true for the women dancers, who all look exceedingly put together (perfect make-up and hair, etc.) throughout the video. Then too, given the innovative choreography of the earlier section, I was surprised by the almost generic wheelchair choreography in the next part, in which we see the able-bodied dancers assist, roll, and tilt the chairs, while Jonathan French and Celeste Dandeker perform a series of decorative arm movements in them. The marked difference between Toole's dancing and that of Dandeker and French struck me as reinforcing a notion that being in a wheelchair is physically less interesting than being outside one. Ironically enough, even though one is a man and the other is a woman, both of these dancers are defined within the exegesis of the film as much more passive and feminized than Toole. While *Outside In* liberates our notions of physical difference by giving us the opportunity to see different bodies in action, it has not sufficiently fractured the iconographic codes in which the wheelchair signifies disability.

Although companies such as Candoco are producing work that stretches the categories of dance and dancing bodies, I feel that much of their work is still informed by an ethos that reinstates classical conceptions of grace, speed, agility, and control within the disabled body. Even though it is true that groups like Candoco and Dancing Wheels that integrate disabled and nondisabled dancers have surely broadened the cultural imagination about who can become a dancer, they have not, to my mind, fully deconstructed the privileging of a certain kind of ability within dance. That more radical cultural work is currently taking place within the contact improvisation community.

Giving a coherent description of contact improvisation is a tricky business, for the form has grown exponentially over time and has traveled through many countries and dance communities. Contact improvisation at once embraces the casual, individualistic, improvisatory ethos of social dancing in addition to the experimentation with pedestrian and task-like movement favored by early postmodern dance groups such as the Judson

Church Dance Theater. Resisting both the idealized body of ballet as well as the dramatically expressive body of modern dance, contact improvisation seeks to create what Cynthia Novack calls a "responsive" body—one based in the physical exchange of weight.[13] Unlike many genres of dance, which stress the need to control one's movement (with admonitions to pull up, tighten, and place the body), the physical training of contact improvisation emphasizes the release of the body's weight into the floor or into a partner's body. In contact improvisation, the experience of internal sensations and flow of the movement between two bodies is more important than specific shapes or formal positions. Dancers learn to move with a consciousness of the physical communication implicit within the dancing. Curt Siddall, an early exponent of contact improvisation, describes the form as a combination of kinesthetic forces: "Contact Improvisation is a movement form, improvisational in nature, involving the two bodies in contact. Impulses, weight, and momentum are communicated through a point of physical contact that continually rolls across and around the bodies of the dancers."[14]

But human bodies, especially bodies in physical contact with one another, are difficult to see only in terms of physical counterbalance, weight, and momentum. By interpreting the body as both literal (the physics of weight) and metaphoric (evoking the community body, for example), contact improvisation exposes the interconnectedness of social, physical and aesthetic concerns. Indeed, an important part of contact improvisation today is a willingness to allow the physical metaphors and narratives of love, power, and competition to evolve from an original emphasis on the workings of a physical interaction. On first seeing contact improvisation, people often wonder whether this is, in fact, professional dancing, or rather a recreational or therapeutic form. Gone are the formal lines of much classical dance. Gone are the traditional approaches to choreography and the conventions of the proscenium stage. In their place is an improvisational movement form based on the expressive communication involved when two people begin to share their weight and physical support. Instead of privileging an ideal type of body or movement style, contact improvisation privileges a willingness to take physical and emotional risks, producing a certain psychic disorientation in which the seemingly stable categories of able and disable become dislodged.

Disability in professional dance has often been a code for one type of disability—namely, the paralysis of the lower body. Yet in contact improvisation-based gatherings such as the annual DanceAbility workshop and the Breitenbush Jam, the dancers have a much wider range of disabilities—including vision impairments, deafness, and neurological conditions such as cerebral palsy. Steve Paxton, one of the originators of the form, creates an apt metaphor for this mélange of talents when he writes:

A group including various disabilities is like a United Nations of the senses. Instructions must be translated into specifics appropriate for those on legs, wheels, crutches, and must be signed for the deaf. Demonstrations must be verbalized for those who can't see, which is in itself a translating skill, because English is not a very flexible language in terms of the body.[15]

My first physical experience with this work occurred in the spring of 1992 when I went to the annual Breitenbush Dance Jam. Held in a hot springs retreat in Oregon, the Breitenbush Jam is not designed specifically for people with physical disabilities as are the DanceAbility workshops, so I take it to be a measure of the success of true integration within the contact improvisation community that people with various movement styles and physical abilities come to participate as dancers. At the beginning of the jam, while we were introducing ourselves to the group, Bruce Curtis, who was facilitating this particular exercise, suggested that we go around in the circle to give each dancer an opportunity to talk about his or her own physical needs and desires for the week of nonstop dancing. Curtis was speaking from the point of view that lots of people have special needs—not just the most obviously "disabled" ones. This awareness of ability as a continuum and not as an either/or situation allowed everyone present to speak without the stigma of necessarily categorizing oneself as able or disabled solely on the basis of physical capacity.

Since that jam, I have had many more experiences dancing with people (including children) who are physically disabled. Yet it would be disingenuous to suggest that my first dancing with Curtis was just like doing contact improvisation with anybody else. It was not—a fact that had more to do with my preconceptions than his physicality. At first, I was scared of crushing his body. After seeing him dance with other people more familiar with him, I recognized that he was up for some pretty feisty dancing, and gradually I began to trust our physical communication enough to be able to release the internal alarm in my head that kept reminding me I was dancing with someone with a disability (i.e., a fragile body). My ability to move into a different dancing relationship with Curtis was a result not only of contact improvisation's open acceptance of any body, but also of its training (both physical and psychic), which gave me the willingness to feel intensely awkward and uncomfortable. The issue was not whether I was dancing with a classical body or not, but rather whether I could release the classical expectations of my own body. Fortunately, the training in disorientation that is fundamental to contact improvisation helped me re-create my body in response to his. As I move from dancer to critic, the question that remains for me is: does contact improvisation reorganize our viewing priorities in the same way that it reorganized my physical priorities?

Emery Blackwell and Alito Alessi both live in Eugene, Oregon: a city specifically designed to be wheelchair accessible. Blackwell was the president of Oregonians for Independent Living (OIL) until he resigned in order to devote himself to dance. Alessi, a veteran contacter who has had various experiences with physical disabilities (including an accident which severed the tendons on one ankle), has been coordinating the DanceAbility workshops in Eugene for the last five years. In addition to their participation in this kind of forum, Blackwell and Alessi have been dancing together for many years, creating both choreographic works, such as their duet *Wheels of Fortune,* and improvisational duets like the one I saw during a performance at Breitenbush Jam.

Blackwell and Alessi's duet begins with Alessi rolling around on the floor and Blackwell rolling around the periphery of the performance space in a wheelchair. Their eyes are focused on one another, creating a connection that gives their separate rolling motions a certain synchrony of purpose. After several circles of the space, Blackwell stops his wheelchair, all the while looking at his partner. The intensity of his gaze is reflected in the constant vibrations of movement impulses in his head and hands and his stare draws Alessi closer to him. Blackwell offers Alessi a hand and initiates a series of weight exchanges that begin with Alessi gently leaning away from Blackwell's center of weight and ends with him riding upside down on Blackwell's lap. Later, Blackwell half slides, half wriggles out of his chair and walks on his knees over to Alessi. Arms outstretched, the two men mirror one another until an erratic impulse brings Blackwell and Alessi to the floor. They are rolling in tandem across the floor when all of a sudden Blackwell's movement frequency fires up and his body begins to bounce with excess energy. Alessi responds in kind, and the two men briefly engage in a good-natured rough-and-tumble wrestling match. After a while they become exhausted and begin to settle down, slowly rolling side by side out of the performance space.

Earlier I argued that, precisely because the disabled body is culturally coded as "grotesque," many integrated dance groups emphasize the classical dimensions of the disabled body's movements—the grace of a wheelchair's gliding, the strength and agility of people's upper bodies, etc. What intrigues me about Blackwell's dancing in this duet is the fact that his movement at once evokes images of the grotesque and then leads our eyes through the spectacle of his body into the experience of his particular physicality. Paxton once wrote a detailed description of Blackwell's dancing which reveals just how much the viewer becomes aware of the internal motivations as well as the external consequences of Blackwell's dancing:

> Emery has said that to get his arm raised above his head requires about twenty
> seconds of imaging to accomplish. Extension and contraction impulses in his
> muscles fire frequently and unpredictably, and he must somehow select the right

impulses consciously, or produce for himself a movement image of the correct quality to get the arm to respond as he wants. We observers can get entranced with what he is doing with his mind. More objectively, we can see that as he tries he excites his motor impulses and the random firing happens with more vigor. His dancing has a built-in Catch-22. And we feel the quandary and see that he is pitched against his nervous system and wins, with effort and a kind of mechanism in his mind we able-bodied have not had to learn. His facility with them allows us to feel them subtly in our own minds.[16]

Steve Paxton is considered by many people to be the father of contact improvisation, for it was his workshop and performance at Oberlin College in 1972 that first sparked the experimentations which later became this dance form. Given Paxton's engagement with contact improvisation over the last four decades, it makes sense that he would be an expert witness to Blackwell's dancing. Paxton's description of Blackwell's movement captures the way in which contact improvisation focuses on the becoming—the improvisational process of evolving which never really reaches an endpoint. Contact improvisation can represent the disabled body differently precisely because it does not try to re-create the aesthetic frames of the classical body or traditional dance contexts. Despite their good intentions, these situations tend to marginalize anything but the most virtuosic movements. Contact improvisation, on the other hand, by concentrating on the becoming of a particular dance refuses a static representation of disability, pulling the audience in as witness to the ongoing negotiations of that physical experience. It is important to realize that Alessi's dancing, by being responsive but not precious, helps to provide the context for this kind of witnessing engagement as well. In their duet, Alessi and Blackwell are engaged in an improvisational movement dialogue in which both partners are moving and being moved by the other. I find this duet compelling because it demonstrates the extraordinary potential of bringing two people with very different physical abilities together to share in one another's motion. In this space between social dancing, combat, and physical intimacy lies a dance form whose open aesthetic and attentiveness to the flexibility of movement identities can inform and be informed by any body's movement.

Needless to say, my involvement with contact improvisation—training, teaching, and researching the form—for most of my adult life—has primed me to see these liberatory possibilities in this work. That training has also allowed me to reimagine my own physicality in the midst of a disability. Although I would not want to minimize the excruciatingly painful process of dealing with a sudden and severe mobility impairment—the exhaustion, intense and unrelenting pain, not to mention the aggravating bureaucracy of American medical institutions—I was grateful that I never once thought to give up dancing. Contact improvisation helped me imagine other ways of moving; other ways to be fully present in my body. Although I still struggled with my own preconceptions about how to dance, and although I still found it difficult to accept the limitations and boundaries of my changed physical possibilities, I was deeply grateful for the model that the DanceAbility work gave me. Yet perhaps more important than helping me to imagine how to dance with my disability, contact improvisation helped me continue to re-conceive dancing even as I began to regain my range of motion and strength in my back. Suddenly I was not interested in getting—as one self-help book put it—"back into shape," for I did not want to simply return to dancing as I had experienced it before. Rather, I wanted to acknowledge this powerful legacy of disability, to keep it marked on my body.

Many of our ideas about autonomy, health, and self-determination are based on a model of the body as an efficient machine over which we should have total control. This is particularly true of the current medical establish-ment, which is based upon an arrogant belief that doctors should be able to fix whatever goes wrong, returning us all as quickly as possible to that clas-sical ideal. Talking over with doctors all the possible interventions into my condition made me realize that I was not sure I wanted to take part in such a system. Indeed, these medical personnel never seemed to notice the irony in their contradictory advice, suggesting, on the one hand, that I should retire from dancing (at the ripe old age of thirty-four), and, on the other hand, claiming that they could fix me up "as good as new" with the latest technological advances in surgery. What they could never envision is that the experience of disability was tremendously important to me—through it I began to really understand my own body and recognize that no matter how limited, mine were strategic abilities.

I refused the surgery and made a dance.

NOTES

1. Mary Russo, "Female Grotesques: Carnival and Theory," in *Feminist Studies/ Critical Studies,* ed. Teresa de Lauretis (Bloomington: Indiana University Press, 1986), 219.

2. Of course, it is important to recognize that almost every category of cultural identity predicated on the body (gender, class, race, sexuality, age, as well as ability) fits into this classical/grotesque divide.

3. Gus Solomns Jr., "Seven Men," *Village Voice,* March 17, 1992.

4. Melinda Ule-Grohol, *Dance Movements in Time* (Cleveland: Professional Flair, 1995), 1.

5. Ynestra King, "The Other Body," *Ms.,* March/April 1993, 74.

6. One might argue that this is no mere historical coincidence, but rather a very specific social backlash against proactive groups working on disability issues. For further discussions of how society molds bodies into its own ideological images see

Susan Bordo, *Unbearable Weight: Feminism, Western Culture, and the Body;* Emily Martin, *Flexible Bodies: The Role of Immunity in American Culture from the days of Polio to the age of AIDS.*

7. King, 74.

8. Adam Benjamin, "In Search of Integrity," *Dance Theatre Journal,* 1993, 45.

9. Ibid., 44.

10. Chris de Marigny, "A Little World of Its Own," *Ballet International,* June 1993, 29.

11. De Marigny, 29.

12. I am indebted to Jodi Falk for lending me a copy of the British TV program *Here and Now* that contained a spot on Toole's retirement. In her presentation at the 1996 CORD conference, Falk quoted a June 1996 review of Candoco that lamented his departure, calling the rest of the company a "competent but unremarkable bunch of dancers." See Jodi Falk, "Questioning the Dancing Body," 1996 CORD Conference Proceedings.

13. Cynthia Novack, *Sharing the Dance: Contact Improvisation and American Culture* (Madison: University of Wisconsin Press, 1990), 186. For references to Judson Dance Theater see Sally Banes's work on the era, especially *Terpsichore in Sneakers* and *Democracy's Body: Judson Dance Theater 1962–1964.*

14. Curt Siddall, "Contact Improvisation," *East Bay Review,* September 1976, cited in John Gamble, "On Contact Improvisation," *Painted Bride Quarterly* 4, no. 1 (Spring 1977): 36.

15. Steve Paxton, "3 Days," *Contact Quarterly* 17, no. 1: 13.

16. Ibid., 16.

Dancing in and out of Africa

Dance Research Journal 32, no. 1 (Summer 2000).

The photograph was striking, no doubt about it: a black man in profile, his eyes squinting into the sun, his mouth open, his dreadlocks spouting out of the ponytail on top of his head. The bareness of his neck and shoulders, combined with the urban trendiness of his coiffure placed him as the synecdoche for the ninth International Festival of New Dance in Montreal (FIND) entitled *Afrique, Aller/Retour.* This image marked all of the official festival publicity, including the stationary for press releases. In addition, it was the central image for the large festival posters that adorned billboards and building walls all over Montreal. This was the first visual cue I received about this international festival of new dance, which was dedicated to showcasing contemporary African dance and dancers. Like any self-respecting critic, I immediately felt as if this image, although wonderfully seductive, was politically suspect. Combined with a festival named *Afrique, Aller/Retour* (which was oddly translated as "Africa, In and Out"), I was prepared to deconstruct the neocolonialist basis of this latest importation of African culture, especially as several of the commissioned works were advertised as collaborations between European choreographers and African dancers (never vice versa). I mean really, who but Europeans get a round-trip ticket "in and out" of Africa? What happens, I wondered, to these dancers after the European choreographers are done with them?

Fortunately, over the course of my stay at the festival—which included a symposium exploring the theme of cultural hybridity featuring talks by dance critics, cultural theorists, and dance artists—I became aware of a silver lining to this international festival. In spite of the corporate marketing and institutional hierarchies, there was still room for real artistic dialogue and critical exchange. In general, the performances I saw staged two different perspectives on intercultural sharing. In some pieces there was a desire to explore what we might term a cultural pastiche, where two movement styles inhabit the same stage environment, and yet the traditions coexist without merging or changing in any fundamental way. In contrast to this collage paradigm, there were other performances in which the dancing was both culturally grounded and intriguingly hybrid at the same time. For example, *Pour Antigone,* by French choreographer Mathilde Monnier placed five African dancers on the stage with five European dancers. Monnier had visited Burkino-Faso in the early 1990s and had been inspired to create a dance based on the Antigone myth about the responsibility for grieving and the conflict between individual needs and civic order. Interestingly enough, Monnier found that the African dancers were much more comfortable expressing grief publicly than the European dancers, who tended to see intense grief as a private emotion. The effect of this evening-length movement interface was less one of a meeting and exchange than one of channel flipping. Much of the dancing was performed in small groups of two or three, with some extended solos, and the dancers rarely communicated across their own movement traditions. Indeed, eventually the European dancers seemed almost entrapped by their own abstract, angst-ridden, movement for movement's sake, especially given the joy with which some of the African dancers moved.

Ironically, it was a collaboration between two of Monnier's dancers that provided one of the most moving examples of a contemporary hybrid of African and European dancing. *Figninto, ou L'Oeil Troué* was created for three male dancers and two musicians by Seydou Boro and Salia Sanon. The performers' dancing encompassed both African-based movements and the idiosyncratic gestures and stillnesses that punctuate a European postmodern dance aesthetic. There were exceptional moments of choreographic beauty when a barrage of fast, tumbling movements would suddenly arrive at an epic stillness, or when the awesome speed of the dancing would shift into a slower, more timeless rhythm. During his talk at the symposium, Salia Sanon elaborated on his experience working with Monnier. At first, he reported, he did not like working in silence, or devising his own gestural sequences. Trained in Africa, he automatically thought of dancing in terms of the music. But, he added, sometimes dancers in Africa can feel as if they are only visual accompaniment to the "real" art of music. Eventually, he found a certain expressive freedom in being able to leave the music and explore the possibility of rhythmic and physical stillness.

Another highlight of the festival was Zab Maboungou's solo, *Incantation*. Maboungou is a Congolese-Canadian choreographer who describes her work as contemporary African dance—a denotation that rests uneasily with stereotypes about the place and function of ethnic dance in the Eurocentric dance scene in Montreal. Although Maboungou is a well-known choreographer who has lived and choreographed in Montreal for many years, this was the first time her work was presented by FIND. As she steps from the darkness into the light onstage, Zab Maboungou immediately introduces the viewer to the aesthetic priorities in her dancing by focusing our attention on the intricate dialogue in her body between the rhythms of the drums and the motion of her dancing. Sometimes she surfs over the beat by drawing out a sustained arching of her upper torso. Sometimes she rides the sound of the drums—slowly sinking and rising as her shoulders punctuate the drummers' shifting cadences. There is thoughtfulness to her moving; a self-reflexivity that reminds me a lot of contemporary American choreographers such as Dana Reitz. Often in *Incantation* she strikes a movement percussively, but allows the reverberations to continue through her body. Calling out vocally as well as with her dancing, she moves through different spaces onstage as if they held special energies—places where movement experiences get called forth.

I began this short report with a deconstructive reading of an image. Despite my reservations about that image and its uses with the publicity of the festival, I will say that the administration of the International Festival of New Dance knows how to develop audiences for dance. For me, Montreal is a kind of dance paradise. Besides having over a dozen suitable venues for dance, complete with the requisite artists' café, Montreal has succeeded in making dance the hippest scene around. Over one-third of the greater Montreal population sees at least one dance event during the festival—an amazing statistic. The opportunity to see as many contemporary African companies as I saw during one week in Montreal was extraordinary for me. Witnessing the incredible diversity of work that blurs the boundaries of traditional and experimental, African and European, opened my eyes to the increasingly global context of contemporary dancing.

32

Rates of Exchange

Movement (R)evolution conference, University of Florida, Spring 2004.

On January 18, 2004, my father died. I begin this essay by evoking his death, not in order to gain sympathy, nor even to create a personal and rhetorical bridge to the question of burial in *Antigone*, but rather to provoke a reflection on the limits of visibility. As anyone who has ever lost an important figure in their life knows, the shock of someone's absence draws out the ironic reiteration of that person's presence. We mourn the physical loss at the same time that we sense an invisible companionship. We bury the dead, and create a myth of their life, weaving the traces of their existence into an epic tapestry of influence and inspiration such that he who is no longer visible lives on in us.

Corporeality also exceeds the visible. Dancers know this. Although we base our work in the material conditions of the body, we are not limited by them. Expressivity requires an engagement beyond the pedestrian and with the ephemeral. From the skin into the soul. Our willingness to work at the edge of what Marcia Siegel called "the vanishing point" gives us an interesting perspective on the temporality of existence. And identity. Movement quickly becomes a metaphor for everything that does not stand still, including life itself. Perhaps, this is why death calls forth dancing—it leads us beyond the visible world.

Contemporary dancing, because it carries the intriguing possibility of being both very abstract and literal, can frame a dancer's cultural identity differently. If we look at examples from a variety of choreographers, we can document the libratory possibilities of movement forms in which the lived body slips in and out of cultural stereotypes. Some contemporary choreography (such as Bill T. Jones's latest formal work) focuses the audience's attention on the highly kinetic physicality of dancing bodies, minimizing the cultural differences between dancers by highlighting their common physical technique and ability to complete the often strenuous movement tasks. Other dances (such as those by the all-female troupe Urban Bush Women) foreground the social markings of identity on the body, using movement and text to comment on the cultural meanings of those bodily markers. By foregrounding the way that identity is figured corporeally, by challenging which bodies are allowed which identities, and by fracturing the voyeuristic relationship between audience and performer, contemporary dance can help us see bodies differently.

In 1993, Mathilde Monnier made a dance about death and loss, about social repression and individual agency. She chose a cast of five African dancers and five Anglo-European dancers, inaugurating another chapter in the ongoing saga of colonial exchange. With the myth of Antigone as the meeting place for two very different movement styles, two very different cultures, and two very different kinds of resources and access, Monnier made a dance. The story of this coming together is told by one of the dancers, Seydou Boro in his documentary 2004 film, *La Rencontre*. But the implication of this retelling calls up very different meanings than did the live performance as I first witnessed it in 1999. This essay, then, reviews these discrepancies between the performance and the film order to try and flesh out what is made visible and what is left unseen in this contemporary vision of intercultural sharing.

I realize, of course, the irony of beginning a talk about the limits of the visible immediately following a film that seeks precisely to make visible an encounter between artists from different cultures. Although they were once referred to as "moving pictures," let us not forget that films have radically different agendas than dances. Movement eludes the gaze of the camera, rendering meaning more fluid. By virtue of the editorial selection, film tends to stabilize meaning, in/stilling a dominant narrative.

La Rencontre is framed by two questions and their answers. These questions—Does contemporary dance have any meaning in Africa? Is there a future for contemporary dance on a continent where dance still has so many religious and secular connotations?—are voiced over an image of a long, thin shadow moving slowly through a variety of Giacometti-like poses. The figure, we later realize, is Mathilde Monnier, and it is her work in Africa that references the definition of "contemporary" used throughout the film. The core of the film charts the creation and remounting of *Pour Antigone*. In long and medium shots, we follow Monnier through the streets of Burkino Faso as she retraces her steps and describes the naissance of this intercultural collaboration. Individual interviews with participants (including various dancers, composer/musician, and set designer) segue into shots of performance footage of *Pour Antigone,* as the process evolves over the course of the film into the choreographic product.

The film reenacts the genesis of this dance by overlaying spoken narratives about its creation onto footage of various workshops taught by Monnier at the moment of her restaging of this work in Africa six years after its premiere in the West. Although the film charts the beginnings of this work, it was produced at its end. In fact, *La Rencontre* constitutes a cinematic eulogy for that mythic moment of initial artistic contact between Africa and

Europe, between traditional and contemporary, between black and white. By the time the film was released, Monnier had since moved onto other projects, most notably as the director of the Centre Chorégraphique National de Montpellier, as had many of her dancers. The film serves as a metaphoric bridge, creating a link from Europe to Africa via an introduction of "contemporary" compositional strategies. This evolution is rendered in the shift of performance footage from *Pour Antigone* to *Figninto*—a collaboration between Salia Sanon and Seydou Boro, two dancers from the original cast of *Pour Antigone* who have since formed their own company. In the film's final frames, these men sit comfortably around a coffee table, articulating the various cross-cultural influences on their own aesthetic—in effect, becoming poster boys for the new contemporary African dance.

La Rencontre, Rencontre. Reencounter. This is a word at once obsolete in the English language and yet used with some frequency in French. Originally it suggested a negative encounter; a sense of meeting someone or something hostile; of running up against something, an enemy or some kind of resistance, unexpectedly. These days, it is most often used to evoke a friendly encounter, an exchange of pleasantries, or ideas. Still, there rests a hint of residual tension in the word, especially considering its root, *contre,* means *against* in French. It is this element of tension as it was staged in the full-length performance that I find missing in the film. Although Monnier speaks of her desire to shake up (*déstabilizé*) her own artistic process by going to Africa, and Salia mentions the unsettling effects—being *perturbé*—of first dancing without music, for the most part, the film elides any sense of intercultural friction, or messiness.

I first witnessed *Pour Antigone,* as well as *Figninto,* at the 1999 International Festival of New Dance (FIND). The theme that year was Africa: In and Out. In the previous piece, I deconstructed the colonialist trope of that unfortunate title, so I will spare us that diatribe on capitalist multicultural art marketing at the cusp of the millennium. Instead, I would like to focus my comments on how these dances staged two different perspectives on intercultural sharing. I am hoping to illuminate (once again, this question of visibility) their uneven rates of exchange.

Pour Antigone was presented in a large theater in Montreal. In the press releases, Monnier made it very clear that she was not interested in the fusion of European postmodern movement and traditional African dance. On one hand, this strategy allowed for each individual to retain his or her own physical subjectivity. On the other hand, it produced, in the words of one critic, an uncompromising meeting in which "The geometric construction of the Western dance body in comparison to the vivacious integrity of African performance is here made painfully clear" (Johannes Odenthal, *Ballett International*). The result was a very odd disconnection between the performers, leading to a double sense of existential aloofness and cultural claustrophobia in which the differences between African (joyful, connected) and European dancers (angular, angst ridden) were bizarrely highlighted.

La Rencontre foregrounds discussions of what the African dancers and choreographers learned from the experience of working with Monnier. Using the metaphor of a tree that needs to be deeply rooted in order to grow into the world, the African dancers emphasize again and again how their work is still connected to the traditional dances they know, even as they articulate how they have been enriched by this recent exposure to contemporary European choreography. By contrast, the European dancers rarely reflect (at least on camera) on what they have learned from this experience, except for one candid soul who jokingly (or not) hoped the African dancers would not immediately take away all the dance jobs. Of course, this point of view reflects the filmmaker's perspective, but at the same time, I wonder that it does not also reinforce a patronizing one-way dynamic of First World/Third World exchange. At one point in the film, Monnier reveals a particularly odd myopia, when she declares that, "we know what traditional African dance looks like ... But we don't know what contemporary [presumably European] dance looks like." But more importantly, I want to underline what I feel is missing in *La Rencontre*—the other half of the exchange. It is short-sighted to limit the discussion to what African choreographers have and can learn from European or American choreographers. Why not also try to articulate what these artists are learning from contemporary African work, even if those influences are not easily visible?

As we thread our way through the multitude of issues concerning cultural contexts and international exchanges at the beginning of the twenty-first century, let us also allow the reverberations of the dancing we see to sound in our bodies and in our souls. Let us imagine the sequel to *La Rencontre*—one in which the spirit of African dancing helps to guide contemporary European choreography into a more holistic, two-way exchange with the world.

33

Moving Contexts

Dance and Difference in the Twenty-first Century

Intercultural Communication and Creative Practice: Music, Dance, and Women's Cultural Identity, ed. Laura Lengel (2005).

Local Intertexts

It is a balmy summer evening as I emerge from *The Sensuous and the Sacred* exhibit of Chola Bronzes at the Cleveland Museum of Art. These ancient bronze images of deities call forth my memories of sacred statues and richly decorated shrines in the south of India, where I traveled to teach and lecture in January 2003. From India to Cleveland; from Cleveland to India. These points of interchange carry infinite artistic possibilities; and yet they are never unmarked by their respective political and economic landscapes. It was warm in Madurai when I arrived, and we gathered in an outdoor compound shaded by palm trees and lush shrubbery. Here some twenty young men and women launched their bodies and their minds into a radically different movement paradigm. By the grace of body language and an amazing interpreter, they followed me through three days of training in contact improvisation—a contemporary form of American dance based on the physical exchange of weight between two (or more) people. Most of these students had never touched a member of the opposite sex before. Yet they were open to the situation and excited about the possibilities of a new movement form. The seeds of my workshop in India were most likely planted almost two decades ago when I saw the great classical Indian dancer Sanjukta Panagrahi perform and first began thinking about dance in an Indian context. I know the ripples from this workshop are still being felt halfway across the world. This essay charts the intellectual and physical trajectory of that seminal experience (as well as later exchanges) to try and elucidate the often tangled issues of cultural representation and somatic reverberation that surface when we engage our dancing bodies across difference.

I realize, as I enter my forties, that I have been dealing with these issues for quite some time now. Like many dancers who came of age in the 1980s, I supplemented my modern dance classes with workshops in a variety of dance styles. Ironically, it was at that historic bastion of modern dance, the American Dance Festival (ADF), that I first experienced the visual and physical power of non-Western dance. Two moments stand out from that summer: my participation in Chuck Davis's African repertory classes and my encounter with butoh in the form of Dairakuda-Kan's performances of the *Sea-Dappled Horse.* As I took up the challenge of learning to move differently, I recognized—through sore muscles and an enduring sense of awkwardness—the complexity of how cultures are both always already inscribed and yet continually reembodied.

Chuck Davis's African American Dance Ensemble is based in Durham, North Carolina, and although selected members travel with Chuck Davis on an annual trip to research and study dance in Africa, the company maintains an extensive outreach program within the Durham community and performs throughout the country. In addition, the company spends the summers in residence at the American Dance Festival. An enormously friendly teacher, Chuck Davis has the gift of making one laugh at oneself and feel at ease—even if you are one of the forty, predominately white, modern dancers trying to pick up the bodily polyrhythms and hand and feet coordinations of a West African. In his teaching, as well as in his company's performances, Chuck Davis attempts to give his audience a sense of the community context in which the African dances that he stages would be originally performed.

The dance I was in was part of a West African village's harvest celebration and for our final, outdoor performance, the rhythmic dance combinations which we had practiced over and over were eventually incorporated into a larger frame of a village setting complete with baskets and our own handmade, tie-dyed costumes. Chuck Davis never suggested, of course, that this student performance approached an "authentic" reconstruction of the original event. There was, however, an implicit belief that this theatrical business of village life would help us see and feel the dances' original context more fully. Although I might now want to probe that assumption more thoroughly, the way in which Chuck Davis repeatedly situated dancing within life experiences certainly helped to create a sense of community among the class members and musicians, which produced a radically different engagement with the dancing than most of the other classes I took that summer.

In retrospect, however, I realize that the ideological referent for Chuck Davis's repertory class was an oddly pastoral and romanticized version of indigenous dancing—that our attention was focused on something we could never quite know, but were attempting to experience anyway. We never discussed what it meant that we were learning these dances in the midst of the American Dance Festival. Indeed, what was the effect of this double physical translation of a dance form from its African source through Chuck Davis's body and onto ours? It is this complex slippage of cultural contexts that both fascinates and troubles me. In the past two decades—without leaving the American continent—I have seen a wide range of dances from around the world and have taken master classes and some intensive workshops in butoh, bharata natyam, capoeira, African and Australian dance, and the hula. Some of these forms have influenced the kinds of movements I enjoy doing, and some have intrigued me intellectually. What I find most compelling, however, is the ways in which these forms continue to shift through the global influences of migration and reinvention.

Perhaps it is the conscious acknowledgment and manipulation of the points of intersection between multiple (and contradictory) cultural influences in butoh that has made my experiences with this dance form so compelling. At ADF, I remember sitting in the dark theater at the beginning of the show, being bombarded with obnoxiously loud static. All of a sudden, there was dead silence and then a flash of bright white lights revealed twelve figures standing, arms spread-eagled, in a semicircle onstage. Naked and arranged in crucifix poses, they were covered from head to toe in a white chalky substance. The men's heads were shaven and the women's long, dark hair was frizzed out in unruly manes that framed their gruesome faces. A rope looped from mouth to mouth, held in place by teeth clenched around red cloth. The next seventy-five minutes took the audience along a journey through the dark side of Akaji Maro's (the company's founder and director) consciousness. In one sequence, for instance, a man on stilts with a stunning, floor-length, and richly embossed kimono slowly seeped his way downstage maintaining a deeply solemn focus all the while a live cock, whose feet were tied to his hat, was frantically beating his wings and calling out in a desperate effort to free himself. Teeming with grotesque sexual temptresses and demented authority figures, this dark world cycled through contradictory moments of hopefulness and hopelessness until suddenly the frenzied action was gone, the stage was bare, and the audience was left in stunned silence.

One of the reasons why I find some butoh work so compelling is the way that its images at once enact and deflate the cultural legacies of Japanese social traditions and Western economic commodification. Influenced by both German expressive modern dance and the traditional Japanese theater arts, butoh appropriates these performance techniques but radically alters their theatrical contexts to create a constant sense of cultural fragmentation. Even though the resulting images are often dissonant, grotesque, or even violent, the performers maintain a deliberate presence and physical integrity—a bodily commitment to the act of performing that practically borders on the religious. Negotiating the minefield of split cultural subjectivities, butoh artists have built their own worlds out of the cultural rubbish of the Eastern and Western superpowers. Predicated on a deep physical engagement with the unknown, butoh carries its own kind of inner logic and offers us a view into the moving reality of multicultural survival.

When I was in my twenties, I was more interested in watching and making dances than in thinking about the intercultural implications of these two brief experiences. Many years, thousands of dance classes, a dozen or so choreographic projects, and several graduate degrees later, I took up these issues again when I attended the 1990 "Peoples of the Pacific" Los Angeles Festival. This massive event was orchestrated by Peter Sellers in a moment of extraordinary hubris and multicultural evangelistic fervor. To begin with, there was the opening ceremony of the festival—an outdoor event billed as an "international sacred ritual featuring Korean Shamans, Hawaiian dancers, Australian Aborigines, Native Americans from the Southwest, Eskimos, and dancers from Wallis and Futuna." In addition, I saw the Javanese Court Music and Dance Company perform traditional works in a nontraditional setting, a collaborative performance of the *Mahabharata* by both kathak and bharata natyam dancers (many of whom were trained within Indian-American communities in the United States), and John Malpede's LAPD (Los Angeles Poverty Department: a multiracial theater group of homeless people)—all in the space of one weekend.

Moving through representation faster than either MTV or the fashion industry, the performing bodies at the L.A. festival piled representations on top of representations in a virtual tornado of cultural signification. Although I felt that many of the performances were meant to celebrate and give visibility to "ethnic" or "traditional" forms of dance, I could not help wondering if the overarching frame of the L.A. festival was not, in fact, reinscribing these terms in such a way to preserve a static notion of cultural identity which would remain safely marginalized within the colonialist power dynamics of American culture. Unfortunately, the L.A. festival never found a way to address these complicated issues of aesthetic values; the politics of differing performance contexts; the questions of reconstruction and revolution within tradition; the differences between ritual, communal, folk, and theatrical forms of performance; and the complexity of audience-performer relationships in cross-cultural exchange. Despite extensive program notes and educational opportunities, there was clearly no way one could possibly pin down an "appropriate"—much less an "authentic"—perspective on these performances, and I wondered if, having traveled across the Pacific to this monster of late capitalist art engineering, many of these "traditional" forms would ever again carry the same meanings, even in their original contexts.

In this moment of global intersection, cultures are rarely stable or knowable containers, and many dancers are choosing to downplay the formal, more abstract, elements of choreography in order to present their dancing bodies as sources of gendered, racial, and sexual identities that can disrupt traditional visions of cultures and respective contexts. Indeed, for both economic and political reasons, *dis*location has become a central theme among many choreographers. These dance artists are working in the spaces in between national or ethnic cultures, in a place that Guillermo Gómez-Peña calls "the fissure between two worlds." Of course, this kind of creative movement across cultural boundaries can pose real challenges for producers, critics, and viewers alike.

Because it carries the intriguing possibility of being both very abstract and very literal, dancing can frame the dancer's cultural identity differently. Some contemporary choreography focuses the audience's attention on the highly kinetic physicality of dancing bodies, minimizing the cultural differences between dancers by highlighting their common physical technique and ability to complete the often-strenuous movement tasks. Other dances foreground the social markings of identity on the body, using movement and text to comment on (indeed, often subvert) the cultural meanings of those bodily markers. Tracing the layers of kinesthetic, aural, spatial, as well as visual and symbolic meanings in dance can help us to understand the complex interconnectedness of personal experience and cultural representation so critical to contemporary cultural theory.

The slippage between the lived body and its cultural representation, between what I call a somatic identity (the experience of one's physicality) and a cultural one (how one's body—skin, gender, ability, age, etc.—renders meaning in society) is the basis for what I consider some of the most interesting explorations of cultural identity in dance. Much of the choreography I have witnessed over the past several decades questions or challenges which cultures belong to which bodies. The fluidity of these exchanges can be either wonderfully liberating, or it can work to reaffirm colonialist dynamics often embedded in First World-Third World interactions. Although it is of the body, dance is not just about the body; it is also about subjectivity—about how that body is positioned in the world as well as the ways in which that particular body responds to the world. By foregrounding the way that identity is figured corporeally, by challenging which bodies are allowed which identities, and by fracturing the voyeuristic relationship between audience and performer, contemporary dance can refute traditional constructions of the body. As we shall see, their work addresses the (dis)connections between physical bodies and their cultural identities, refiguring the relationship between the "eyes" of the audience and the "Is" of the dancers in order to open up new ways of moving and being in the world.

Her knee lifts in a step that gets caught in mid-air, suspended while the under beat of the drums gradually coaxes its way through her torso and out her shoulders, arms, and wrists until it reaches a final parting caress in her hands. Then another, and another, each step rising like the tide through her body while she tilts her head to listen and wait for another impulse to move. Her eyes are lulled by the soothing rhythms of the drums and her face seems almost sleepy as it shifts from one side to another. A deep breath pulls her out of her reverie and her chest rises up, swelling with a call that fills the space with the sound of her voice.

I wrote this description of Zab Maboungou's dancing after seeing the beginning section of *Reverdance*—an evening-length solo work. As she steps from the darkness into the light onstage, Maboungou immediately introduces the viewer to the aesthetic priorities in her dancing by focusing our attention on the intricate dialogue in her body between the rhythms of the drums and the motion of her dancing. Sometimes she surfs over the beat by drawing out a sustained arching of her upper torso. Sometimes she rides the sound of the drums, slowly sinking and rising as her shoulders punctuate the drummers' shifting cadences. There is a certain thoughtfulness to her moving; a self-reflexivity suggested in her program notes. "*Reverdance* is a celebration of movement which emphasizes the intimate over the flamboyant; nuances of internal adventure unravel through a progression of pieces, a saraband of small metamorphoses emerging from alternating melodies . . ." *Rever* is French for "to dream," and yet Maboungou does not translate *rever* in the English version of the title (which sounds like both reverdance and riverdance): a choice that serves to underscore both the dreamlike quality of her dancing and the continuous flow of the motion (like a river) throughout her body.

I saw an excerpt from *Reverdance*, while I was in Montreal for the bi-annual International Festival of New Dance (FIND). Maboungou's showing was part of an alternative festival of local Quebec dance (fondly called the OFF-FIND) and it included a discussion with the artist afterwards. Zab Maboungou is a Congolese-Canadian dancer who describes her work as "contemporary African dance"—a denotation that, as we shall see, rests uneasily with stereotypes about the place and function of traditional ethnic dance both in the Eurocentric as well as the Afrocentric dance communities. In the discussion of *Reverdance* that follows, I use Clifford Geertz's notion of a "thick" description—an analysis that elucidates the multiple layers of meaning in cultural performances—to demonstrate how *Reverdance* resists the stereotypical production values of what often get presented as "African" dance in the New World. In the example that follows, I argue that her work *re*fuses and *con*fuses the polarization of contemporary and traditional labels in African dance, provoking a debate about the politics of naming in dance.

Visually, *Reverdance* presents us with many of the iconic signs of African dance. There are musicians onstage who set the atmosphere for the dancing with their drumming. The dancer is barefoot, wearing a raffia skirt and an elaborate raffia necklace with shells and beads. She is clearly of African descent, with medium-brown skin and a short Afro. Her movements are multi-focused and multi-rhythmic, composed of the isolations of the shoulders, central torso, and the hips. And yet, the deep internal focus of her solo and the subtle shifts of emotions differ radically from the African dance that usually gets presented in Canada and the United States. Typically, the dancing is spectacular, aerobic, and frequently acrobatic, with the movement paralleling the musical accents of the drumming. The drums dictate the tempo and the steps, with each change signaled by the drummers. The atmosphere is most often exuberant, with the sense of dancerly one-upmanship encouraged by those on the sidelines.

Maboungou's dancing, however, seems to have a much more dialogic relationship with the music, and she often sustains a gesture across many beats. Her movement is rarely punctuated in an emphatic or forceful manner. Rather, the rhythms seem to mull around in the center of her body—her hips in conversation with her shoulders, or her belly responding to the movements of her arms. Sometimes, such as in the section of *Reverdance* entitled *Savanes* (Savannah) she dances in silence, continuing the music through her vibrating body. It is this striking difference in performative intent from what often gets marketed as "African" dance that, I argue, opens up a space for Maboungou's own experience of that identity to become visible. Because Maboungou refuses to enter the popular construction of an African woman dancer, her audience cannot easily plug her into a stereotype. The looping of similar movement with subtle variations in attack or rhythm in Maboungou's dancing illustrates the double (and doubling) effect of repetition. The fact that Maboungou is always in motion, that she is always at once creating and dissolving images, allows her both to enact an identity and refuse its stability. Her dancing is about the process of becoming, not the "what" one has become. The gap created by this difference forces the viewer to look again, asking us to follow the nuances in her very personal experience of that identity.

Maboungou's choreography—her dancing signature—resists any simple categorization. While the cultural basis for her dancing is primarily African, her performances also evoke for me the shifting musicality of Isadora Duncan as well as the internalized focus and unpretentious attitude of Yvonne Rainer's postmodern dance. Because her presence vibrates between various cultural and aesthetic identities, Maboungou has, until recently, eluded popular and critical attention.[1] Her dilemma is one many contemporary minority artists face. Splayed between different communities, these artists must negotiate a minefield of strategic alliances and shifting identities. Because her work is so individual and departs from typical mainstream notions of what constitutes "African" dance, the African communities in Montreal have had trouble seeing her work as a cultural resource of traditional dance. At the same time, because she uses the vocabulary of African dance, the Eurocentric avant-garde dance scene in Quebec does not include her as one of their contemporary choreographers. Ironically, rather than her innovations serving to broaden our notions of what constitutes African dancing, the opposite effect takes place, with people questioning whether her work is really authentic or not.

Africanists have long debated whether it is more important to focus on the similarities and continuities across various African cultures as well as those in the African diaspora, or whether we should be recognizing the real differences not only between African experiences in the New World, but also between the diversity of African cultures on the continent. A book like Asante's *African Culture: The Roots of Unity,* published in 1985, argues stridently for a sense of connection among all African peoples. Later works, particularly those by African-American feminists in the late 1980s and 1990s are more willing to recognize the dialectic of continuity and discontinuity, particularly concerning issues of gender and sexuality. This is, of course, an enormous debate that I cannot begin to do justice to in this context. Dance scholars such as Brenda Dixon Gottschild and Kariamu Welsh-Asante are uncovering the Pan-Africanist foundations of much Western dance. This is important work in the dance field, but we must be careful not to assume uniformity in the name of unity. Indeed, we must also call attention to the ways in which only certain aspects of African dance (celebratory, acrobatic, presentational, energetic, etc.) get marketed as "African." This deconstructive analysis will allow us in turn to realize the ways that dance by African peoples can consciously resist the construction of these stereotypes, opening up the possibility for a cross-cultural dialogue of multiple influences in contemporary African dance.

What is at stake here is not just what gets defined and presented as traditional African dance, but also how the spectator/performer relationship is constructed through the representational structures of the performance. How do we engage with Maboungou's dancing? Often, for instance, companies such as the Chuck Davis Dance Company will try to create the theatrical illusion of a community setting, but this serves more as a frame for their highly spectacular dancing than as an indication of the aesthetic priorities of their work. As with any commercial staging of an indigenous form of dance that has roots in a rural, communal, or ritualized setting—be it Native American, classical Indian, or African dance—the director/choreographer must make decisions about ethnic visibility and cultural identity. The Chuck Davis Dance Company is dedicated to showcasing the extraordinary heritage of dances from West Africa for a variety of Euro-American and African-American audiences, and it has a laudable and extensive outreach organization that seeks to give African-American youngsters an appreciation of their cultural backgrounds. As a resident company at the American Dance Festival—a six-week-long summer workshop that draws hundreds of dancers each year—the Chuck Davis Dance Company has also exposed many people (including me) to their technique and repertory of African dance. In their performance, director Chuck Davis serves as a sort of master of ceremonies, welcoming his audience in the name of peace, love, and respect for everyone. He then introduces each dance and often gives a short contextual background for the work. His company and companies like them have created an important visibility for African and African-American dance and I want to make clear how much I admire their work.

Nonetheless, all this usually takes place within a presentational format that I find problematic. Although the movement forms and the casual theatrical business surrounding the dancing are quite different from the status quo of American concert dance (in which there is rarely any verbal interaction between the audience and performers, or even among the performers themselves), I find that the representational structures of traditional gazes are not really challenged in these situations. That is why performances like these can easily slip back into a racist ideology that frames the dancers as spectacles of the "other"—as black bodies that are inherently exuberant and naturally rhythmic. I am not suggesting that this racist gaze is monolithic or necessarily invoked in all of these performances. Much depends on the venue, the marketing, and the audience. I have witnessed the building of *communitas* in the theater during a Chuck Davis performance that radically displaced this gaze, but I have received enough press releases advertising Latino, African-American or Native American companies with adjectives such as colorful, sensuous, exciting, and even exotic to recognize how easily it can be reinscribed.

What struck me in the first minute of watching Maboungou's dancing was how she constructed a performance that resisted a colonial gaze that I find often gets repositioned in the more presentational styles of African-American dance. The excerpts of *Reverdance* that I saw took place in an intimate studio setting where there was no proscenium arch to separate the audience's space from that of the performer. The makeshift lighting that illuminated her dancing body spread out to include the audience. In addition, her physical presence seemed to ride a fine line between an open generosity and a self-centered focus. We were, after all, able to see the minute details of her movements rippling through her torso, and yet it was clear from her internal focus, subdued face, and three-dimensional (rather than exclusively frontal) use of space, that we were witnessing her experience in such a way that insisted on its own integrity.

When Maboungou refuses to address the audience in the usual presentational format, when she does not hit any recognizable shapes or iconographic movements, or when she insistently returns to repeat a choreographic phrase with only slight variations, she emphasizes a similar process of "becoming" that fractures any static notion of her identity as an African woman dancer and choreographer. The experience of watching her enter a movement phrase again and again, each time with a different emphasis, forces the audience to witness the reality of her experience within that motion, fracturing the power dynamic in traditional gazes where the object of sight is there for the viewer's pleasure, not their own. Maboungou's "becoming" thus resists commodification as any one image, and the lights fade out with Maboungou still in motion.

As Maboungou's dancing body moves through the double moment of representation and experience that is the basis of live performance, her audience has to interpret the visible signs of race and ethnicity in light of her somatic experience. Following her bodily rhythms, their gazes are pulled away from any static image of who she is, or what she represents. Because she moves both with and through our preconceptions of African dancing, she is revising how we come to know that term, giving us an example of how dancing can at once recognize and move across ethnic identity. In Maboungou's performance, cultural representation flickers in and out of somatic identity like a high-frequency vibration, dissolving the boundaries of categories such as nature/culture, body/mind, and private/public, self/other. This interconnectedness of bodies and identities creates what I consider the transformative power of live performance. Let us make the most of it.

NOTE

1. Conversation with the artist, Montreal, October 1995.

34

Three Beginnings and a Manifesto

Conversations across the Field of Dance Studies, Fall 2007

I

It is mid-August and I am sitting on a porch by a lake in Maine. I am here at Bearnstow—a dance retreat run by Ruth Grauer and Bebe Miller in the good old modern style of combining nature and art. The sun has just come out after two days of heavy rain; interrupting my thoughts on the history and future of dance studies with the seduction of a fresh day. I catch myself reflecting on a conversation that I had last night with two smart young dancers. I liked them; they were strong, hearty women equipped with degrees from good colleges and the kind of optimism that four years of rent-free studio space can foster. After dancing, they cornered me. The fireplace at my back; their sweaty, excited faces pressing in on me, I was questioned about graduate schools. Here was one vision of the future, I thought, and I was genuinely at a loss about where to send them. You see, they had both come from progressive liberalarts institutions where dance theory and dance practice had already been so well integrated that they did not want to choose between an MFA and an MA course of study. Gourmands, they wanted their dancing and reading too. Where was the graduate program that had amazing technical and compositional instruction AND fabulous intellectual training—a place that allowed them to be feisty and thoughtful? It seemed as if they had to choose one approach over the other. I understood their impatience.

II

Summer's almost over. The joint SDHS/CORD conference at the Centre National de Danse in Paris on rethinking theory and practice has come and gone, and I am helping to compile the proceedings—an incredible outpouring of over one hundred papers in French and English. The field of dance studies is clearly thriving and expanding. Looking over these wonderful papers written from a wide variety of critical perspectives, I take a moment

to reflect on the many ways in which the old paradigms are being reconfigured, including the relationship between intellectual inquiry and physical
practice. But I have also done enough departmental reviews at various colleges and universities over the past few years to know that teaching faculties
and curricular programs can be resistant to this kind of change. Yes, we all
want to integrate theory and practice, but then the worries that with only
twenty-four hours in the day one aspect of dance studies will become diluted
begin to creep up on us.

III

I walk into the vast studio and head over to the seminar table in one corner.
This is Warner Main Space at Oberlin College—one of the largest and most
beautiful dance studios in the world (Steve Paxton said so). Filled with light,
its wooden floor, walls, and ceiling hold the legacy of over a century of modern dance, and today, for the first time, I have set up a classroom in it. I am
teaching a first-year seminar entitled Bridging the Body/Mind Divide, and
I decided to fashion a space that did just that. Soon, fifteen eager freshman
will enter, probably bewildered by the need to take off their shoes and cross
over this big wooden oval. The possibilities presented by this configuration
of studio and seminar, of philosophical texts and somatic study both thrill
and scare me. I feel as if I have been preparing for this moment all my academic life. I am tired of switching back and forth, of being the "bookie" type
among dancing colleagues and the "dancey" type among academics. It is a
grand experiment, and I am intrigued by the fact that for a whole semester,
every dance class in that space will confront the "other" legacy of learning,
while my first-year seminar (not a dance course) will become accustomed to
the dual acts of reading and moving. I do not know where this experiment
in undergraduate teaching will lead, but I am looking forward to exploring
with these fifteen first-year students the interconnected realms of embodied
knowledge and critical thinking.

Manifesto

This is a call for a radical reconfiguring of dance curricula, especially on
the graduate level. Recognizing that all thinking dwells in its own corporeal
space and that all physical practices have ideologies behind them, I would
like to see new dance studies curricula devised that integrate both kinds of
articulations (physical and theoretical) within the space of one degree. This
is not simply a question of adding a dance history or theory course to an
MFA course of study, nor is it about giving (some) credit to practice in a doc-

toral degree. Rather, I am suggesting we think about completely refiguring the terms of the whole equation, throwing out old models of the separation of skills such that we train for the doing and thinking about—the making and writing together. What would it be like to teach technique, history, and composition together? (It would require, to begin with, that various teachers begin to talk with one another about the relevance of what they are teaching—a potentially awkward, but useful, conversation.) This might help us keep dance studies meaningful in these challenging times, offering a place (a big open space, with a seminar table and bookshelves on one end) in which the two young dancing scholars I met at Bearnstow can continue their education without feeling as if they have to sacrifice one aspect of their connection to dance in order to do so.

35

Improvisation as Radical Politics

Dance Research Journal 35, no. 1, 2003.

If Richard Bull and Cynthia Jean Cohen Bull (that is, Cynthia Novack) were both alive and dancing these troubled days, they would no doubt be responding to the current political crisis by staging an evening of improvisational dance at their Warren Street Performance Loft in downtown New York City. Maybe their traditional Saturday-evening performance would be a special event culminating a day of various performative actions connected with the recent antiwar demonstrations in urban centers across the world. I can envision the piece that they might have made with their longtime collaborator, Peentz Dubble: a multilayered synthesis of sound collage (no doubt Richard Bull would have enjoyed sampling and deconstructing the various pro-war declarations of George W. Bush), combined with improvised text and movement critiquing the government's readiness to justify imperialist aggression. Perhaps there would be various kinds of physical collisions—a certain clipped gestural franticness. Eventually, this chaotic field would crystalize into a haunting stillness. Either during the performance or in conversation afterwards, Bull would most likely invoke his first antiwar dance, *War Games,* created in 1968 in protest of the Vietnam War. In his witty and ironic manner, he would enter the debate over SUVs staged in the *New York Times,* commenting dryly on the fact that the Loft's performance space is barely big enough to park two of these tanks on wheels, ironically suggesting that we pay attention to the fact that four-wheel drives are replacing the arts in the twenty-first century.

Imagining an improvisational dance created posthumously—calling up the dancing ghosts of Bull and Novack—might seem an odd way to begin a book review, but it is due to Susan Foster's intriguing blend of history and homage in her latest book *Dances That Describe Themselves: The Improvised Choreography of Richard Bull,* that I am able to invoke the improvisational spirit of Bull's work. Written in memoriam for her good friend Cynthia Novack (who, before her death, had started a book on Bull—her dance partner and husband), Foster's book intersperses commentary from Novack's writings on Bull, as well as observations from dancers who worked with Bull, throughout Foster's own analysis of the cultural context that shaped his contributions to the dance field. This is a most personal form of scholarship; which is not to say that it is overly subjective, but rather that it carries the weight of untimely deaths. In the beginning of the book, Foster describes her approach as participant-observer, and there are sections throughout the book (some of the most lively debates) when she successfully morphs into one of Bull's most fabulous personas to channel the voice of the "Dance That Describes Itself." At times performative, at times thoughtful, this book is built over a river of loss and love that runs throughout much of Foster's writing. Foster's personal connection to Richard and Cynthia does not stop her, however, from bringing her intellectual acumen into play—stretching a history of Bull's work into an examination of the historical roots, aesthetic networks, cultural influences, and theoretical implications of late twentieth-century improvisational dancing.

First with his colleagues and students at New York University and SUNY-Brockport, and later under the auspices of the Improvisational Dance Ensemble at the Warren Street Performance Loft, Richard Bull crafted an approach to improvisation based on exposing and then manipulating the process of composing a dance. Bull's work provides an enlightening counter example to common assumptions that situate improvisation in opposition to composition. The notion that improvisation is a spontaneous creative expression of individual physical pleasure, drawing on "intuitive" experiences of the body, is usually promulgated by dance educators not terribly interested in improvisational as a performance genre. Compositional decisions are made continuously when performing improvisation with a group, coordinating space, rhythm, and text. As Foster argues throughout the book, Bull brilliantly deconstructed the implied binary of form versus freedom, critical analysis versus spontaneous discovery, mind versus body, to formulate a sophisticated dialectic of structure and invention within his improvisational scores. In this sense, Anne Flynn's comments about her participation in Bull's 1970 piece *Making and Doing* are quite telling: "I never really understood why people viewed improvisation as mindlessly doodling around. Dancing in Richard's pieces demanded an incredibly high degree of concentration and taxed short-term memory . . . The consequences of not paying attention to everything around you were severe. You'd be out there fully exposed for your lapse in concentration until someone rescued you. I learned to move less and remember more."[1]

In the first two chapters—"Genealogies of Improvisation" and "Making and Doing"—Foster performs a revisionist history of postmodern dance by tracing the interconnectedness of Bull's ongoing involvement and interest in jazz with his developing approach to improvised choreography. Drawing on the work of critics such as Brenda Dixon Gottschild and Amiri Baraka, Foster excavates the often unacknowledged influence of African-American cultural history on white artists. Jazz music, for instance, provided Bull with an example of the interdependency of set and open forms, showing him how structure could provide a communal space within which each individual was able to create a personalized variation. Jazz became a model for Bull's desire to create group activities that projected at once a sense of cohesiveness (we are making this dance together) and expansion (but how we get there depends on what each of us contributes this time around). Honing these liberatory possibilities into an aesthetic approach to dance making, Bull constructed improvisational scores as a way to explore the social.

In these chapters, Foster elucidates the cultural differences in how white and black artists used the improvisational strategies coming out of the African-American cultural legacy of survival and resistance. Along with an analysis of various key works by Bull and his collaborators, she discusses the interrelatedness of artists as diverse as Louis Armstrong, Merce Cunningham, the Living Theater, Carolee Schneeman, Second City, Eleo Pomare, Danny Nagrin, Dianne McIntyre, and the Grand Union, among others. While it is intellectually exciting to read a history of the experimental performances of the 1960s and 1970s that builds critical connections between the black arts movement and white avant-garde performance, the elaborate web of comparing and contrasting so many different groups in the midst of a discussion of Bull's work can become unwieldy, creating a certain amount of organizational gridlock and analytical repetition.

In the next chapter, "Economies of Community," however, Foster deftly weaves the history of the Warren Street Performance Loft into a structural analysis of the changing economy of dance making and production from the late 1970s to the 1990s. During this time, Foster asserts, the "landscape of art production" shifted dramatically. Pressured by changes in funding structures and the introduction of corporate sponsorship, artists in the 1980s were forced to create elaborate administrative infrastructures and to package their work in easily marketable ways. Tracing the development of contemporary New York City dance venues such as Dance Theater Workshop (DTW), the Kitchen, PS 122, and Movement Research, Inc., Foster demonstrates how small, informal performance spaces such as Bull's Warren Street Performance Loft (and improvisation in general) lacked the slick profile needed to thrive in the increasingly corporate world of dance production. It was particularly difficult for artists working in improvisation to market a "product" which was, in fact, a "process" that necessarily changed from performance to performance. Elusive, movement improvisation resists commodification; for many of us, that is part of its charm. Even though the Improvisational Arts Ensemble changed its name to Richard Bull Dance Theater in 1985 in an effort to compete effectively in this kind of marketplace, they were unable to really capture the kind of critical attention needed to generate further funding. Nonetheless, the Warren Street Performance Loft became an alternative space for many kinds of improvising, and Bull continued to make and produce work throughout the 1980s and the 1990s.

While the intellectual analysis in these chapters is historically important and critically sophisticated, the soul of Bull's work is found elsewhere—in the margins and in the immortal persona of *The Dance That Describes Itself* (TDTDI). In the introduction and then again in the interlude toward the end of the book, this voice serves to disrupt and dismantle (sometimes just to "dis") the smooth academic tone of the author. Originally invented in 1973 (and revised in 1974 and 1977), TDTDI is a phantom that "possesses" dancers both verbally and physically in order to stage an existential inquiry into the nature of dance. Brought back to life in contrasting font by Foster, the dance takes on a voice in the text that is playful and irreverent, frequently butting in to comment on Foster's assertions and deliver alternative views. "This is all very well and good, but don't think I don't notice you trying to take control of this text, reasserting your reasonable analysis of a transcendent experience."[2] The pleasure of this voice, of course, is that it captures an aspect of Bull's eccentric imagination and it is wonderfully contagious! Early on, Foster relates how SUNY dancers internalized "the dance" to the point that it metamorphosed (in the midst of a scholastic crisis) into *The Dance that Keeps Itself from Flunking Out*. Not only dancers, but also readers can easily become possessed by TDTDI; by the end of the introduction, I too felt that I had been embodied by this persona.

Unfortunately, however, *The Dance That Describes Itself* (having made quite an impression) appears only occasionally in the next few chapters. When it does reappear during the "Interlude: Epistolary Choreographies by the Dance That Describes Itself" our dancing friend seems interested in many of the same questions that inspire Susan Foster's best kind of intellectual analysis. Written in the voice of TDTDI, this smart (but alas, no longer "smart-ass") interlude stages improvisatory encounters between critical theories and various contemporary forms of social dancing. Sure enough, Foucault, Bourdieu, Bakhtin, and de Certeau get to mix it up with the likes of aerobics, breakdancing, and raves. This feisty duet between dance and theory is one of Foster's greatest moments, and as thoughts and movements push and pull one another, she posits the transgressive potential of thoughtful dancing. "The process of making the dance in performance foregrounds our awareness, as performers and as viewers, of the continual attentiveness that is required in order to keep the dance happening. Like democracy, the dance must be made, struggled over, negotiated, reconciled, and reconfigured in perpetuity."[3] Improvisation as Radical Politics. Beginning at the site of a loss, Foster travels back through history to record how the extraordinary dancing of those who have passed away can be reanimated, living on through the pages of a book to describe itself and inspire us all.

1. Susan Foster, *Dances That Describe Themselves: The Improvised Choreography of Richard Bull* (Middletown, CT: Wesleyan University Press, 2002), 70.

2. Ibid., 7.

3. Ibid., 236.

36

Space and Subjectivity

Dance Chronicle 32, no. 9, 2009.

In her seminal essay, "Throwing Like a Girl: A Phenomenology of Feminine Bodily Comportment, Motility, and Spatiality" (1980), feminist philosopher Iris Marion Young connects female bodily uses of space and force to women's social status. Attending to the intricacies of embodied experience, Young identifies three traditional modalities of women's physical being in the world: ambiguous transcendence, inhibited intentionality, and discontinuous unity. Basically, this is fancy language for "throwing like a girl." That is to say, not using one's whole body (using only the forearm instead of the whole torso, shoulder, and arm), not believing you can do it, and not following through (giving up halfway through the throw). Given the ubiquitous exercise regimes most contemporary women subject themselves to, it may be hard to imagine a pre-gym era. But, in fact, it is not that long ago that defined upper-body muscles were considered unfeminine (and working class), and a woman's social grace depended upon the primness of her posture. The dynamic between cultural inscription and individual resistance has long informed women's relationships with their own bodies, and both feminist scholars and dance theorists grapple with the tensions produced by the intersection of cultural habit and movement innovation. How women came to claim their physical subjectivity is also an important part of the history of modern dance.

In her intriguing book, *Rhythmic Subjects: Uses of Energy in the Dances of Mary Wigman, Martha Graham and Merce Cunningham,* Dee Reynolds retraces some of that history in chapters on Mary Wigman and Martha Graham, and then continues into the present by discussing work by Merce Cunningham and new digital technologies. Like Iris Marion Young, Dee Reynolds is interested in the conjunction of experience and representation. The key concept in Reynolds's fascinating interdisciplinary and multilayered approach is energy—a slippery term that is alternately illuminating and vague. "Energy is connected with rhythm through expenditure and economy. Innovative dance rhythms are grounded in changes in energy expenditure through new 'economies' of energy, which can manifest the subject's resistance to constraints and transform the 'self.'"[1] In her introduction,

Reynolds refers to the Greek root of the world, *en* (in) and *ergon* (work) to define energy as "the capacity to perform work."[2]

Yet because her subject is dance (an ambiguously "productive" activity at best), Reynolds also defines energy in movement terms as combinations of force and space. Throughout the book she charts the overlapping of movement invention and cultural transformations within Wigman's, Graham's, and Cunningham's dance techniques and choreography. This concept of energy allows her to connect the "micro" details of movement analysis to the "macro" picture of historical and social contexts. Dee Reynolds is a cultural theorist with a focus on French modernity (her first book was on Symbolist aesthetics and early abstract art) and she writes in an early footnote that, while she is not a dance practitioner, she has studied at the Laban Centre and taken classes in various movement techniques. Understandably, her preferred movement analysis is Rudolf Laban's effort/shape work. In her introduction, Reynolds compares her methodology to one that Jane Desmond calls for in the latter's edited volume, *Meaning in Motion:* "To keep our broader levels of analysis anchored in the materiality and kinesthesia of the dancing body, we need to generate more tools for close readings, and more sophisticated methodologies for shuttling back and forth between the micro (physical) and macro (historical, ideological) levels of movement investigation."[3]

Reynolds's chapter on Mary Wigman, "Opening Rhythms: Spatial Energies in Mary Wigman," is one of her best, partially because Wigman's work lends itself perfectly to an effort/shape analysis and partially because Reynolds uses the burgeoning "body culture" of early twentieth-century Germany to develop her discussion of "kinesthetic imagination." ("Because kinesthetic imagination can be activated through virtual [e.g., empathetic] as well as actual movement, it may be experienced by spectators of dance as well as by dancers themselves."[4]) In this chapter, Reynolds weaves Wigman's conflicted relationships with the modernist aesthetics and restrictive politics of Germany into an analysis of her use of weight, space, and force. Reynolds deftly situates Wigman's reception by the Nazis—for whom she tried to work, but who ultimately dismissed her work as "too philosophical"— as well as her audiences. Discussing the evolution of Wigman's "absolute" dance, Reynolds articulates how Wigman used dynamic space to resist the cultural norms of a constrained and eroticized female body.

The chapter begins with an epigraph by Laban: "Besides the motion of bodies in space there exists motion of space in bodies."[5] Like many of her generation, Wigman was schooled in Dalcroze rhythmic gymnastics, but she turned down an offer to run a Dalcroze school in Berlin in order to work with Laban. Under his tutelage, Wigman expanded her reach as a dancer and began to create short movement studies. In Germany at the beginning of the twentieth century, the term energy connoted a (quasi-mystical) sense of life force that vibrated in people and animated the world. Connecting this cultural fascination with vitalism to Wigman's integrated use of space, Reynolds quotes an extraordinary passage, written by Wigman, in which she describes the dynamic exchange between world and artist. "Like lightning, perhaps just for one second he is caught up in and flooded with the wave of the great current of life, which extinguishes him as an isolated existence and makes him a present of participation in the whole."[6]

In her dancing, Wigman was able to mobilize space beyond her own kinesphere. Spinning, for which she was famous, Wigman could alternately create the centrifugal force and then ride it, at once creating the whirlpool and then enjoying the pleasure of being caught up by it. The breath-like rhythmic phrasing of Wigman's work followed this sequence of ebb and flow, projecting the body into space and then sustaining that movement by bringing a spatial awareness into the body. The resulting representation reflected what Reynolds describes as a "striking conjunction of individuality and universality."[7] By highlighting the shared sensibilities, including neuromuscular pathways, established by a cultural moment in which the body was privileged as a salvational force, Reynolds builds an argument about metakinesis. "Wigman's foregrounding of kinesthetic (and here synesthetic), rather than primarily visual appeal, encouraged the spectator to respond through kinesthetic empathy rather than through objectification of the dancer as an erotic female figure."[8]

Unlike Wigman's fluid exchanges with space, Graham's movement innovations were focused on attack and arrest to provide a vision of a "fierce" female energy. In her chapter on Graham entitled "Virile Rhythms," Reynolds situates this energy as distinctly American, urban and modernist, even masculinist. "Tightness and hardness were entirely characteristic of the effort qualities of Graham's early work, whose vector of energy projection from inside to outside corresponded with contemporary Americanist and masculinist discourses, and constructed a paradoxically "masculinist" feminism, predicated on rhythms of empowerment."[9] This new energy was based on acceleration and consumption, where the body is less likely to find the ecological equilibrium of launching and riding space and more likely to be in conflict with the space, or trying to overcome it. Although movement in Graham's technique is repeatedly initiated in the core and moves to the periphery (from the pelvis to the arm or leg), it does not return from the space back into the body in the same way that Wigman's movement did.

Thus we have the ideological basis for Graham's famously bound flow— her "contraction and release" that is based less on the pastoral ebb and flow of breath rhythms and more on the punch of urban life. One of the most important aspects of Graham's early use of energy was her play with weight and solidity—something that gradually became lost as successive generations of Graham dancers became lighter and more fluid. Reynolds quotes a comment by Dorothy Bird, a first-generation Graham dancer: "Martha told us that when we move, the audience must feel the muscles thrusting against the resistance of our weight."[10] The resulting representation, Reynolds argues, is one of an embodied presence of power and strength. She describes Graham's epic *Frontier* (1935) as an example: "Once again, Graham succeeded in conveying a female person who was both feminine and assertive, female and representative of a male constituency, a 'frontierswoman' who encapsulated the (legendary) experience of the 'frontiersman.'"[11]

Having spent a considerable amount of time discussing the physical experiences and metaphysical images of empowered women in Wigman's and Graham's choreography, Reynolds's chapter on Cunningham, "Punctual Rhythms: Life Energies in Merce Cunningham," has to do some tricky and unexpected footwork to shift the emphasis from her analysis of representations of women as subjects to arguing for Cunningham's representations of dancers as embodying a sort of postmodern mobile subjectivity. In many ways, this intellectual dance (with help from Jacques Derrida and Pierre Bourdieu) is modeled on what she is claiming for Cunningham's work— unexpected shifts of spatial and movement directions, the playfulness of a process based on chance procedures, the nonhierarchical use of body parts, and the decentered visual fields. Unlike earlier chapters, Reynolds tends to flip between historical and aesthetic contexts and discussions of Cunningham's movement innovations without really highlighting the connections between the two. Sometimes, however, there are intriguing glimpses of their interconnectedness.

Early on, for instance, Reynolds suggests that "climates of homophobia, conformism, false projections of intimacy and determinism were among the factors that favored the development of movement strategies through which embodied identities became at once more fluid and flexible and more autonomous and private."[12] But this kind of cultural analysis never gets developed, partially because right at the moment she seems to be about to get somewhere with an argument (something about queer mobility—slipperiness of performance identities?), she quickly shifts directions and drops the subject. What is curious in this chapter, given the kinds of thorough analyses in the earlier ones, is that Reynolds so often uses Cunningham's and Cage's own words to talk about what they do. This, even after relating a skeptical comment by Carolyn Brown (whose recent memoir, *Chance and Circumstance,* should make any analysis of Cunningham's work more complicated with regard to issues of hierarchy and gendered dynamics) that "You shouldn't believe everything that is said to you."[13] While I find some of Reynolds's connections intriguing (applications of Derridean *différance* and discussion of Maurice Merleau-Ponty), I still find it hard to parse some of her liberatory claims for Cunningham's choreography with the kinds of traditionally gendered partnering and very traditional notions of virtuosity and line that comprises the backbone of Cunningham's choreography.

Like many in my generation, I spent the last two decades of the twentieth century training in various dance techniques, including Graham and Cunningham in college and Wigman-inspired classes in graduate school (by Helmut Gottschild, one of the Wigman dancers whom Reynolds interviews). When I first moved to New York City, I studied at the Cunningham studio. And I spent a lot of that time thinking about representations of subjectivity in dance. For me, the intersection of cultural theory and movement analysis that Reynolds is charting in her book resounds both physically and intellectually. I believe wholeheartedly in her project: exploring how energy—the somatic elements of space and force—shapes human experiences of subjectivity in movement. The catch, though, is that while the kinesthetic imagination of a movement vocabulary can lead to one set of meanings, how that technique is mobilized within choreography can carry vastly different meanings depending on the other representational frames involved. Thus, even though I relished the multidimensionality and excitement of executing the challenging phrases taught in the Cunningham studio, I was often astonished to see how little of that experience was translated within the formalist aesthetics and technological frameworks of Cunningham's set work. What starts as a quirky and postmodern movement curiosity can often look like pretty standard virtuosity by the time it gets onstage. Nonetheless, I appreciate Reynolds's willingness to deal with the contradictions that arise when one engages both a close reading of movement techniques and a broader analysis of choreography. In its careful attention to both kinesthetic imagination and cultural context, *Rhythmic Subjects* gives us an important blueprint for a true dancing theory.

NOTES

1. Dee Reynolds, *Rhythmic Subjects: Uses of Energy in the Dances of Mary Wigman, Martha Graham and Merce Cunningham* (Hampshire, England: Dance Books, Ltd., 2007), 1.

2. Ibid., 3.

3. Jane Desmond, *Meaning in Motion* (Durham, NC: Duke University Press, 1997), 2.

4. Reynolds, 1.

5. Ibid., 43.

6. Ibid., 67.

7. Ibid., 83.

8. Ibid., 87.

9. Ibid., 97.

10. Ibid., 108.

11. Ibid., 135.

12. Ibid., 141.

13. Ibid., 149.

37

Strategic Practices

Dance Research Journal 44, no. 2, 2012.

Improvisation is an elusive subject. Despite much late twentieth-century and early twenty-first-century dancing being deeply intertwined with a variety of improvisational practices, there is a regrettable paucity of books dealing with this slippery and yet seductive topic. Even though there has been a veritable explosion of dance scholarship over the past three decades, the written texts dealing with movement improvisation are still limited to various how-to manuals for dance educators, or books that deal with one particular individual without situating their work within a historical and aesthetic context. There are, of course, a few memorable exceptions, such as Susan Foster's delightful and brilliant exegesis on the work of Richard Bull (*Dances That Describe Themselves: The Improvised Choreography of Richard Bull*), but these are few and far between.

Fortunately 2010 was a banner year for dance improvisation, producing two new books: Melinda Buckwalter's *Composing While Dancing: An Improviser's Companion* and Danielle Goldman's *I Want To Be Ready: Improvised Dance as a Practice of Freedom*. Melinda Buckwalter is a dancer, writer, and contributing editor to *Contact Quarterly*. She has personally studied with many of the twenty-six dance artists whose teaching and performance work she documents in her "improviser's companion." Danielle Goldman is an assistant professor at The New School, and her contribution to the literature on improvisation is an academic text that began as her dissertation in the Performance Studies department at New York University's Tisch School of the Arts. Both books reflect the specific orientations of their respective writers: one is interested in getting more people moving and improvising; the other is interested in building an intellectual analysis of the notion of "freedom" in dance improvisation via a series of case studies. Understandably, these books are directed to different audiences and it is unlikely that there will be much crossover between those two readerships. This is unfortunate, for I feel that it is high time we close the gap between the language of practitioners and that of theorists in order to begin a dialogue within improvisation that includes both the kinetic pleasures of the moving body and the valuable insights that critical theory can bring to practice.

On its back cover, *Composing While Dancing* promotes itself as a "practical primer to the dance form." By introducing the life work of twenty-six artists whose teaching and performing focuses primarily on improvisation, Buckwalter highlights the importance of this multifaceted exploration in contemporary dance. Her user-friendly how-to approach is underscored not only in the enthusiastic tone of the writing—punctuated by exclamations such as "If you aren't already, start improvising!"[1]—but also in the manual-like organization of the information. In addition to sections dealing with various approaches to space, time, music, shape, and image, there are short biographies of the artists, a glossary of terms, and a section at the end of each chapter featuring practices for future research. These simple step-by-step instructions—"How is time passing for you right now? Think up a movement practice for yourself that might shift the way you feel time. See if it works . . ."[2]—are surrounded by tidbits of personal and poetic reflections in her self-described "Field Notes" and "Interludes."

The bulk of each chapter is composed of short segments documenting the practices that fit within its respective thematic rubric. For instance, in the chapter titled "Dancing Takes Shape," we are exposed to glimpses of the work of Anna Halprin, Deborah Hay, Eiko and Koma, Steve Paxton, Richard Bull, Keith Hennessy, Nina Martin, Penny Campbell, Susan Sgorbati, Mary Overlie, Lisa Nelson, Prapto, and Barbara Dilley—all in twenty pages of text. Needless to say, none of these mini-discussions (sometimes a mere two paragraphs) are able to develop into nuanced, complex, or critical evaluations of an artist's work or a comparison of different approaches to the exploration of music, for example. A number of these artists show up in many other sections as well, making for an oddly erratic flip-book of information and a certain amount of repetition. It is hard to get a sense of the complexity of someone's work by reading two or three paragraphs in four different chapters. For instance, Nina Martin's work with improvisational ensembles is touched on in chapters 1–5 and 7, while Pooh Kaye is mentioned only briefly in a section on using objects in improvisation. Given the truncated nature of those two paragraphs representing Kaye's film and performance work, one wonders why Kaye was included at all, until a glance at the biography section reveals that she and the author collaborated on a duet while Buckwalter was in graduate school at Bennington College.

The author's choice of the artists included is explained in her introduction: "The dancemakers included here are not an exhaustive list of those working in the field of improvisation by any means; the selection represents the web of my relatively local activities, mostly confined to the East Coast of the United States. My selections represent only specific cross-sections of the artists' work."[3] Here, personal preference stands in for the writer's methodology in peculiar and opaque ways. Given the glaring omission of any African-American improvisers such as Dianne McIntyre or Ishmael Houston-Jones within this book, the short section in the introduction, "Gaining Cultural

Perspective," presents an obfuscated apology for not bothering to research further than the author's proverbial neighborhood. Also, the uneven and sporadic discussions of the central figures such as Nina Martin, Lisa Nelson, and Steve Paxton make it difficult to develop any sense of continuity within the work of individuals who are discussed at some length. As a book, *Composing While Dancing*'s structure is awkward, and I feel that the list-like delivery of information would be better served in a website format, where hyperlinks could facilitate reading about an individual artist's work across chapters based on thematic concerns.

For me, the most compelling chapters in *Composing While Dancing* were the later ones, "The Eyes" and "Performing Science." I was particularly interested in the rich discussion of Lisa Nelson's work in a subsection entitled "The Kinesthetics of Seeing." As a long time coeditor of *Contact Quarterly,* Lisa Nelson is one of the most important, yet frequently under-recognized figures in the development of contemporary improvisation. Her work in video and her focus on how we learn to see movement has influenced multiple generations of dancers, improvisers, and choreographers. The descriptions of her "Tuning Scores"—her signature approach to spontaneous composition—open up a much-needed discussion of representational images that balances the book's emphasis on sensation and improvisational process.

I also appreciated that *Composing While Dancing* was, as the author explains, "researched with my body." The field notes sections in each chapter were particularly evocative. In these, Buckwalter reflects on her own experience learning from many of the artists profiled. I was especially drawn to her discussions of the moments when a particular approach to improvisation created a bit of friction for her and rubbed against her kinesthetic preferences. For instance, in speaking of Nina Martin's "Ensemble Thinking Workshop," she writes:

> However, a few dancers from somatic studies backgrounds (like myself) had trouble separating the compositional dialogue from the developing of movement material; the two were entwined in our training . . . I was reserved but willing to go for the ride, and though I found it difficult at times, I was curious about how the other side of the coin liked to work.
>
> And it did end up working for me. I found that I had to let go of my comfort zone at first, but what I knew deeply still served me. Martin's work offered me a way of getting up to speed—if reluctantly—and taught me, most importantly, how to shift gears.[4]

Improvisation as a negotiation of friction, of uncomfortable or difficult situations—what Danielle Goldman characterizes as "tight places"—is the central theme of *I Want To Be Ready*. In this book, Goldman refuses the all too common assumption that movement improvisation, by removing the most obvious structures of technique or composition, leads to an expressive freedom unfettered by society or history. Instead, Goldman claims improvisation's potential as a strategic practice of intervention into these power regimes, describing it as "a full-bodied critical engagement with the world, characterized by both flexibility and perpetual readiness."[5] Following Houston Baker's use of the term "tight place," she asks, "Who moves and who doesn't?" in order to highlight the ways in which one's sociohistorical position affects one's mobility.

Through a series of case studies that, once again, were chosen on the basis of personal preference ("Early in this project, . . . I decided to write only about improvised dancing that I wanted to spend time watching"[6]), Goldman argues that improvisation constitutes a technology of selfhood precisely because of its appetite for movement in the presence of constraints. *I Want To Be Ready* looks at examples of this response-ability from different social and theatrical performances in the second half of the twentieth century. She analyzes the improvised dancing at New York City's Palladium Ballroom in the 1940s and 1950s, the connections between the 1960s nonviolent protest techniques and certain aspects of the training in contact improvisation, various collaborations between dancers and jazz musicians, and Bill T. Jones's return to improvisation in his *The Breathing Show*.

Although improvisation is a woefully under-studied field, the books that do exist represent the Judson Dance Theater and Grand Union, Steve Paxton and the development of contact improvisation, and that generation of like-minded dancer/improvisers, from multiple perspectives. Even Bill T. Jones's improvisational work has received a fair amount of press. But little has been done with movement improvisation's relationship with music, or the group of dancers working in collaboration with jazz musicians in the 1960s and 1970s. Therefore it was with a sense of relief (finally) and a great deal of scholarly curiosity that I read chapter 2, "We Insist! Seeing Music and Hearing Dance," which focuses on the performing and teaching work of Judith Dunn and Bill Dixon, as well as that of Dianne McIntyre's group, Sounds in Motion.

In this chapter, Goldman rewrites the narrow and often whitewashed history of postmodern improvisation that begins with the members of Robert Ellis Dunn's famous choreographic workshops at the Cunningham studio. Along with Steve Paxton, Yvonne Rainer, Trisha Brown, Simone Forti, Deborah Hay, Elaine Summers, and the like, Judith Dunn (who was married to Bob Dunn at the time) was also attending Bob Dunn's composition classes and dancing with the Cunningham Company. Soon, however, she met Bill Dixon—a multifaceted African-American musician working with various writers, poets, and media artists in the black vanguard. Besides performing together in a number of different venues, Dixon and Dunn taught together extensively, including at Bennington College, where Dixon founded the Black Music Division.

Dianne McIntyre's work with musicians and dancers in her company Sounds in Motion has also been underrepresented in the history of improvisation and dance history in general. Fortunately, this is beginning to change, mostly because McIntyre keeps on making work well into her seventh decade. Goldman's elucidations of how McIntyre negotiated the racism of modern dance as well as the politically charged sexism of the time (which equated blackness with masculinity) show how connected the strategic skills of improvisation were with McIntyre's ability to survive in a context that often excluded her. In addition, the descriptions of McIntyre's seminal collaboration with Abbey Lincoln and Max Roach help bring a new attention to this less well-known chapter of American dance.

Dianne McIntyre moved back to Cleveland from New York City about a decade ago, and since then I have had the pleasure of getting to know this fierce and determined doyenne of African-American dance in person. Seeing McIntyre continue to perform improvisation and choreograph for others at the age when most people have retired (her most recent premiere was the choreography for a new choreo-poem by Ntazake Shange), made me fully appreciate Goldman's comment in the book's conclusion that: "Improvised dance literally involves giving shape to oneself and deciding how to move in relation to an unsteady landscape. To go about this endeavor with a sense of confidence and possibility is a powerful way to inhabit one's body and interact with the world."[7]

I read these two books on improvisation while teaching physical mindfulness and contact improvisation for seven weeks in Greece (the first three weeks in Athens among the demonstrations). Certainly Goldman's ideas about improvisation as a negotiation of "tight places" resonated in this context of austerity and revolt. Sometimes space was materially tight, with thirty-three people crammed into a small studio; at other times it was psychically tight, because many of the participants were fighting a feeling of apathy. Working with various communities of professional and student dancers, it was clear to me that improvisation opened up spaces that were more meaningful in the present context than some of the more traditional modern and ballet dance techniques which still dominate in many dance schools in Greece. Indeed, the skills embedded in many techniques of contemporary improvisation provide important strategies for making connections between our physical experiences of dancing and how we live in the world. In that sense, I found the thoughts of anthropologist Angeles Arrien cited in the last pages of Buckwalter's *Composing While Dancing* particularly useful when introducing a round-robin at an Athens Contact Jam. I suggested that we follow her cardinal rules:[8]

1. Show up.
2. Pay attention.
3. Tell the truth.
4. Don't get attached to the results.

As both these books make clear, this is excellent advice for dancing, as well as living, in the twenty-first century.

NOTES

1. Melinda Buckwalter, *Composing While Dancing: An Improviser's Companion,* (Madison: University of Wisconsin Press, 2010), 5.
2. Ibid., 73.
3. Ibid., 4.
4. Ibid., 72.
5. Danielle Goldman, *I Want To Be Ready: Improvised Dance as a Practice of Freedom* (Ann Arbor: University of Michigan Press, 2010), 5.
6. Ibid., 139.
7. Ibid., 146.
8. Buckwalter, 157.

38

Resurrecting the Future

Body/Image/Technology

Screendance Conference, American Dance Festival, July 2006.

I feel compelled to begin with a confession. I am, by nature, a technophobe. Physically addicted to moving in real time and space, politically committed to supporting live performance, I tend to resist screens of all kinds. I mean it: I am so bad I still write first drafts with a pen and paper. When I began my book on Loïe Fuller, little did I imagine that the research for the last chapter would bring me—of all people—to a conference on Screendance at the American Dance Festival. Yet, as we shall see, Fuller's innovative use of light and motion (the two essential elements of any screendance) prefigured many twenty-first-century experiments with these same elements. In addition, the critical reception of her work in the late nineteenth and early twentieth centuries parallels in enlightening ways contemporary dialogues about dance and technology. At the core of these discussions lies the complex relationship between physical expression and visual abstraction, between body and image in dance.

Loïe Fuller's early works such as the *Serpentine Dance* and *Fire Dance* embody a central paradox of dance as a representation of both abstract movement and a physical body. Her dancing epitomizes the intriguing insubstantiality of movement caught in the process of tracing itself. Surrounded by a funnel of swirling fabric spiraling upwards into the space around her and bathed in colored lights of her own invention, Fuller's body seems to evaporate in the midst of her spectacle. Because of this, many scholars cover over the kinesthetic and material experience of her body in favor of the image, rather than reading that image as an extension of her dancing. Descriptions of her work get so entangled with artistic images or poetic renderings of her serpentine spirals and multicolored lights that they easily forget the physical labor involved. Then too, there are all those apologies and side notes about how Loïe Fuller did not have a dancer's body, or any dance training really, as if the movement images were solely dependent on the lighting, as if it were all technologically rendered. (One typical example: "The influence of Loïe Fuller upon the theater will always be felt, particularly in the lighting of the scene and in the disposition of draperies. *But she was never a great dancer. She was an apparition.*"[1] There is an odd urgency in my responses to these commentaries; my whole body revolts with the somatic knowledge that something else was going on.

What was going on, of course, was a performance that confused conventional ways of looking at dance, one that turned on a completely new movement vocabulary based on a series of strategic movement impulses. Not only did Fuller's work eliminate the poses and aesthetic placement of limbs in steps and gestures, but it also used the body sequentially. Working with suspensions and momentum, Fuller initiated a twist in her torso that swirled through the upper body to lift the fabric. She then rode that motion, recognizing through trial and error when she needed to move again. If she moved too soon, the suspension was cut short and the expansive billowing of fabric was truncated. Similarly, if she hesitated, the fabric gained too much momentum in its descent that made it that much harder to get back up into the air. This was a little like riding a bike—knowing exactly when to pedal and when to coast. Because Fuller quickly mastered the complex figure-eight coordination necessary to keep one side or another of her costume billowing in the air, it was the serpentine figures in the air, rather than her body, that became the focus of the audience's gaze. As Giovanni Lista makes clear in his comments on Fuller's early choreography:

> The veil becomes the space for the lines until it is no more than the surface on which, as in Art Nouveau, the pure lines appear. The dancer's body is completely absent, all the while being absolutely present as a force creating waves of lines. It is at precisely this moment that her vital soaring is closest to her being: a pure energy revealing and inscribing the movements of life, the manifestations of the spirit, and the very impossibility of representing it through depictions of nature.[2]

This description of Fuller's dancing as figurative lines drawn in space presents us with a historical example of the intriguing vacillation between absence and presence, body and image at play in much contemporary screendance.

Like any new genre of art, Fuller's innovations required a different method of looking. In his essay, "Torque: The New Kinaesthetic of the Twentieth Century," Hillel Schwartz delineates similar patterns of perceiving movement in many aspects of early twentieth-century life:

> Motion pictures, like modern dance, corporeal mime and, soon, the schools of naturalistic or Stanislavskian acting, demanded much more than a simple reading of one discrete attitude after another. They demanded a reading of the body in motion and an appreciation of the full impulse of that motion.[3]

Loïe Fuller's dancing has been described by many twentieth-century scholars as a precursor to film—a way of placing lights on a moving screen, rather than moving images on a stationary screen. What interests me most in this context, however, is how the early twentieth-century audience eventually learned to see expressive emotion in the midst of continuous motion. Watching Fuller's dancing, spectators were led to attend not to the poses at the end of a musical phrase, but rather to the motion between phrases; not to the decorative arrangement of arms and legs, but to the sequence of movement from center to periphery and back again. I believe that this ability to stream back and forth from core to periphery and from figure to ground is a critical aspect of watching movement onstage at the beginning of the twentieth century, as well as on-screen at the beginning of the twenty-first century:

> In the terrible bath of fabrics fans out, radiant, cold, the performer who illustrates many spinning themes from which extends a distant fading warp, giant petal and butterfly, unfurling, all in a clear and elemental way. Her fusion with the nuances of speed shedding their lime-light phantasmagoria of dusk and grotto, such rapidity of passions, delight, mourning, anger; to move them prismatic, with violence or diluted, it takes the vertigo of a soul as if airborne on artifice.[4]

This famous depiction of Fuller's dancing by Stéphane Mallarmé could easily be mistaken for a description of *Le Lys de la Vie*—Fuller's first foray into cinema. Produced in 1921, with the assistance of her artistic collaborator and life partner, Gab Sorère, this film expands upon many of Fuller's earlier theatrical experiments, even as it weaves these visual effects into a cinematic narrative. *Le Lys de la Vie* was a children's story written by Queen Marie of Romania, a close friend of Loïe Fuller, and was first staged in Paris in 1920 as a movement theater piece. It was later reprised onstage at the Metropolitan Opera House in October 1926 as a tribute to Queen Marie, who was then visiting America.

Le Lys de la Vie is a classic fairy tale of unrequited love, complete with a heroic quest that comprises the entire second half of the narrative. For the film, the staged choreography and effects were transposed to the landscape of southern France, where idyllic gardens, sun-dappled woods, and the ocean provide the backdrop for this story of two princesses competing for the love of a handsome prince in search of a wife. The prince's sudden illness prompts Corona, the more adventurous one, to journey across wild and fantastic lands in search of a magical "Lily of Life." She is aided in her quest by the fantastic creatures of the forest, who immediately recognize the purity of her soul. She finds the miraculous flower and revives the prince who, alas, falls in love with the sister. In despair, Corona runs off to the woods and dies of a broken heart, but her body is retrieved by the fairies and carried off, presumably to join their world.

Hailed as a "miracle cinématographique" *Le Lys de la Vie* interrupts this rather banal narrative with spectacular special effects—many of which had not been used previously in the cinema. In addition to her usual repertoire of lighting options, including underlighting and sophisticated shadow-puppet effects, Fuller spliced negative images directly into the film, creating intriguing juxtapositions of light and dark, as well as breathtaking images of another world. She also played with slow motion, creating that suspended atmosphere by instructing her dancers to move slowly as the cinematographer cranked the film as fast as possible. Reviewers were enthusiastic, describing her work as enchanting, dreamlike, a miracle of grace, and a masterpiece. Tellingly, M. Borie writes in *La Liberté*: "Miss Loïe Fuller finds an intensity of effect and expression in a pastoral simplicity that highlights her thoughts and gestures, as well as her use of light and visual perspective, it captures the eye and the imagination of the spectator. Here, she obtains effects that have never been seen before . . . Miss Loïe Fuller has created a poem written with light and shadow, a poem that comes from an art so noble and so pure that none can rest insensitive to its crystalline beauty."[5]

We have arrived at a crossroads here. Given more time, I would love to discuss how a later film, *La Féerie des Ballets fantastiques de Loïe Fuller,* which was completed in 1934 after Fuller's death, pushed Fuller's cinematic innovations even further, disrupting the cinematic gaze in ways that prefigured the feminist film analyses of the 1980s. Similarly, I could talk about how Fuller's experimental techniques had a profound influence on the French avant-garde cinema—particularly in the work of René Clair and that of Germaine Dulac. Or, I could follow up on Julie Townsend's intriguing assertion that *Le Lys de la Vie* is the "most explicit development of the 'queer' in Fuller's work."[6] All these possibilities are fascinating, and provide important perspectives on the cultural currency of Fuller's allure. At present, however, inspired by M. Borie's reading of Fuller's film as a poem, I have decided to return to Mallarmé's evocations of Fuller's work in order to explore a central theme in screendance—the paradoxical absence of body, yet presence of figure. Specifically, I want to consider a critical question for mediated dance: When the body is absent, what constitutes its movement signature? And how do we learn to read that signature as a cipher for a (once) live body?

> To understand that the dancer *is not a woman dancing,* for the juxtaposed causes that she *is not a woman,* but a metaphor summarizing one of the elementary aspects of our form, sword, cup, flower, etc., and *that she does not dance,* suggesting, by ellipsis or élan, with a corporeal writing that would necessitate paragraphs of prose in dialogue as well as description to express, in the rewriting: poem disengaged from all writing apparatus.[7]

It would be easy to dismiss this famous passage by Mallarmé as erasing the material body of the female dancer. As a metaphor, she floats in space, disconnected from the hand that writes. But today, I am interested in asking, what does she leave behind? For Mallarmé, the reflection on the other side of the French intransitive verb *is*—that is to say, "not a woman dancing," is disrupted by an intriguing prepositional phrase, "with a corporeal writing" (*une écriture corporelle*). Thus, even as she is disembodied, the dancer leaves a signature, like a ghost writing from beyond the page. I am interested in this idea of "corporeal writing," both in terms of Fuller's legacy, and in terms of visual iconographies common in screendance, particularly those generated by motion capture technologies. Before I elaborate on the comparisons of this *écriture corporelle* with something like *Ghostcatching*, however, let us consider another kind of trace left by Loïe Fuller.

On June 11, 1916, Loïe Fuller inscribed the first page of her new autograph book with her own "corporeal writing." Entitled *The Ghosts of My Friends*, this leather-bound volume instructs its readers to "sign your name along the fold of the paper with a full pen of ink, and then double the page over without using blotting paper." The result, when turned vertical instead of horizontal, is a Rorschach-like image that is, quite literally, an embodied signature. For, although they are not mimetically representative, these insignias do look, in some weird way, like little skeletons. The symmetry of these figures and their loops and strokes resemble limbs and ribs, and it is fairly easy to distinguish shoulder girdles and pelvises. The friends who signed Fuller's book include August Rodin, Rose Beuret, Flora Haile, May Cobbs, and Rudolph Valentino. Now, although these writings do not represent in any direct way the bodies of the signers, they do figure as little traces of an embodied signature. Fascinating hieroglyphs, their obliqueness is impossible to translate, but incredibly seductive—they are images that stay with you, crying out for interpretation.

I would like to suggest that this early twentieth-century exercise in ghostwriting is a precursor of contemporary experiments like *Ghostcatching*—the 1999 collaboration between Bill T. Jones, Paul Kaiser, and Shelley Eshkar. At the heart of this comparison lies the whole question of a dancing signature, the question about whether there is such an identifiable trace for each body that remains after the body is gone, and, if so, how do we capture it? My research suggests that many of the discussions of *Ghostcatching* focus on the tension between Jones's usual focus on the cultural markers of identity on his body, and the visual abstraction of his virtual "ghosts." In her essay on *Ghostcatching*, subtitled "An Intersection of Technology, Labor and Race," Danielle Goldman quotes Jones as he addresses an audience of university students and asks: "Do you see the sexual preference of the person, the race of the person, the gender of the person, and then, can you see what they're doing?"[8] This kind of double vision that Jones identifies is especially crucial in performances like his 2002 solo, *The Breathing Show*, in which he juxtaposes his bodily presence—his breath, voice, movements, and sweat—with the visual traces of his virtual self. But what happens, we must ask, when all that is left are those virtual lines of light and motion? How can we reembody them? Or do we even want to?

To address this question, I would like to return to Mallarmé's notion of a corporeal writing and ask what it would mean to "read" *Ghostcatching* not with nostalgia for what has been lost, but rather with sensibility for what might be gained in the translation between body and line. Felicia McCarren points to this intriguing possibility when she suggests: "The dance comes closer to the Mallarméan poetics of an ideal theater by making-present, rather than visually representing . . . It provides the spectator with the opportunity to imagine, rather than simply to see."[9] I believe that this notion of making present without representing is crucial for us today, for it calls for a more active witnessing. In an essay on *Ghostcatching* evocatively titled "Absent/Presence," Ann Dils echoes this sentiment when she explains how, in the midst of all the co-motion sponsored by Jones's traces and their spawns, she felt that her own role as spectator was "unusually active."[10]

Similarly, because her dancing presented an ongoing transformation of shapes that never solidified into literal representations, Fuller asked her audience to look differently, to follow the contours of her bodily writing without stabilizing its meaning. If we take our cue from Mallarmé's reading of her dancing as script, we can begin to look at contemporary works like *Ghostcatching* with another kind of lens. We can learn to follow those moving signatures in a way that carries kinesthetic perception at its core, thus implicating both the past and the future in a new visual economy.

NOTES

1. J. E. Crawford Flitch, *Modern Dancing and Dancers* (Philadelphia: J. B. Lippincott, 1912), 72.

2. Giovanni Lista, *Loïe Fuller: Danseuse de la belle époque* (Paris: Editions Stock, 1994), 288.

3. Hillel Schwartz, "Torque: the New Kinesthetic of the Twentieth Century," in *Zone 6 (Incorporations),* ed. Crary and Quinter (New York: Urzone, 1992), 101.

4. Stéphane Mallarmé, *Oeuvres Complètes* (Paris: Bibliotheque de la Pleiade, 1945), 596.

5. Program from l'Arsenal archives.

6. Julie Ann Townsend, "The Choreography of Modernism in France: The Female Dancer in Artistic Production and Aesthetic, 1830–1925," PhD diss., University of California, Los Angeles, 2001, 152.

7. Mallarmé, 304.

8. Danielle Goldman, "Ghostcatching: An Intersection of Technology, Labor and Race," *Dance Research Journal* 35, no. 2 (Winter 2003): 71.

9. Felicia McCarren, "Stephen Mallarmé, Loïe Fuller, and the Theater of Femininity," in *Bodies of the Text,* ed. Ellen Goellner and Jacqueline Shea Murphy (New Brunswick, NJ: Rutgers University Press, 1995), 221.

10. Ann Dils, "Absent/Presence," in *Moving History/Dancing Cultures,* ed. Ann Dils and Ann Cooper Albright (Middletown, CT: Wesleyan University Press, 2001), 468.

39

F
   A
      L
      L
         I
         N
            G . . . ON SCREEN

International Journal of Screendance, Spring 2011.

> The expression, "fall from grace," becomes an impossible statement when
> falling itself is experienced as a state of grace.
> —NANCY STARK SMITH

By the time she wrote these words as part of an editor's note for the fall
1979 issue of *Contact Quarterly*, Nancy Stark Smith had been practicing
falling for seven years. From 1972 and the beginning performances of contact improvisation at the John Weber Gallery in New York City until 1979,
her body had learned to experience the momentum of a descent without
clenching up or contracting with fear. She had internalized the trained reflexes of extending one's limbs to spread the impact over a larger surface
area and was able to adapt instinctually to seemingly endless variations of
the passage from up to down.

    This essay traces falling—that passage from up to down—on screens and
in contemporary dance by looking at examples of screendance from the last
three decades of the twentieth century in order to think about the meaning
of falling at the beginning of the twenty-first century. The genesis of my
inquiry comes from a larger project on contemporary embodiment called
Gravity Matters. In what follows, I focus specifically on the representation
of falling as a state of being suspended between earth and air, the finite
and the infinite. I am interested in how falling on screen can help us see the
moments of a fall that are often unaccounted for in live performance, and
how the visualization of that "gap" can be theorized. As Nancy Stark Smith
suggests:

Where you are when you don't know where you are is one of the most precious spots offered by improvisation. It is a place from which more directions are possible that anywhere else. I call this place the Gap . . . Being in a gap is like being in a fall before you touch bottom. You're suspended—in time as well as space—and you don't really know how long it'll take to get "back."[1]

Because screendance is able to visualize that suspension in time as well as space, it may, in fact, help us to think about aspects of falling off the screen, in situations where gravity really does matter.

What I share with my screendance colleagues whose writing is included in this inaugural issue of the *Screendance Journal* is an interest in delineating the interconnected spheres of screen technologies and dance. Indeed, the parallel development of early cinema and modern dance at the beginning of the twentieth century highlights their mutual influence. As many books and articles attest, both art forms shaped new ways of seeing the kinesthetic dimensions of a visual experience. Oddly enough, at the turn of the twentieth century, even as new technologies of editing and distribution were making screendance ubiquitous, an anachronistic nostalgia for the presence of a live unmediated body took hold in some areas of the dance field and set up an unfortunate opposition between "real" dancing bodies and their filmed images. My research in both early and late twentieth-century dance has convinced me that this attitude does not account for the important and fruitful exchanges of movement information between the two genres. I believe that screens can influence how we think about live bodies just as the dancing bodies have revolutionized movement on camera. One of my purposes here is to chart the ways that film and video help dancers see what they are doing, making visible moments of a fall that were previously unavailable to analysis. This iconography of the space in between up and down is elaborated by an approach to falling on screens that shifted historically from act (in the 1970s), to impact (in the 1980s), to suspension (in the 1990s), to a leveling out of the difference between up and down (in the 2000s).

The evolution of Nancy Stark Smith's falling paralleled the development of contact improvisation. In 1972, when a crew of assorted college students and dancers (including Smith) were experimenting under the guidance of Steve Paxton, contact improvisation looked like an exercise in throwing and catching bodies that mostly crashed to the ground on the large wrestling mat. By 1979, the form had evolved into a major influence on contemporary dance, with a professional group of teacher/performers and an ever-expanding collection of skills—falling being a primary one. During the weeklong tenth-anniversary series of performances at St. Marks Danspace in New York City (1983), the signature virtuosic moves of contact improvisation—spinning shoulder lofts and falls that looped to the floor only to cycle back up into the air—were much in evidence.

Interestingly enough, much of this early work was documented by Steve Christiansen on video (open reel half-inch) and the edited complications of this material in *Chute* (1975) and *Fall After Newton* (1987) are well-known and widely distributed. Although each video has spoken narration by Steve Paxton describing the development of contact improvisation, they differ radically from one another, both in terms of content and editing. *Chute* is essentially a ten-minute distillation of seventy-five hours of practice for the first contact improvisation concert in June 1972. The video is grainy black-and-white footage shot close to the dancers. In this early collection of different exercises we see a bunch of young people trying out the possibilities of launching one's body into the arms of a partner. These experiments with catching, falling, and dancing in physical contact often end up in awkward positions or clunky splats. The overall feeling of the work has a palpable sense of curiosity; a frankness with failed attempts that seems to say, "Well, that didn't work, let's try again."

Fall After Newton, in contrast, is elaborately and smoothly edited. The video traces eleven years of contact improvisation through an almost exclusive focus on Nancy Stark Smith's dancing. The preface to the transcript of Paxton's authoritative narration (included in the commercial video) explains: "The great fortune of having video coverage of performances from the very beginning offered the possibility of examining one dancer's development and looking for corresponding growth in the dance form itself." The video begins with over a minute of Smith perched on Paxton's shoulders as he spins quickly. This long sequence from 1983 sets up the implicit narrative of virtuosity as both the text and the editing also showcase Smith's spectacular dancing, particularly her falling. As the viewer is treated to an extraordinary series of smoothly layered shots of Smith falling from the shoulders of Curt Siddall, Steve Paxton, and Danny Lepkoff, Paxton notes: "Higher momentum brings new areas of risk. In order to develop this aspect of the form we had to be able to survive it." Smith's falls are looped together into one long sequence with regular pauses and then in slow motion, before returning to real time.

The final section includes several slow repetitions of a particularly intense fall where Smith lands directly on her back. Although the fall is slowed down to demonstrate Paxton's narration ("During this very disorienting fall, Nancy's arms manage to cradle her back, and this spreads the impact onto a greater area. And she doesn't stop moving. That helps to disperse the impact over a slightly longer time"), the viewer can still see the impact reverberate through her body, even as she rolls (now in real time) out of it and keeps dancing. Paxton's unintentionally patronizing comment "She doesn't seem bothered," elicits snorts and laughter from my students every time I show the video. And yet the slow motion repetition, combined with Paxton's articulation of how to survive that moment of disorientation, really helps my students visualize the possibility of expanding their attention within a fall. As Smith relates in her editor's note: "When I first started falling by choice, I noticed a blind spot. Somewhere after the beginning and before the end of the fall, there was darkness." Working from image backwards to sensation, viewers can learn from her example how to stay in the light.

The slow-motion falling on screen that is a hallmark of *Fall After Newton* has a precedent in televised sports. From the early days of the *Wide World of Sports,* where the "thrill of victory" was always paired with "the agony of defeat"—a shot of a skier or runner wiping out in spectacular manner— to the almost animation-like effect of high-definition instant replays, mediatized sporting events have always broadcast slow-motion falls. More and more these shots, like the slow-motion gunshots in popular movies, transform something essentially awful into abstractly beautiful effect. In sports, however, the camera usually returns to the live action with scenes of the player being carted off the field and pans to the worried look on the coach or girlfriend, before cutting to a beer commercial. Slow-motion replays are now habitual in professional sporting events, especially in basketball, where even at a live game most of the viewers are watching the enormous screens to see what "really happened" in those split seconds before the foul. Early on in the development of the work, Steve Paxton once compared watching contact improvisation to watching sports, where you watch with a relaxed attention until some exciting move pulls you to the edge of your seat.

This comparison between sports and dance and their media legacies is more than coincidental, of course. During the late 1980s and the 1990s, certain genres of contemporary dance (what I tend to call the Euro crash-and-burn aesthetic) highlighted a physically virtuosic, intensely driven body. Édouard Lock's company, La La La Human Steps, from Montreal, is one well-known example of this approach to the human body this side of the Atlantic. His main dancer is Louise Lecavalier, who has the profile and attitude of a prima ballerina-cum-rock star, and it is her extraordinary dancing that drives his increasingly "mega" media extravaganzas such as *Infante c'est destroy.* Produced in 1991 (choreography is much too plebian a term for what actually transpires onstage), this dance and rock event toured internationally for several years.

Throughout this nonstop seventy-five-minute spectacle, Lecavalier's body—both its hardened aerobic energy and its filmed image—is continuously on display. Pitted against the pounding sounds of Skinny Puppy, Janitors Animated, David Van Tiegham, and Einsturzende Neubauten, her dancing uses the driving beat of the music to stretch dance movements to the outer limits of physical possibility and endurance. Over and over again Lecavalier launches her body across the stage, flying through the air like a human torpedo. She gets caught by another dancer, thrashes around with him for a while, then vaults out of his arms, only to rebound back seconds later. Her body spends more time catapulting horizontally than it does moving vertically. Sometimes she is caught and guided to the floor by her partner (as in Smith's falls), but most of the time her body is so tightly coiled that she practically bounces off the floor and back into another lateral vault.

In another context, I have analyzed with some care the heavy metal iconography and gender dynamic of *Infante c'est destroy*.[2] I return to this work now with a slightly different intent. For the purposes of this essay, I am curious about the contrast between Lecavalier's dancing and the filmed images of her naked body falling slowly through the space in the second half of the show. After we have seen Lecavalier and her various sidekicks slam their bodies relentlessly around the stage (think of the physical equivalent of a heavy-metal guitar solo), an enormous screen slowly descends across the front of the stage. At first, the film shows Lecavalier clothed in a medieval suit of armor, complete with sword (à la Jeanne d'Arc), and then later falling naked through a vast, bleak space. There is no coherent narrative in this short surreal film. Jump cuts inexplicably move her from a figure of power (the knight) to a woman bleeding, to a Christ-like transcendence. She is aggressor, victim, and saint, all the while imaged in larger-than-life celluloid.

Yet in the moments when she is falling through space, there is an otherworldly calm that envelops the audience. These moments are completely detached from the events onstage. Although her blonde hair and alabaster skin are recognizable, Lecavalier's body is transformed on the film. She floats peacefully on screen, supported by the digital technology that allows her image to transcend gravity. She is falling on screen, but falling in such a suspended atmosphere that she seems to be evaporating. Then she lands. Shot from underneath a glass floor, the impact is clear. We see her land on all fours; breasts bouncing, hair flailing. The shot is repeated, several times. Although the slow-motion editing mutes the jarring effect of her return to gravity, the audience still experiences a visceral reverberation of that jolting sensation whose effects are nonetheless clearly visible. What makes this sequence particularly eerie is the fact that we do not see the chain of events that led from her floating to landing. We see her suspended, but we do not see the real momentum of her fall—only the seconds before impact. It is like the story of Adam and Eve without the apple. The image of her strong yet vulnerable naked body resting in air one minute and then hitting the ground the next is both disturbing and bizarrely beautiful.

The American equivalent of La La La Human Steps is Elizabeth Streb's company, Ringside. Over the past twenty-five years, Streb has been involved in making pieces that focus the audience's attention on how a human body (or bodies) interacts with various kinds of equipment such as poles, balls, hoops, plexiglass walls, a board on wheels, a coffin-like box suspended sideways in the air, two 4 x 8 birch plywood panels, trapeze harnesses, various kinds of adult-sized jungle gyms, and a trampoline that can catapult people up to thirty feet in the air. Streb's dancers hurl themselves through space, slamming their bodies into the various pieces of equipment. Although the fierce physicality and built-up muscularity, as well as the way her dancers vault through the air is analogous to the dancing in La La La Human Steps, Streb's work is much plainer, with a lot less theatricality, a lot less "attitude," and a lot less pretension than Lock's mega spectacles. Typically in a Streb concert, one walks into the theater while the technicians are testing and adjusting the equipment. The dances start with the dancers casually walking on stage, shaking a limb here and there to loosen up, and preparing themselves as if for a race or some kind of sports event. Once they have arranged themselves and glanced around to see if everyone is ready, the dancers launch into whatever physical challenge is being attempted in this particular dance.

More recently, Streb has been working with layering the movement tasks that are a signature of her work with real-time video projections. Her 2003 piece, *Wild Blue Yonder,* which was commissioned as part of a 100th anniversary celebration of the Wright Brothers's first flight, juxtaposes the real flight of the dancers swan diving off a large trampoline and landing on a thick gym pad with the manipulated images of their shadows. Like many of Streb's works, this dance focuses on bodies flying and falling though the air. The physical stamina of her dancers is breathtaking, and yet the relentless repetition of their stunts tends to dull the impact of those extraordinary feats.

Wild Blue Yonder begins with the dancers entering the performance space and lining up on a ledge in between the scrim and the trampoline. As they jostle and adjust their spacing, the audience sees glimpses of their shadows projected against the twilight blue scrims. First one, and then another, and another dancer jumps off the ledge and onto the large trampoline which catapults them up high into the air. Arms spread out to their sides, the dancers swam dive down, bracing themselves at the last moment as they hit the crash pad. Their acts are spectacular, but it is the image of the dancers' shadows—those black alter egos—that is most riveting to watch. Suspended in the air for a moment, they really do look like airplanes.

Bit by bit, the dancers speed up—launching themselves one right after the other like the finale of the Fourth of July fireworks. As more and more bodies take to the air, their shadows become erratic and unpredictable, often staying on the screen long after the live body has landed. Sometimes the shadows will introduce a new movement motif, a flip, or a pike turn, until eventually the images on-screen take on a life of their own. This choreography of shadow and video image is infinitely more fanciful and varied than that of the live dancers, who must inevitably contend with the call of gravity that brings them abruptly back to the earth. Unfortunately, we never get to see images of this experience suspended in time, for the projected bodies never land, they only fade away. Predictably, the curiosity that fueled the Wright Brothers's ambition to fly keeps the audience gazing at the shadows floating in the sky, while the live bodies drop out of sight.

The context of my investigation of falling on screens is a deeper inquiry about the culture of falling post 9/11. Seeing *Wild Blue Yonder* makes me wonder: Have the disturbing images of free-falling bodies dropped out of our sight? Are we overly comfortable with a technology that can suspend falling indefinitely such that we never are confronted with that final negotiation with gravity? What would it mean to use the technology of screens not to divert our attention from those spectacular falls at the beginning of the twenty-first century, but rather to examine the spaces in between that past and our future? In other words, how can we use screendance to teach us how to land a fall safely—both physically and culturally? Ideally, I would be able to point to a recent screendance that realized a vision of falling that was both suspended and grounded. But that screendance has not yet been invented.

NOTES

1. Nancy Stark Smith, "Editor Note" in *Contact Quarterly* (Spring/Summer 1987): 3.

2. See "Techno Bodies," in *Choreographing Difference: The Body and Identity in Contemporary Dance* (Middletown, CT: Wesleyan University Press, 1997).

40

The Tensions of *Techné*

On Heidegger and Screendance

International Journal of Screendance 2, no. 1 (Spring 2012).

I entered the Screendance network from a slightly oblique angle. On the one hand, I was more unschooled in contemporary examples of screendance than many of my colleagues, and I certainly was much less addicted to YouTube searching and my computer in general. On the other hand, I came to the table with a curiosity about the historical and theoretical intersections of bodies and machines throughout the twentieth century and a fair dose of feminist film theory. Thus, as people around me chatted about so-and-so's new film, or the latest politics of the latest curator at the latest screenings, I was busy looking out for the ways in which the act of filming dance was implicated in the screened representation and how the ubiquity of screens in contemporary dance affects how we watch movement. That is to say, I have become interested not only in what we are seeing (a particular filmmaker's signature, the long shots, the jump cuts, the choreography, etc.), but in how the very structure of our seeing (both on and off the screen) has been affected by filmic technologies. As we enter the second decade of the twenty-first century, I believe that we must think seriously about the implications of the increasing presence of screens in the dance field as a whole. In other words, how has looking at dance on screen made us look at dance on stage differently?

At first, I must admit that I was a wee bit put off by what I perceived as the lack of attention to theoretical perspectives in discussions about screendance that I was witnessing in and around the various festivals. But then I began to see that maybe my role in the Screendance network and the *International Journal of Screendance* was to call for more intentionality about how screendance helps construct our vision of twenty-first-century dancing bodies. There are, of course, multiple tensions between live performance and mediated images, many of which relate to the radically different economies of their respective circulation and exchange. But I believe that these material and conceptual tensions can be very productive if we are willing to examine their interconnectedness. *Attention, intention, tension*: these words are in the forefront of my mind when I begin to think about the relationship between dance and technology.

In his 1954 treatise, *The Question Concerning Technology*, philosopher Martin Heidegger connects the terms technology and technique with their etymological root, *technē*—an ancient Greek concept that refers at once to the skills of the artisan and the visionary power of the artist. Heidegger also links *technē* to episteme: a way of knowing the world. Thus dance techniques and media technologies are not simply about the capacity of machines (or even the dancer's body as machine); they also concern how we come to know the world. For Heidegger, this knowledge is not a passive recognition of what already exists, but rather a method of "bringing forth," a "revealing" of a truth. He writes:

> Thus what is decisive in *technē* does not lie at all in making and manipulat-
> ing nor in the using of means, but rather in the aforementioned revealing. It
> is as revealing, and not as manufacturing, that *technē* is a bringing-forth . . .
> Technology comes to presence in the realm where revealing and unconcealment
> takes place, where *aletheia*, truth, happens.[1]

Although his philosophical language is dense, and his use of gerunds is at times delightfully peculiar, what I appreciate in this essay is the idea that technology could render, rather than efface, presence—be it theatrical presence, or a more existential being-in-the-world.

My decision to curate a cluster of short responses to Heidegger's essay was prompted by a discussion in an editorial board meeting last June. There, we were brainstorming which historical and theoretical essays might inspire or provoke a cluster of interesting responses. I turned to Heidegger, knowing, of course, that many people react fairly strongly to both his theoretical insights and the legacy of his association with National Socialism in Germany. And yet, despite the awkward fit of history (a lot has happened in the last fifty-seven years) and discipline (philosophy), I felt this essay had helped me to articulate the inherent interconnectedness between dance and technologies, including the ways that dance techniques are, in fact, examples of affective technologies of the body. Rereading the essay years later, I recognized that even back in the 1950s, Heidegger had thought through how often habit can masquerade as knowledge, and the intertwined issues concerning power, desire, and imagination that are embedded within our relationship to technology. Right at the beginning of his essay, Heidegger elucidates the importance of being intentional about this relationship when he writes:

> I never experience our relationship to the essence of technology so long as we
> merely conceive and push forward the technological, put up with it, or evade it.
> Everywhere we remain unfree and chained to technology, whether we passion-
> ately affirm or deny it. But we are delivered over to it in the worst possible
> way when we regard it as something neutral; for this conception of it, to which

today we particularly like to do homage, makes us utterly blind to the essence of technology.[2]

I asked four people who work as artists, screendance makers, and scholars to respond to Heidegger's *The Question Concerning Technology* from the perspective of their own interests in the field. What follows is a sequence of writings that both speak to Heidegger's essay and each other in unexpected and interesting ways. Prompted by Heidegger's use of etymology to think past the obvious, Ann Dils traces the roots of the words "screen" and "dance." These histories provide a slightly difference perspective on the term screendance which Ann uses as an opportunity to look again at *Ghostcatching*—a collaboration between Paul Kaiser, Shelley Eshkar, and Bill T. Jones about which she had written over a decade ago. In his essay, "The Sorrow and the Pithy," Kent de Spain provides a trenchant overview of Heidegger's main points, weaving into his analysis a tongue-in-cheek, but also very hopeful, commentary on the problems and possibilities of working in the folds of movement and screens. Lisa Naugel and John Crawford write about their collaboration with Active Space and the ways in which memory and illusion are called forth by their use of the latest interactive technologies. Finally, Tom Lopez channels the ancestral spirits of *technē* and *poïesis:* two of Heidegger's favorite terms. In Tom's multivocal writing, these "twins" are put into dialogue across the divide of time and space, each one commenting and cross-referencing (sometimes contradicting) the other's words. I cannot stop feeling as if Heidegger would be pleased to read these musings sponsored by his essay. I thank my colleagues for taking the time out of their busy lives to share their thoughts on "the tensions of *technē*."

NOTES

1. Martin Heidegger, *The Question Concerning Technology and Other Essays* (New York: Harper & Row, 1977), 13.
2. Ibid., 4.

41

Falling

Performance Research 18, no.4 (August 2013).

Falling is predicated on a slippage through time and space. Marked by the trajectory between up and down as well as before and after, falling refers to what *was* while moving toward what *will be*. This is true whether you fall on ice or fall in love. Crossing over literal and metaphoric states of being in the world, falling opens a threshold between the past and the future. Falls knock us off our feet, confusing our sense of the world's order. These radical shifts in orientation register in our connective tissue as well as our psyche. Falls can be traumatic to be sure—disorienting at the very least. But because they stretch across a liminal space in which the present is suspended, falling can also inspire new orientations, including ones that challenge our expectations of economic stability and social success.

I have been thinking a lot about falling these days: falling buildings, falling planes, falling economies, falling governments, but most particularly falling bodies. Over the course of the first decade of the twenty-first century, we have witnessed a series of spectacular and horrible falls that have had both global and local repercussions. From the sudden and horrific collapse of the World Trade Center towers to the economic recession and its resulting slippages in employment, from the cyclical plunges in housing values to the periodic crashes of the stock market (not to mention the latest fiscal cliff), we live in a state of almost constant anxiety about things falling apart and our bodies reflect that.

In this essay, I want to explore the interconnected realms of the theoretical and the practical. That is to say, I will trace both the cultural rhetoric surrounding falling and the physical experience of moving from up to down. What do these two different perspectives on falling have to say to one another? Or, perhaps more precisely, what can the intentional practice of falling teach us about how to survive personal and social crises? I ask these questions not only to underline the importance of embodied experience in talking about historical events, but also because I want to think seriously about the physical practices that might help us survive this cultural moment. Instead of nervously trying to avoid falling in a world in which so many aspects of our social, political, and economic environment are being turned upside down, I believe we need to learn how to fall intentionally. Taking a lesson from the contemporary movement form of contact improvisation, we can practice ways in which to move with and through the descent, channeling the vertical momentum of a fall into the horizontal expression of a roll. The experience of falling can teach us a great deal about resiliency—physical as well as emotional and even economic resiliency—helping us, in turn, to mitigate the vague panic that seems to have permeated almost everyone's being these days.

As a cultural metaphor, falling carries a pretty heavy symbolism in the West. Whether we are talking about the hubris of Icarus or the evil of Satan, the collapse of stock markets or the public stumbling of the latest politician to lose his integrity on the Internet, falling is generally seen as a failure, a defeat, a loss, or a decline. In short, a fall charts a passage from the lofty heavens of stardom to the grit of the earth. Socially, it is a perilous journey: not only do boys, angels, and men fall, of course, but women have also been doomed by this cultural hegemony of the vertical. In an overly determined slippage that quickly shifts from literal to metaphoric, women are dubbed "fallen" when they lose their virginity (and therefore their chastity and moral innocence). This gendered scenario is no doubt connected to that first spectacular fall from Paradise—for a woman's fall from vertical to horizontal retraces in one fell swoop the physical, cultural, and spiritual damnation of Eve (or one of her many updated prototypes). In most situations, falls are always already falls from grace.

Interestingly enough, the first definition for the word *fall* in my *American Heritage* dictionary is largely removed from the cultural baggage that implicates failure in a fall. Here fall is simply: "to move under the influence of gravity." Now this is a phrase that dancers and choreographers can relate to—for we know in our bones that every movement is, in fact, a dance with gravity. Even the most traditionally trained ballerina is aware of the fact that stillness (especially on pointe) is never a static balance, but rather a dynamic play with the forces of gravity. Those of us who work in contemporary dance forms learn very quickly to rely on our proprioceptive sensibility to prime the body for a variety of responses to gravity.

At its core, movement is a series of falls—some small, some more spectacular—that propel the body through time and space. Using gravity, we can attune our sensibilities to the more subtle of those displacements. This kinesthetic tuning gives us an awareness of the physical possibilities in which a body can be both grounded and open to moving in any direction. If we shift the orientation of the West's vertical hegemony, falling can become not just an ignominious ending, but rather the beginning of other possibilities. In an editor's note to the Healing issue of *Contact Quarterly,* Nancy Stark Smith suggests just such an alternative view when she writes: "The expression 'fall from grace' becomes an impossible statement when falling itself is experienced as a state of grace."[1]

By the end of the twentieth century, the signature virtuosic moves of contact improvisation—spinning shoulder lofts and falls that looped to the floor only to cycle back up into the air—were much in evidence at jams around the world. And yet it is instructive to reexamine the dynamic of these early days of contact improvisation when falling still registered as an existential experience and not simply another movement skill. In describing this transition from fear to form, Nancy Stark Smith writes:

> The more I fell, the more familiar the sensation of dropping through space became, the less disoriented I was during the fall. Staying awake from the first moment of balance loss, I found that falling was itself a dynamic balance. One in which the forces at play—gravity, momentum, and mass—were all operating in their natural order and if my mind was with me, I could gently guide that fall toward a smooth landing. Confidence came with experience and soon enjoyment took the place of fear and disorientation.[2]

Disorientation is a word that insists on its opposite for meaning. To be disoriented is to be undone; thrown off-balance. But it also hints at a deeper knowledge. We rarely think about where we are until we have been lost. In order to understand what orients us, we need to experience disorientation. In the conclusion to her meditation on shifting orientations in *Queer Phenomenology*, Sara Ahmed writes:

> Moments of disorientation are vital. They are bodily experiences that throw the world up, or throw the body from its ground. Disorientation as a bodily feeling can be unsettling, and it can shatter one's sense of confidence in the ground or one's belief that the ground on which we reside can support the actions that make a life feel livable. Such a feeling of shattering, or of being shattered, might persist and become a crisis. Or the feeling itself might pass as the ground returns or as we return to the ground.[3]

Thrown off-balance, the body skews our sense of direction in ways that may reframe our politics of location or the cultural organization of space. Falling offers a new slant, so to speak, on the binary of up and down. Indeed, we might even posit, following Ahmed's work in phenomenology, that falling insists on a shift of orientation—a different perspective from which we might learn, even once we return to the ground. In order to experience this difference in falling, however, it is important not to shut off sensation, including the sensation of losing one's ground. Embracing disorientation is not the same as feeling totally comfortable with it. Part of the productive tension in this line between panic and total ease is the edge created by a "beginner's mind"—the willingness to feel awkward and lost without undue panic. As Nancy Stark Smith notes in her early discussion of falling: "This is not to say that disorientation, confusion and dis-ease have no place in the geometry of balance. They, in fact, stimulate the balancing mechanism. Stimulate us to ask questions . . ."[4]

Of course, disorientation is not necessarily a radical gesture. It can also provoke a conservative reaction, as can falling. Take, for instance, the panicked response of the U.S. government to the falling of the World Trade Center towers on September 11, 2001. That terrible fall was seen as a failure on many levels and created a great deal of disorientation and fear, especially in the United States. What got lost in the process of transforming fear into patriotism was the potential for disorientation to mobilize new positions or guide us towards an understanding of our previous moorings. As Sarah Ahmed notes: "The point is not whether we experience disorientation (for we will and we do), but how such experiences can impact on the orientations of bodies and spaces, . . . The point is what we do with such moments of disorientation, as well as what such moments can do—whether they can offer us the hope of new directions, and whether new directions are reason enough for hope."[5]

Being attentive to spatial disorientation comes from a physical practice that includes getting used to being upside down, spinning, falling in every direction (especially through one's back space), as well as moving with momentum—sometimes with one's eyes closed. Phenomenologist Maurice Merleau-Ponty describes disorientation as "the vital experience of giddiness and nausea."[6] I believe this "vital" experience has psychic, not to mention physical, implications. Personally, I find that by working with disorientation, my body can open up to places and ideas that my mind has a hard time finding on its own, including other ways of thinking about falls and falling. Accepting the opportunity that disorientation provides, we can look for new directions not only in which to fall, but also within the fall itself, enjoying the moments of expansion between the up and the down. For in this slanted trajectory, we can experience two directions at once—finding the suspension across space while at the same time feeling gravity's pull into the ground. Nancy Stark Smith refers to this moment as a "gap."

> Where you are when you don't know where you are is one of the most precious spots offered by improvisation. It is a place from which more directions are possible that anywhere else. I call this place the Gap . . . Being in a gap is like being in a fall before you touch bottom. You're suspended—in time as well as space—and you don't really know how long it'll take to get "back."[7]

For Smith, that suspension between two known points (up and down) opens up multiple possibilities and different orientations. For me this "gap" allows for a suspension of one kind of cultural paradigm (that falling is failure), such that other meanings might take its place.

La Chute (The Fall) is a series of photographs by Denis Darzacq of young men (and one woman) caught in midair.[8] Shot between 2006 and 2007, these images capture falling bodies a foot or two (sometime mere inches) from the ground. In his artist's statement accompanying the portfolio, Darzacq describes this work as a meditation on the individual in an urban environment, with particular reference to both 9/11 and the plight of the working-class poor in the outskirts of Paris. In these photographs, young men from predominantly immigrant communities of the Parisian banlieus are shot against a backdrop of generic concrete buildings—what Darzacq calls the "soulless" architecture of many public-housing projects. Catching a body suspended in between the launch and the recovery, Darzacq is able to infuse the potent image of youthful vitality with an air of existential vulnerability.

The juxtaposition of this kind of energized physicality—part parkour, part capoeira and part circus—floating in midair underscores the marginalized position of urban youth. At the same time, the intensity of the experience of flying and falling vacates any posturing or gestural attitude we might associate with urban youth subcultures. Many of the photographs do not even show facial expressions. Nonetheless, the off-kilter, splayed, and irregular arrangements of flailing arms and legs create a sense of individual personalities. The trajectory of the fall is interrupted by the click of the camera, and the resulting freeze gives us a pause in which to consider their experience. Ironically, many viewers of this series think that the image has been manipulated; that it is not a "real" action shot. They cannot even imagine the elastic potential of this space in between sky and earth, fall and recovery.

The tension that this suspension creates was made clear to me in a short film by Marie-Clotide Chery documenting a photo shoot with Darzacq and a group of young people from the outskirts of Paris. At one point, the photographer is encouraging a young French man of African descent to try some moves again without stopping himself or being overly self-critical. Darzacq tells him: "Remember this is photography, not video."[9] This comment about a choice at the moment of shooting (instead of at the moment of editing) is further developed in a later scene where another participant is reviewing images of himself. This young man mentions how in order to launch himself into space he envisions the movement as a whole, from the preparation through to the recovery. When he sees his body suspended in the photograph, he realizes that "the rest doesn't matter." Which is not to say that the context does not matter. On the contrary, Darzacq "freezes" their movement in order to expose their subjectivity. His work is deeply motivated by a culturally progressive agenda—making visible an experience that is often overlooked.

In Darzacq's work, the narrative of falling is suspended. His photographic frame operates as both interruption and absorption. By prolonging a movement midair, these images give us an opportunity to think about moments in between the beginning and an ending of a leap. The denouement may seem inevitable, but it is not necessarily predetermined. Indeed, Darzacq's *La Chute* makes visible what Erin Manning, referencing Deleuze, terms "the elasticity of the almost." "The body-elastic is the body of the between, the body of the almost, when the movement is on the verge, actual but almost virtual, hanging, pulsing, spiraling."[10] Like Nancy Stark Smith, Manning imbues this gap or suspension with improvisational possibilities. She thinks of it as an interval, a moment of poignant openness that has otherworldly ("almost virtual") potential. It is this mutual experience of an interval that structures the magical synchrony of moving together, whether it is two dancers in a tango or contact duet, the faller and the fall, or the meeting of a young person's leap of faith and a photographer's ability to capture that brief suspension of disbelief.

All suspensions come to an end, of course, and what matters then is how we hit the ground. Defined abstractly as "the property of a material that enables it to resume its original shape or position after being bent, stretched or compressed," resiliency in people is usually determined by a mix of historical circumstances, sociocultural background, familial disposition, and individual attitude. For the young urban movers documented in Darzacq's photographs, this skill is measured in the ability to continue with a next move; the ability to find the ground through a shoulder, back, hip, or hand in order to push off and back to their feet. In front of the camera, they try the same move over and over again, launching themselves through the air and hitting the ground like a bouncing ball. Their physical resiliency is awesome—a testament to the vast potential of human survival. But does physical flexibility always yield a psychological elasticity as well? What do these images of suspension, Smith's idea of the "gap" or Manning's notion of "the elasticity of the almost" tell us about the falls that result in the loss of livelihood, social status, or a loved one's life?

In his contribution to the *Women and Performance* issue on falling, Jason King notes how fragile the concept of social mobility is in the African-American community. "Falling is downward mobility, descent . . . Slipping, stumbling, and tripping are all performances of disorientation, de-anchoring, rootlessness; they precursor the fall or the slide (the gliding fall) or the tumble (the rolling fall) or the flop (the thudding fall)."[11] In the midst of this very real fear of losing socioeconomic status, however, is a parallel focus on resiliency. "Every opportunity to fall becomes an opportunity to rise."[12] Citing examples from history and popular (Tina Turner), poetic (Maya Angelou), and political (Malcolm X) cultures, King points out how much the black community invests in the rhetoric of verticality. Shifting the directional emphasis of "get-up, stand-up" (after recognizing, via Michelle Wallace, its inherent masculine bias), King proposes that we keep the activist nature (keep moving) but rethink the Christian insistence on the vertical as necessarily virtuous. "Disorientation, the fall, is reorientation, the rise is the fall; climax is denouement."[13]

While we often interpret resiliency to mean getting right back up to where we were before the fall (bouncing back), it can also suggest a certain flexibility—one in which the possibility of reorientation after disorientation leads one into different directions, or even a different notion of directionality. In this refiguring of the politics of verticality, I join Judith Halberstam whose book *The Queer Art of Failure* encourages the improvisational possibilities of what she calls "low theory." "Under certain circumstances falling, losing, forgetting, unmaking, undoing, unbecoming, not knowing may in fact offer more creative, more cooperative, more surprising ways of being in the world."[14] Here we return to the potential of contact improvisation to help us understand something critically important.

When I first began teaching dance technique and contact improvisation in the mid-1980s, my students were hungry for the physical experience of disorientation and the intellectual sensibilities of deconstruction. They loved to spin and fall, and they clearly connected these wild displacements of the body with an open attitude about who they were and what they wanted to do. Nowadays, I am struck by the shifting needs of young people's bodies. Generally, they do not want to be pushed too hard, or thrown off-balance. Their identities are less fluid. Specifically, I believe that the experience of growing up in a post–9/11 America has created a real fear of falling; a fear of losing stability in a world that is already so chaotic. I am also aware of how many of my undergraduate students (who grew up in the wake of 9/11) feel a bizarre sense of dis/location as their lives become increasingly implicated in the weightless exchanges on the Internet. Seeing my students struggle with this disembodied inertia, I am interested in exploring how we might reimagine earlier paradigms of location and place while still incorporating gravity as an essential sensibility. I guess I am really interested in asking: what are the dual practices of mobility and gravity that make sense for our time?

Although a lot of professional work in contact improvisation focuses on the virtuosity of the up—awesome spinning lifts that sail around the room— to my mind the truly radical potential of contact improvisation at this historical juncture lies in the physical training that celebrates the down, dwells on the floor, revels in the process of rolling, sinking, and crawling. Through these kinesthetic experiences that orient toward gravity, contact improvisation can lead us into a resiliency that not only helps us survive the inevitable falls of life, but also rescues us from the relentless ascension and striving for success that marked the late twentieth century. This practice could help us recognize what the body already knows, that falling can guide us to a state of grace—if we are willing to take the risk.

1. Nancy Stark Smith, "Editor's Note," *Contact Quarterly* 5, no. 1 (1979): 3.

2. Ibid.

3. Sarah Ahmed, *Queer Phenomenology* (Durham, NC: Duke University Press, 2006), 157.

4. Smith, 3.

5. Ahmed, 158.

6. Merleau-Ponty, as cited in Ahmed, 157.

7. Nancy Stark Smith, "Editor's Note," *Contact Quarterly* 12, no. 2 (1987): 3.

8. Denis Darzacq, 2006, La Chute portfolio (www.denis-darzacq.com/portfolios .htm) and video (www.youtube.com/watch?v=5HonzF8LbLE).

9. www.youtube.com/watch?v=5HonzF8LbLE.

10. Erin Manning, *Relationscapes: Movement, Art, Philosophy* (Cambridge, MA: MIT Press, 2009), 114.

11. Jason King, "Which Way is Down?," *Women and Performance* 1, no. 1 (2004): 27.

11. Ibid., 29.

13. Ibid., 43.

14. Judith Halberstam, *The Queer Art of Failure* (Durham, NC: Duke University Press, 2011), 2–3.

Afterword

This collection of my writing is dedicated to my students. In the two decades that I have been teaching at Oberlin College, the students in my classes have jumped on me, rolled over me, pushed me, and resisted my weight in ways that ultimately supported the direction of my academic career. Throughout courses new and untested, or tried and true, they have always been accepting and encouraging; joining me on an adventure that crosses back and forth over disciplines and learning styles, theory and practice. My students inspire me. We may not always agree, but I rarely feel disinterest or apathy from them, and I cherish the heat of each encounter. I am deeply gratified when I get an email several hours after class has ended (or even one month or many years) detailing how an insight from the course materialized in their daily lives.

From time to time, I teach workshops to professional dancers or pre-professional students outside of a college setting and these interactions, although brief, can also be powerful and rewarding. Often when I travel abroad, I give an academic talk and then teach a movement class, and in those situations I relish the fact that I model the possibility of connecting dancing and critical thinking. Indeed, I enjoy the surprise on these students' faces when, having been introduced as a "mature" dance scholar, I then break out my healthy kinesthetic appetite for momentum and force in the studio. I learn and teach by moving and being moved, and I hope to continue that engagement with other bodies as long as I can.

Of course, my life has not always been so integrated. I spent a lot of my twenties and early thirties nervous that I was perceived as being neither fully a dancer nor fully a scholar. Like many people who cross over a cultural binary (whether it is a gendered, racial, or class-based one—we are all implicated in this body/mind divide), I often felt like I did not fit in anywhere. I was too intellectual and analytic for the dance (particularly the contact improvisation) scene and too body-centric for academics. At some point, I made my peace with my dancer/scholar identity, eventually turning it into a point of pride. As I look over the pieces collected here, I realize that they carry the different reverberations of that journey into self-acceptance.

Everybody's life is an improvisation, but for those of us who work with movement improvisation there is a lot more attention to how this practice in navigating unforeseen moments structures our lives. Improvisation, particularly contact improvisation and the many somatic practices that revolve around its physical training, has been the lifeline that has helped me to survive professional disappointment and physical injury, family trauma, and various lapses of imagination. As many essays in this collection make clear, I am committed to the disorientation and open-endedness that improvisation sponsors. I feel that I thrive best in the spaces in between the lines—be they the lines between theory and practice, dancing and writing, or the lines between twenty-year-old students and a fifty-year-old professor. Every time we enter the space between the lines of our expectations, we are making ourselves vulnerable by staking out the possibility of failure. Yet I believe that this improvisational impulse—this willingness to put yourself out there in the space of a contact improvisation round-robin, a dance studio, or in writing—is essentially a generous gesture.

One of the mantras that I frequently repeat in class is one I heard a long time ago from Nancy Stark Smith à propos improvisational dancing: replace ambition with curiosity. I think that is a good life motto. I realize, however, that it can be tough to keep embracing curiosity, especially in a cultural moment when so many things seem tentative and fragile. But the alternative for me is to stop moving into that open space of possibility, and that is not a choice I am prepared to make. So, it is with a sense of curiosity about the next step that I turn from writing to dancing, as I leave my desk and venture over to our weekly contact improvisation jam in Warner Main to engage with the politics and poetics of corporeality once again. Thankfully, I am not alone.

Acknowledgments

The Cleveland Reader, "Joseph Holmes, Sizzle and Heat," first published in April/
May 1992. Reprinted by permission.

Contact Quarterly, "The Mesh in the Mess," first published in winter 1987,
"Mining the Dancefield: Spectacle, Moving Subjects and Feminist Theory," first
published in Spring/Summer 1990. Reprinted by permission.

Conversations Across the Field of Dance Studies, "Three Beginnings and a Manifesto by Ann Cooper Albright," first published in fall 2007. Reprinted by
permission.

Dance Chronicle, "Space and Subjectivity," first published in no. 32, 2009. Reprinted by permission.

Dance Research Journal, "Dancing in and out of Africa," first published in vol. 32,
no.1, 2000, "Improvisation as Radical Politics," first published in vol. 35, no. 1,
2003, "Matters of Tact: Writing History from the Inside Out," first published in
vol. 35, no. 2, 2003, "Situated Dancing: Notes from Three Decades in Contact
with Phenomenology," first published in vol. 43 no. 2 fall 2011, "Strategic Practices," first published in vol. 44, no. 2, winter 2012. Reprinted by permission.

Dialogue Magazine for the Arts, "In Dialogue with *Firebird*," first published in
May/June 1992, "Performing Across Identity," first published in November/
December 1991, "Dancing Bodies and Stories They Tell," first published in
March/April 1993, "Embodying History/ The New Epic Dance," first published
in March/April 1994, "Desire and Control: Performing Bodies in the Age of
AIDS," first published in March/April 1996.

Duke University Press, "Auto-Body Stories: Blondell Cummings and Autobiography in Dance," first published in *Meaning in Motion: New Cultural Studies of
Dance*, edited by Jane Desmond, 1997. Reprinted by permission.

Frontiers: A Journal of Women Studies, "Writing the Moving Body: Nancy Stark
Smith and the Hieroglyphs," first published in vol. X, no. 3, 1989. Reprinted by
permission.

International Journal of Screendance, "Falling on Screen," first published in vol. 1,
no. 1, Spring 2010, "The Tensions of Technē: On Heidegger and Screendance,"
first published in vol. 2, no. 1, Spring 2012. Reprinted by permission.

Journal of Dance and Somatic Practices, "Training Bodies to Matter," first published in vol. 1, no. 1, 2009. Reprinted by permission.

Michigan Quarterly Review, "Strategic Abilities: negotiating the disabled body in
dance," first published in vol. 37, no. 3, summer 1998. Reprinted by permission.

Movement Research Journal, "Through Yours to Mine and Back Again: Reflections
of Bodies in Motion," first published in Fall 1993, "Researching Bodies: The
Politics and Poetics of Corporeality," first published in Spring 2004, "Physical
Mindfulness," first published in Spring 1998. Reprinted by permission.

Oxford University Press, "The Tanagra Effect: Wrapping the Modern Body in the
Folds of Ancient Greece," first published in *The Ancient Dancer in the Modern
World*, 2010. Reprinted by permission.

Perfomance Research, "Falling," first published in 2013. Reprinted by permission.

Praeger, "Moving Contexts: Dance and Difference in the 21st Century," first published in *Intercultural Communication and Creative Process: Music, Dance and Women's Cultural Identity*, 2005. Reprinted by permission.

Protée, "Open Bodies: Changes of Identity in Capoeira and Contact Improvisation," first published in vol. 29, no. 2, 2001. Reprinted by permission.

Research and Dance Education, "Channeling the 'Other': An Embodied Approach to Teaching Across Cultures," first published in vol. 4, no. 2, 2003. Reprinted by permission from Taylor and Francis (www.tandfonline.com).

Wesleyan University Press, "Femininity with a Vengeance: Strategies of Veiling and Unveiling in Loie Fuller's Performances of Salomé," first published in *Traces of Light: Absence and Presence in the Work of Loïe Fuller*, 2007, "Embodying History: Epic Narrative and Cultural Identity in African-American Dance," first published in *Moving History/Dancing Cultures*, 2001, "Present Tense: Contact Improvisation at Twenty-five," first published in *Taken by Surprise: Improvisation in Dance and Mind*, 2003. Reprinted by permission.

Women and Performance: "Dancing Across Difference: Experience and Identity in the Classroom," first published in Women and Performance, vol. 6, no. 2, 1993, "Pooh Kaye and Eccentric Motions," first published in Women and Performance, vol. 2, no. 2, Issue 4, 1985, "Johanna Boyce," first published in Women and Performance, vol. 3, no. 2, Issue 5, 1986, "Improvisations by Simone Forti and Pooh Kaye/*Blood on the Saddle*/ *Active Graphics II* and *Tangled Graphics*," first published in *Women and Performance*, vol. 4, no. 1, 1988/1989, "Song of Lawino," first published in Women and Performance, vol. 4, no. 2, 1989.

Index

emotion, exploring in contact improvisation, 211, 237–44, 258

empathic kinesthetic perception: in contact improvisation, 211, 237–44, 273; and intersubjective space, 72; Sklar's proposal, 10–11; in Wigman's subjectivity, 345; in writing/dancing history, 178–82, 183–84, 185–87

energy exchange, in physical movement, 166, 167–69, 172, 321–24, 344–47

epic dance narratives: *Bones and Ash*, 151, 164–69, 172, 173n30; *Last Supper at Uncle Tom's Cabin*, 52–53, 151, 153, 155, 156–64, 170–72; New Epic Dance, 50–54, 148–50

Eshkar, Shelley, 358

ethnic identity. *See* cultural identity and representation

Fagan, Garth, 50–52, 54

Fall After Newton, 362–63

falling, 15–16, 56–57, 270, 271–73, 360–66, 370–76

feeling as process/verb, 211, 238–39, 241–42, 243–44

female body: improvisation and empowerment of, 28–30; inhibited intentionality, 4, 276, 343; shifts in presentation, 65–68; as site of repression, 7, 23–24, 64, 188–89; socialization of, 4–5, 7–8; veiling and unveiling of, 121, 124, 129, 192–93; writing the, 83–87, 90

feminine values in Uncle Tom character, 154–55

feminist perspectives: authorial signatures, 62, 98–99, 110; and body/mind separation, 220; Boyce's interaction with, 25–26; and cultural assumption about bodies, 6–7; Cummings, 37–38; and dance as resistance, 31–32; de Lauretis, 7–8; disruption of conventional body representations, 64–75; and double reading of body and text, 182; embodiment's role in, 8–9; introduction/overview, 61–63; in Jones's *Last Supper*, 161; and Kaye's play in performance, 23–24; and phenomenology, 2, 4; in Uchizono's performance of *Désirée*, 46; writing the moving body, 62, 76–90; Young, 4, 13, 276, 343. *See also* autobiography in dance; Fuller, Loïe; gender

Fenley, Molissa, 66

Fifteen Years of a Dancer's Life (Fuller), 119

Figninto, ou L'Oeil Troué (Boro and Sanon), 319, 323

film: dominant cultural narrative's preference in, 322–24; Fuller's innovations in, 205, 356–57; Kaye's play of image and movement, 22–23; Lock's *Infante c'est destroy*, 44–45; Rainer's subjectivity through invisibility, 61–62, 64–65; screendance and live dance, 355–59, 360–69, 373–75; and virtuosic view of dancing bodies, 310

Firebird (Fokine and Stravinsky), 40, 41–42

Flynn, Anne, 339

Fokine, Michel, 40, 41–42

Folies Bergère, 117, 179

Forti, Simone, 27–30, 294

Foster, Susan Leigh, 4, 178, 211, 212–13, 238, 338–41

France, Antole, 201–2

Franko, Mark, 181

freedom, 3, 42, 98

French, Jonathan, 311

Fricke-Gottschild, Hellmut, 140, 146–47

Fuller, Loïe: biographical sketch, 179; body vs. image, 354–58; and Colette, 192–93; films of, 205, 356–57; Greek influence, 201–3; historical tracings, 175–87, 354–58; introduction, 115–20; and Isadora Duncan, 202–3; lighting technology, 123, 128, 180, 184, 354, 357; music visualizations, 204–5; performative identity, 116–18, 121–23, 125–30, 132–36; *Salomé* (1895), 62–63, 115, 116, 118–19, 125–30, 132; and Salomé as stereotype, 124–25; somatic experience of, 175–76, 178–81, 183–84, 185–86; spirituality of light for, 184–85; *La Tragédie de Salomé* (1907), 62–63, 132–36; as writer, 119, 189, 358

Gamble, John, 79

Garafola, Lyn, 143

Garelick, Rhonda, 116–17, 118

gaze: disrupting traditional gender views, 61, 65–66; in *Firebird*, 41–42; Fuller's manipulation of, 119–20, 355–56; objectifying, 40, 44–45, 66, 188–89; racist, 333; shifting dynamic in *Dialogues*, 40–41, 42–43; and slave ownership, 158; and spectator/performer relationship, 10,

ABOUT THE AUTHOR

A dancer and scholar, Ann Cooper Albright is Professor and Chair of Dance at Oberlin College. Combining her interests in dancing and cultural theory, she is involved in teaching a variety of courses that seek to engage students in both practices and theories of the body. She is founder and director of *Girls in Motion*, an award winning afterschool program at Langston Middle School and co-director of *Accelerated Motion: Towards a New Dance Literacy*, a digital collection of materials about dance. The book, *Encounters with Contact Improvisation* (2010), is the product of one of her adventures in writing and dancing with others.